W9-BKP-101

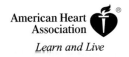

American Heart Association
Learn and Live

The AHA Clinical Series

SERIES EDITOR ELLIOTT ANTMAN

Biomarkers in Heart Disease

This book is dedicated to my wife Zena,
and my children Nicholas, Mikaela,
and Benjamin, for keeping me focused
on what is most important.

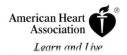

American Heart
Association
Learn and Live

The AHA Clinical Series

SERIES EDITOR ELLIOTT ANTMAN

Biomarkers in Heart Disease

EDITED BY

James A. de Lemos

University of Texas Southwestern Medical Center
Dallas, TX
USA

Blackwell
Publishing

© 2008 American Heart Association
American Heart Association National Center, 7272 Greenville Avenue, Dallas, TX 75231, USA
For further information on the American Heart Association:
www.americanheart.org

Blackwell Publishing, Inc., 350 Main Street, Malden, Massachusetts 02148-5020, USA
Blackwell Publishing Ltd, 9600 Garsington Road, Oxford OX4 2DQ, UK
Blackwell Publishing Asia Pty Ltd, 550 Swanston Street, Carlton, Victoria 3053, Australia

First published 2008
1   2008
Library of Congress Cataloging-in-Publication Data

Biomarkers in heart disease / edited by James A. de Lemos.
     p.   ;   cm. – (AHA clinical series)
  Includes bibliographical references and index.
  ISBN-13: 978-1-4051-7571-5 (alk. paper)
  ISBN-10: 1-4051-7571-0 (alk. paper)
1. Biochemical markers–Diagnostic use.   2. Heart–Diseases–Molecular diagnosis.   I. De Lemos, James A.
II. American Heart Association.   III. Series.
[DNLM: 1. Heart Diseases–blood.   2. Heart Diseases–diagnosis.   3. Biological Markers–blood.   4. Predictive Value of Tests.   5. Risk Assessment–methods.   WG 141 B615 2008]

RC683.5.C5B56 2008
616.1'2075–dc22
                    2007049289

ISBN: 978-1-4051-7571-5

A catalogue record for this title is available from the British Library

Set in 9/12 pt., Palatino by Aptara Inc., New Delhi, India
Printed and bound in Singapore by Fabulous Printers Pte Ltd

Commissioning Editor: Gina Almond
Editorial Assistant: Jamie Hartmann-Boyce
Development Editors: Fiona Pattison and Beckie Brand
Production Controller: Debbie Wyer

For further information on Blackwell Publishing, visit our website:
http://www.blackwellpublishing.com

Contents

Contributors

Editor

James A. de Lemos, MD
Associate Professor of Medicine
Coronary Care Unit Director
University of Texas
Southwestern Medical Center
Dallas, TX, USA

Contributors

Fred S. Apple, PhD
Medical Director Clinical Laboratories
Hennepin County Medical Center
Professor, Laboratory Medicine and Pathology
University of Minnesota School of Medicine
Minneapolis, MN, USA

Christie Ballantyne, MD
Professor of Medicine
Section of Atherosclerosis and Vascular Medicine
Baylor College of Medicine
Center for Cardiovascular Prevention
Methodist DeBakey Heart Center
Houston, TX, USA

Mark Chan, MD
Duke Clinical Research Institute
Duke University Medical Center
Durham, NC, USA

Ron C. Hoogeveen, PhD
Assistant Professor of Medicine
Section of Atherosclerosis and Vascular Medicine

Baylor College of Medicine
The Methodist Hosptial
Houston, TX, USA

James L. Januzzi, MD, FACC
Department of Medicine and Division of Cardiology
Massachusetts General Hospital
Boston, MA, USA

Amit Khera, MD, MSc
Assistant Professor of Medicine
Director, Program in Preventive Cardiology
University of Texas Southwestern Medical Center
Dallas, TX, USA

Michael C. Kontos, MD
Departments of Internal Medicine
Cardiology Division; Emergency Medicine and Radiology
Virginia Commonwealth University
Richmond, VA, USA

Renato D. Lópes, MD, PhD
Fellow
Duke Clinical Research Institute
Duke University Medical Center
Durham, NC, USA

Abelardo Martinez-Rumayor, MD
Department of Medicine and Division of Cardiology
Massachusetts General Hospital
Boston, MA, USA

James McCord, MD
Henry Ford Heart and Vascular Institute
Henry Ford Health System
Detroit, MI, USA

David A. Morrow, MD, MPH
TIMI Study Group
Cardiovascular Division
Department of Medicine
Harvard Medical School and Brigham & Women's Hospital
Boston, MA, USA

Vijay Nambi, MD
Assistant Professor of Medicine
Section of Atherosclerosis and Vascular Medicine
Baylor College of Medicine
Center for Cardiovascular Prevention
Methodist DeBakey Heart Center
Houston, TX, USA

L. Kristin Newby, MD, MHS
Associate Professor of Medicine
Division of Cardiovascular Medicine
Duke University Medical Center
Durham, NC, USA

Thomas E. Noel, MD
Department of Internal Medicine
Cardiology Division
Virginia Commonwealth University
Richmond, VA, USA

Torbjørn Omland, MD, PhD, MPH
Department of Medicine
Akershus University Hospital, Lørenskog
Faculty of Medicine
University of Oslo
Oslo, Norway

A. Mark Richards, MD, PhD, DSc
Christchurch Cardioendocrine Research Group
Department of Medicine
University of Otago
Christchurch, New Zealand

Marc S. Sabatine, MD, MPH
TIMI Study Group
Cardiovascular Division
Department of Medicine
Harvard Medical School and Brigham & Women's Hospital
Boston, MA, USA

W.H. Wilson Tang, MD, FAHA
Assistant Professor of Medicine
Cleveland Clinic Lerner College of Medicine
Cleveland, OH, USA

Richard W. Troughton, MB, PhD
Christchurch Cardioendocrine Research Group
Department of Medicine
University of Otago
Christchurch, New Zealand

Torgun Wæhre, MD, PhD
Department of Medicine
Akershus University Hospital, Lørenskog
Faculty of Medicine
University of Oslo
Oslo, Norway

Preface

It can be argued that a "perfect storm" has been brewing to focus interest on cardiovascular biomarkers. The number and complexity of treatment strategies for patients with acute and chronic cardiovascular diseases have increased substantially, with multiple options now typically available for each major disease state. Biomarkers serve as simple tools to select between alternative therapies, ideally helping to personalize therapy based on better understanding of underlying pathobiology in an individual. As basic investigators unravel the pathophysiological processes underlying specific cardiovascular diseases, not only are potential therapeutic targets identified, but also new biomarkers are discovered. Moreover, the nascent fields of genomics and proteomics promise to be powerful tools for additional biomarker discovery.

Although the potential of biomarkers to enhance cardiovascular care is extremely bright, the practicing clinician is challenged with determining how current and future biomarkers should be used in patient care, which is a fundamentally different process from early marker discovery. *Biomarkers in Heart Disease* is the first title in the *AHA Clinical Series* and is aimed at meeting the needs of clinicians, providing cardiologists, internists, emergency department physicians, laboratorians, and other health care providers with a clear understanding of the role of biomarkers in contemporary cardiovascular medicine. This book focuses both on the strengths and pitfalls of currently available markers, also providing information on the most promising biomarkers that are likely to impact practice in the next few years. The book is divided into four parts, organized around clinical scenarios rather than individual biomarkers. Part I focuses on biomarkers in the evaluation and management of patients with suspected acute and chronic ischemic heart disease, Part II on heart failure diagnosis and monitoring, Part III on the increasingly important area of population screening, and Part IV offers a perspective on where the field is moving in the future. This book will help the practicing physician decide which biomarkers to measure, when to measure them, how to interpret the results, and how to make decisions based on the test result. As such, we hope it will be an invaluable resource to practicing physicians and health care providers.

Each of the chapter authors are international leaders in their respective fields, and it has been an honor to work with such a fabulous group of experts. I would like to thank Dr. Elliott Antman for his mentorship and support through this book as well as throughout my career.

James A. de Lemos, MD

Foreword

The strategic driving force behind the American Heart Association's mission of reducing disability and death from cardiovascular diseases and stroke is to change practice by providing information and solutions to healthcare professionals. The pillars of this strategy are Knowledge Discovery, Knowledge Processing, and Knowledge Transfer. The books in the AHA Clinical Series, of which *Biomarkers in Heart Disease* is included, focus on high-interest, cutting-edge topics in cardiovascular medicine. This book series is a critical tool that supports the AHA mission of promoting healthy behavior and improved care of patients. Cardiology is a rapidly changing field and practitioners need data to guide their clinical decision-making. The AHA Clinical series, serves this need by providing the latest information on the physiology, diagnosis, and management of a broad spectrum of conditions encountered in daily practice.

Rose Marie Robertson, MD, FAHA
Chief Science Officer, American Heart Association

Elliott Antman, MD, FAHA
Director, Samuel A. Levine Cardiac Unit, Brigham and Women's Hospital

PART I

Biomarkers for the Evaluation of Patients with Ischemic Heart Disease

Chapter 1

Protocols for diagnosing myocardial infarction

James McCord

Introduction

In 2005 cardiac markers of necrosis were ordered for over 13 million patients in Emergency Departments (EDs) in the United States [1]. The use and interpretation of cardiac markers are fundamental for the diagnosis of myocardial infarction (MI). Cardiac marker protocols for diagnosing MI must be viewed in the context of the consensus document published in 2007 concerning the redefinition of MI. This consensus document states the rise and fall of a specific cardiac marker, preferably cardiac troponin I or T (cTnI, cTnT) is essential to the diagnosis of MI, in the context of either ischemic cardiac symptoms, electrocardiographic changes, or a new wall motion abnormality on cardiac imaging [2]. This chapter will discuss the candidate markers for diagnosing MI. In addition, different strategies for "ruling-in" and "ruling-out" MI will be reviewed, including multimarker approaches, analysis of change over time in marker levels, and point-of-care testing.

Candidate markers and kinetics

CK-MB

Prior to the introduction of cTnI and cTnT, creatine kinase (CK)-MB was the most common marker of myocardial necrosis used in the evaluation for MI. CK-MB is an 86,000 Dalton isoenzyme that is predominantly located in myocardial cells and is released into the circulation in the setting of MI. However, CK-MB constitutes 1–3% of the total CK found in skeletal muscle, and is also present in smaller quantities in other tissues such as intestine, diaphragm, uterus, and

Biomarkers in Heart Disease, 1st edition. Edited by James A. de Lemos.
© 2008 American Heart Association, ISBN: 978-1-4051-7571-5

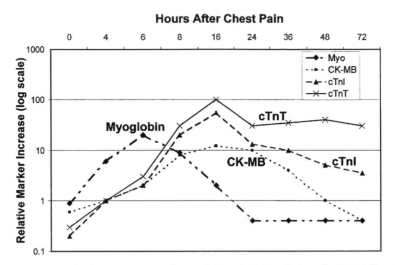

Fig. 1.1 Temporal release patterns of myoglobin, CK-MB, cTnI, and cTnT following myocardial infarction. *Clin Chem* 2007; **53**: 552–574.

prostate [3]. The specificity of CK-MB for diagnosing MI is limited by the fact that it is not unique to the myocardium and is elevated in the setting of muscle trauma. The use of a relative index, which is a function of the level of CK-MB mass relative to total CK activity, improves specificity, but may limit sensitivity [4]. Moreover, CK-MB may be elevated due to clearance abnormalities in renal failure or hypothyroidism. CK-MB becomes elevated in the circulation 3–6 hours after symptom onset in MI, and remains elevated for 24–36 hours (Fig. 1.1).

Cardiac troponin I and T

The troponins (I, C, and T) are a complex of proteins that modulate the calcium-mediated interaction between actin and myosin in myocardial tissue [5]. cTnI and cTnT are 23,500 and 37,000 Dalton molecules, respectively; they have isoforms that are unique to cardiac myocytes, enabling very specific assays using monoclonal antibodies to select epitopes of the cardiac form [6,7]. Most troponin is bound to the contractile apparatus of the cardiomyocyte, but 3% of cTnI and 6% of cTnT exist free in the cytoplasm [8,9]. The initial elevation of cTnI or cTnT detected in the circulation after myocardial necrosis is thought to be a function of the free cytolsolic form, whereas the prolonged elevation is caused by degradation of the contractile pool. The early release kinetics of cTnI and cTnT are similar to CK-MB, allowing detection at 3–6 hours after symptom onset during MI. However, cTnI and cTnT may remain elevated for 4–7 and 10–14 days, respectively.

The cardiac troponins offer numerous advantages over CK-MB for evaluating patients with possible MI. Because cTnT and cTnI do not circulate in measurable levels among healthy adults, a very low cut-off range can be used to define elevation, leading to higher sensitivity than CK-MB. Patients who in the past would have been classified as unstable angina with normal CK-MB values may have minor myocardial necrosis detected by an elevation in cTnI or cTnT [10,11]. Introduction of widespread troponin testing resulted in up to a 25% increase in the detection of MI in patients with normal CK-MB values [12]. With the newer, more sensitive cTn assays the increased frequency of the diagnosis of MI may even be higher, estimated at 28% to 195% depending on the cut-point used [13]. Cardiac troponin measurement yields fewer false-positive results in the setting of trauma, surgery, and renal failure as compared to CK-MB [14,15].

The recommended cut-off value for an elevated cardiac troponin is the 99th percentile of a control reference group at a precision level of $\leq 10\%$ Coefficient of Variation (CV, which is a measure of precision and is defined as standard deviation/mean) [2]. Although these low-level cardiac troponin elevations are very specific for myocardial damage, troponin elevation in itself does not indicate the mechanism of injury. Pulmonary embolism, congestive heart failure, and myocarditis can all lead to cardiac troponin elevation [16]. In addition, diabetes mellitus, left ventricular hypertrophy, chronic kidney disease, and congestive heart failure can all lead to minor cardiac troponin elevation in an asymptomatic, ambulatory population [17].

Myoglobin

Myoglobin is a 17,800 Dalton hemoprotein that is found in all tissues. Myoglobin has been used in the diagnosis of MI because it is an early marker that can be detected 1–2 hours after symptom onset, and remains elevated for up to 24 hours; studies have shown that myoglobin offers high sensitivity for detecting MI in the first few hours after presentation [18]. However, the use of myoglobin as a stand-alone marker has significant limitations including low-specificity for MI in patients with renal failure or skeletal muscle trauma [19]. Also, given that myoglobin rises and falls rapidly in the setting of MI, the level may normalize in patients that present >24 hours after symptom onset [20]. Considering its rapid rise and fall, and limited specificity, myoglobin has usually been used in combination with CK-MB or cTn.

Point-of-care testing

There are several assays that can measure cardiac markers at the point-of-care (POC). These include assays that measure myoglobin, CK-MB, and cTnI or cTnT. As cTn is the preferred cardiac marker for evaluating patients with possible MI, all manufacturers of POC cardiac markers include either cTnI or cTnT. The POC assays can be either quantitative or qualitative and some have corresponding

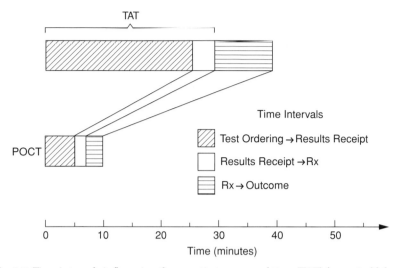

Fig. 1.2 Time intervals influencing therapeutic turnaround time (TAT) for central laboratory (top) and point of care (POCT) (bottom) testing strategies. Rx = therapy. Kost G. *Chest* 1999; **115**: 1140–1154.

central laboratory analyzers that yield similar results. If an institution uses a POC device that does not have a corresponding central laboratory analyzer, this is important to realize as the same specimen will yield different results on POC and central lab tests, and the cut-points for determining abnormal results will be different, which may lead to clinical confusion. Although in general central laboratory systems offer greater precision at low levels of biomarkers, some studies have shown equivalent clinical performance between POC technology and central laboratory assays [21–27]. However, one study of 4447 patients with acute coronary syndrome demonstrated that a significant number of patients that had a positive central laboratory cTnT assay did not have elevated values as measured by a cTnI POC device [28]. Thus, it is critical to know the diagnostic performance of the particular assay that is being used.

The promise of POC testing of cardiac markers is a more rapid turnaround time (TAT) leading to possible faster triage and treatment of patients evaluated for MI. Factors that affect TAT are delays in delivery of the sample to the central laboratory, preanalytical steps necessary to prepare sample, analysis time, and delivery of results to the ordering physician (Fig. 1.2). The National Academy of Clinical Biochemistry (NACB) [29] and the International Federation of Clinical Chemistry (IFCC) [30] have recommended 60 minutes or less from the time that blood is drawn to the reporting of results. The American College of Cardiology/American Heart Association (ACC/AHA) have also recommended a 60-minute TAT, but state 30 minutes is preferred [31].

Table 1.1 Turnaround time (in minutes) for point of care testing compared to central laboratory

Reference #	POCT	Central Laboratory	Time Reduction
Cargher [32]	38	87	49
Lee-Lewandrowski [35]	17	110	93
Collinson [36]	20	79	59
McCord [37]	24	71	47
Singer [40]	15	83	68
Sieck [39]	20	90	70
Gaze [34]	20	85	65
Altinier [38]	17	82	65
Hsu [33]	26	65	39

POCT = Point-of-Care Testing

Numerous studies have shown that when using POC devices the TAT for cardiac marker results can be decreased in the range of 39 to 93 minutes when compared to a central laboratory strategy [32–40] (Table 1.1). This time savings can translate into more rapid triage and medical decision making. In a randomized controlled study in the ED by Murray [41], 93 patients had blood testing at the POC and 87 patients had samples sent to the central laboratory. Blood tests that were available at the POC included electrolytes, glucose, hematocrit, and qualitative CK-MB and myoglobin. Patients were only entered into the trial if all blood tests ordered were available POC. This was a heterogeneous population and did not require that the patient was being evaluated for possible MI. The median length of stay (LOS) of patients in the POC group was 3.5 hours and in the central laboratory group 4.4 hours (p = 0.02). The difference was greater in discharged patients who comprised 75% of all patients: POC 3.1 hours versus central laboratory 4.3 hours (p < 0.001). In a study by Singer [40] of patients evaluated for MI in the ED, 232 patients had cTnI measured in the central laboratory in the initial phase and subsequently 134 patients had cTnI measured at the POC. No other tests were measured at the POC. The median LOS in the POC group was 5.2 hours versus 7.1 hours in the central laboratory group. The time to results reported in the POC group was 14.8 minutes as compared to 93 minutes in the central laboratory group. In addition, the time to call for admission in the POC group was 2.7 hours as compared to 4.7 hours in

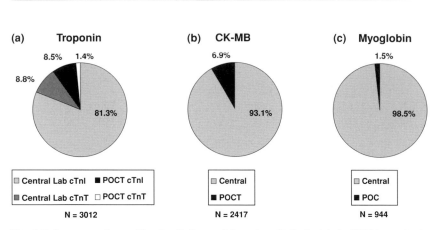

Fig. 1.3 Survey performed by the College of American Pathologists in 2005 to evaluate utilization of central laboratory compared to point of care testing (POCT) for cardiac markers. Wu A. *Point of Care* 2006; **5**: 20–24.

the central laboratory group. Thus, in this study measurement of POC cTnI led to faster medical decision making and decreased LOS. POC testing of cardiac markers has been used in the prehospital setting in ambulances and in remote locations such as cruise ships [42–45]. Although POC testing of cardiac markers is more expensive per unit test, the decrease in LOS may make a POC strategy financially appealing in certain institutions.

Although it is intuitively appealing that the more rapid identification and treatment of non–ST-segment elevation myocardial infarction (NSTEMI) patients by cTn measured at the POC can improve patient outcomes, there are no compelling data to validate the 30–60 minute recommended TAT for cardiac markers. Time to identification and treatment of patients with ST-segment elevation myocardial infarction (STEMI) is crucial as improved patient outcomes are clearly very time dependent [46], but initial decision making is based on electrocardiographic findings rather than biomarker levels. In contrast, although patients with NSTEMI identified by an elevated cTn benefit from glycoprotein IIb/IIIa inhibitors, low-molecular weight heparin, and cardiac catheterization with percutaneous intervention [47–50], there are insufficient data to conclude that these therapies delivered 60 minutes or so earlier, afforded by POC measurement of cTn, improve patient outcomes. Although POC testing of cardiac markers are used in some centers, most institutions measure cardiac markers in the central laboratory (Fig. 1.3). Although it is hoped that POC testing will eventually impact outcomes in ACS, at the present time the most compelling reason to use POC testing is to more rapidly identify high- and low-risk patients, which may lead to shorter LOS. The exact affects of POC testing will likely be specific to certain institutions and depend on factors such as volume, patient acuity, and staffing.

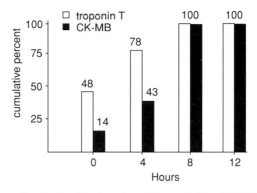

Fig. 1.4 Proportion of patients with elevation of troponin T or CKMB through 12 hours in a chest pain observation unit. Newby. *Am J Cardiol* 2000; **85**: 801–805.

Serial sampling of cardiac markers

Elevations of cTnI and cTnT are not sufficiently sensitive at presentation in the ED and must be measured serially over time to adequately exclude MI. Numerous professional organizations agree that cTn should be measured over at least 6 hours. Although some guidelines state that 6 hours is adequate [51], others suggest 6–9 hours [52,53], or even 6–12 hours [54]. Newby [55] evaluated 383 consecutive patients in a chest pain observation unit that had nondiagnostic electrocardiograms, no high-risk clinical features, and normal CK-MB values at presentation. There were eight (2.1%) patients that had MI. Patients had serum CK-MB and cTnT measured at 0, 4, 8, and 12 hours. All patients who were positive by either CK-MB or cTnT at 12 hours were already identified by both positive CK-MB and cTnT at 8 hours (Fig. 1.4). Hamm [56] evaluated 773 patients with chest pain of less than 12 hours duration and without ST-segment elevation on their electrocardiograms. There were 47 (6.1%) patients with a diagnosis of MI. Samples were taken for cTnI at presentation and at 4 hours. If the patient presented within 2 hours after chest pain onset, then a third sample was drawn at least 6 hours after symptom onset. Therefore, all patients had at least 2 samples, the last being at least 6 hours after symptom onset. Among the 47 patients with MI, 31 (66%) had a positive cTnI at presentation and all 47 (100%) had an elevated cTnI at 4 hours. Herren [57] evaluated a 6-hour "rule-out" MI strategy in 292 consecutive patients evaluated in the ED with nondiagnostic electrocardiograms who presented within 12 hours of symptom onset. All patients had CK-MB measured at arrival. If patients presented <3 hours after symptoms onset, there was a CK-MB measured at 6 hours. Patients that presented within 3–12 hours of symptom onset had a second CK-MB measured at 3 hours after presentation. Patients then had a cTnT measured at 48 hours. Of the 238 patients that had all normal CK-MB values, there was only 1 that had an elevated cTnT of 0.11 ng/dl. On review at 1 month this one patient was doing well with no electrocardiographic evidence of MI. The negative predictive value for MI of serial CK-MB over 6 hours was 99.6%.

The study by Newby suggests there is no reason to measure cTn beyond 8 hours. Although in the Hamm study cTnI was not measured in general beyond 6 hours after symptom onset, there were only 2 adverse events at 30 days (1 death and 1 MI after discharge) in the 602 patients that had negative cTnI, yielding a 0.3% adverse event rate. Thus, an adequate sample set for evaluating patients for possible MI is a sample at presentation and a second at least 6 hours after symptom onset. Patients that present >6 hours after symptom onset may proceed to stress testing, if clinically indicated, with 1 normal cTn value at presentation. With newer, more sensitive and precise cTn assays the necessary time period for serial testing will likely shorten (see next section).

Multimarker strategies and analysis of dynamic change in markers over time

Taking advantage of the different release kinetics of the various cardiac markers, studies of combinations of markers have evaluated the ability to rapidly exclude MI in less than 6 hours. A cardiac marker that rises early in the setting of MI, most commonly myoglobin, combined with one that increases later, CK-MB or cTn, allows MI to be identified more rapidly and, therefore, excluded in less time. A patient who has completely normal myoglobin and CK-MB or cTnI over the first few hours after presentation to the ED could proceed to their final disposition more rapidly. Patients that have only an elevated myoglobin would require serial testing over a longer period to confirm myocardial necrosis. Kontos [58] evaluated 101 patients admitted from the ED for possible MI. Blood samples for CK-MB and myoglobin were taken at 0, 4, 8, 16, and 24 hours. There were 20 MIs. The individual sensitivities for myoglobin and CK-MB at 0 and 4 hours were 85% and 90%, respectively. The combined sensitivity for both markers over 4 hours was 100%. McCord [37] studied 817 patients in the ED where myoglobin, cTnI, and CK-MB were measured at 0, 1.5, 3, and 9 hours. There were 65 patients with MI. The combined sensitivity of myoglobin and cTnI over 90 minutes was 96.9% (negative predictive value 99.6%). Measurement of CK-MB and blood sampling at 3 hours did not improve sensitivity. It should be noted that these studies used CK-MB as the gold standard for MI detection, and thus sensitivity may not be quite as high if a troponin-based standard was used.

A dynamic change (delta) in any cardiac marker can identify a patient earlier in the setting of MI. Various strategies utilizing delta markers alone or in combination with typical abnormal cut-off values have been studied. Ng [59] studied 1285 consecutive patients in the ED. There were 66 (5.1%) patients diagnosed with MI. Myoglobin, cTnI, and CK-MB were measured at 0, 0.5, 1.0, 1.5, 3, and 6 hours. At 90 minutes the combined sensitivity of CK-MB, cTnI, and delta-myoglobin (defined as >25% increase over 90 minutes) was 100%. Kontos

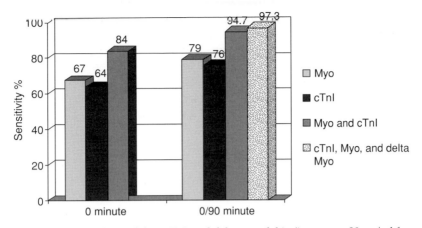

Fig. 1.5 Sensitivity of myoglobin, cTnI, and delta myoglobin (increase > 20 ng/ml from baseline to 90 minutes) to detect myocardial infarction within 90 minutes of presentation. Sallach. *Am J Cardiol* 2004; **94**: 864–867.

[60] evaluated 2093 patients who were admitted to the hospital for possible MI. There were a total of 186 (8.9%) MIs. The combined sensitivity at 3 hours for the combination of CK-MB ≥8.0 ng/mL, relative index (CK-MB × 100/total CK) ≥4.0, or at least a 2-fold increase in CK-MB without exceeding the upper range of normal was 93% over 3 hours. Fesmire [61] studied 710 patients evaluated in the ED who had a baseline CK-MB <2 times the upper limits of normal (12 ng/mL) and blood draws at 0 and 2 hours. A CK-MB was considered positive at 6 ng/mL and a delta-CK-MB was positive if there was a change from 0 to 2 hours of ≥1.6 ng/mL. There were 113 patients diagnosed with MI (68 NSTEMI and 45 STEMI). The sensitivities of CK-MB and delta-CK-MB at 2 hours were 75.2% and 92%, respectively. The specificity of 2-hour delta-CK-MB was 95.3%. These studies, and many others, although of conceptual interest, also employed a CK-MB definition of MI and thus have limited clinical application in the modern era. Few studies have evaluated multimarker or delta-marker strategies in the context of cTn-defined MI.

Sallach [62], in a retrospective reanalysis of a prior study [37], analyzed 817 consecutive patients evaluated in the ED. MI was defined in accordance with the ESC/ACC 2000 guidelines concerning the redefinition of MI and required at least one cTnI >0.4 ng/mL. Blood samples were taken at 0, 1.5, 3, and 9 hours for myoglobin and cTnI. A delta-myoglobin >20 ng/mL increase over 90 minutes was considered positive. There were 75 patients (9%) who had MI. The sensitivities for the various combinations are shown (Fig. 1.5). The combined sensitivity of cTnI, myoglobin, and delta-myoglobin >20 ng/mL was 97.3% at 90 minutes. There were only 2 patients with MI not identified within 90 minutes with this strategy. One patient had intermittent chest pain consistent with unstable angina that led to an MI. The myoglobin rose from 144 ng/mL at 90 minutes to 233 ng/mL (>200 ng/mL abnormal) at 3 hours and cTnI was abnormal at 9 hours. The other patient actually had a decrease of myoglobin >20 ng/mL at 90 minutes, and if this patient was considered positive the early sensitivity would be even higher. This patient likely had a very early peaking myoglobin that was already decreasing. Fesmire [63] reported on 975 patients evaluated in the ED that had blood samples drawn at 0 and 2 hours for cTnI, CK-MB, and myoglobin that had a cTnI at presentation ≤1.0 ng/mL (Abbott Axym). MI was defined as either cTnI >1.0 mg/mL, new significant Q-waves in 2 contiguous leads, cardiac death, or death for unknown reason. They reported that the sensitivity of delta- CK-MB >0.7 ng/mL at 2 hours of 93.2% was higher than delta-myoglobin >9.4 ng/mL of 77.3%.

Improved troponin assays: cut-points, precision, and implications for the role of myoglobin and CK-MB

The recommended cut-point for an abnormal cTn is at the 99th percentile of a reference control group with an acceptable CV ≤10%. [2] Earlier cTn assays had such a high degree of analytical imprecision at low levels that none met the stringent precision requirements at these low levels, so a higher cut-point than the 99th percentile was used to meet the ≤10% CV precision requirement. However, assays have now been developed that are close to or meet the criterion for <10% CV at the low 99th percentile level. Most published studies have used the less precise and less sensitive cTn assays. However, a few studies have investigated the early diagnostic utility of these new sensitive and precise cTn assays. MacRae evaluated the need for measuring cTnI over 6 hours when evaluating patients for possible MI in the ED [64]. The assay used the AccuTnI (Beckman Coulter) with the 99th percentile level of 0.04 ng/mL. This was a retrospective study performed using stored samples from 1996. There were 258 patients enrolled and specimens were collected at presentation and then hourly until 6 hours after symptom onset, and thereafter at 9, 12, 24, and 48 hours. MI was defined as at least 1 sample >0.04 ng/mL and at least 20% change between specimens. There were 92 MIs. There was not a significant difference in the proportion of patients with troponin elevation when comparing patients who had cTnI measured ≥3 hours as compared to ≥6 hours (Fig. 1.6). This study suggests that with the newer, more sensitive, and precise assays that a "rule-out" MI protocol may be able to be reduced from 6 hours to 3 hours. However, these findings need to be corroborated in other studies before any change in current clinical algorithms should be considered.

The diagnostic utility of myoglobin and CK-MB has been studied with the newer cTn assays. Eggers [65] studied 197 consecutive patients in the ED with nondiagnostic electrocardiograms. There were 43 patients (22%) with MI. Blood samples were drawn at time of presentation, every 30 minutes during the first 2 hours, and then at 3, 6, and 12 hours. The samples were analyzed on the Stratus

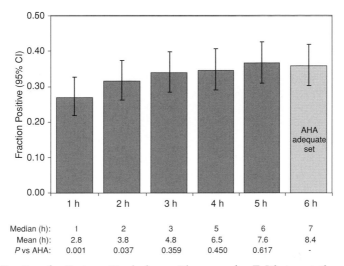

Median (h):	I	2	3	5	6	7
Mean (h):	2.8	3.8	4.8	6.5	7.6	8.4
P vs AHA:	0.001	0.037	0.359	0.450	0.617	-

Fig. 1.6 Fraction of patients positive by hour with an assay for cTnI that meets the precision of $< 10\%$ coefficient of variation (CV) at the 99th percentile (0.04 ng/ml). MacRae. *Clin Chem* 2006; **52**: 65.

CS device (Dade Behring). The 99th percentile for this assay has been reported at 0.07 ng/mL [66] and the 10% CV is 0.10 ng/mL [67]. The cumulative sensitivity was highest for cTnI at 0.10 ng/mL at all time points (Fig. 1.7). Importantly, the measurement of CK-MB or myoglobin did not improve sensitivity. However, the specificities of cTnI and CK-MB at 6 hours were 76% and 88%, respectively. Amodio [68] reported on 516 patients evaluated for possible MI. A cTnI-based definition for MI was used. Blood samples were drawn at presentation and every 6 hours thereafter; cTnI and myoglobin were measured on the Dade Stratus CS. There were 110 patients (21.3%) with MI. The sensitivity of cTnI was reported at very low values, including those below the 10% CV. Although in this study there was not early frequent sampling of myoglobin, the measurement of myoglobin at 6 hours did not improve early sensitivity. Kavsak [69] retrospectively analyzed 228 patients who were evaluated for possible MI in 1996 and had stored samples. Specimens were drawn at presentation and then hourly until 6 hours, and thereafter at 9, 12, 24, and 48 hours after symptom onset. In the original study CK-MB isoforms were measured, and in the reanalysis myoglobin and cTnI were measured on the Accu cTnI assay (Beckman Coulter). The new definition of MI was retrospectively applied to cases after cTnI measurement and the prevalence of MI increased from 46 patients (20%) to 91 (40%). The measurement of myoglobin or CK-MB did not improve early sensitivity.

When cTn assays are available, the routine measurement of CK-MB to evaluate patients for possible MI is unnecessary. However, the measurement of CK-MB still may be helpful in particular situations such as determining reinfarction in

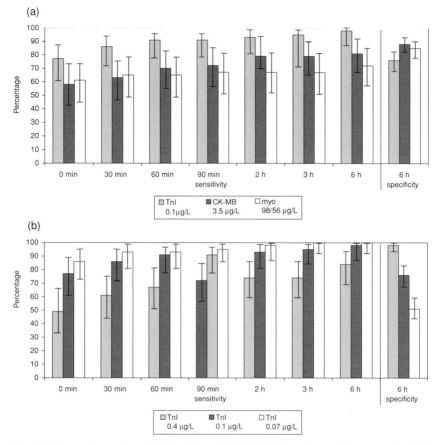

Fig. 1.7 Comparison of sensitivities of myoglobin, CK-MB, and a sensitive assay for cTnI at various cut-points and time intervals. Note the improved sensitivity for the lower cTnI threshold of 0.1 ng/mL early after presentation. Eggers. *Am Heart J* 2004; **148**: 574–581.

patients already with an elevation of cTn. Prior studies performed even before the newer, more sensitive, and precise cTn assays were available suggested that CK-MB did not improve sensitivity for MI detection [37]. An argument for the routine use of CK-MB in evaluating patients with possible MI is lessened further with the 3rd generation cTn assays. Presently many institutions routinely measure CK-MB in combination with cTn. This strategy is unnecessary and a poor use of resources. During the transition period with the new cTn assays, a "reflexive" cTn strategy may be reasonable. The laboratory measures cTn only if the cTn value is normal. However, the laboratory will automatically run and report CK-MB if the cTn is even mildly elevated. This enables the clinician to have at their disposal a CK-MB value when attempting to sort out a patient with any level of cTn elevation. Several institutions use this strategy presently (e.g., Mayo Clinic, Henry Ford Hospital). Similarly, a few recent studies suggest that myoglobin measurement in a multimarker strategy may not improve early sensitivity as low levels of cTn can be detected early after MI by these more sensitive cTn assays. The diagnostic utility of myoglobin, or change in myoglobin, early on in the setting of MI needs to be investigated further in the context of the new cTn assays.

A change over time in low-level cTn levels may assist in the identification of MI, particularly among patients who have equivocal historical or ECG evidence to support MI. A dynamic change in low-level cTn levels over time would suggest acute active myocardial necrosis and distinguish these patients from those that have chronic elevations. Low-level cTn elevations can be detected in asymptomatic ambulatory patients with a history of diabetes mellitus, heart failure, renal insufficiency, or left ventricular hypertrophy [17].

Although low-level cTn detection may enable more rapid detection of MI, and therefore a faster "rule-out" MI process, low-level cTn detection has lower specificity for MI. Minor cTn elevation may be seen in multiple clinical scenarios where there is myocardial damage but not a clinical scenario of MI (pulmonary embolism, myocarditis, heart failure, and many others). With the ultra-sensitive cTn assays the frequency of abnormal cTn values in patients without MI will increase in the ED. In the era of ultra-sensitive cTn assays historical and electrocardiographic findings will be even more important in assessing patients for possible MI. If further studies of the new cTn assays demonstrate no incremental diagnostic utility of myoglobin, then the door is open for other multimarker strategies to be developed that include novel markers of ischemia together with highly sensitive cTns (see chapter 5).

References

1 Nawar EW, NR Xu J. National Hospital Ambulatory Medical Care Survey: 2005 Emergency Department Summary. *Advance Data from vital and health statistics* 2007: 1–32.

2 Thygesen K, Alpert JS, White HD, Jaffe AS, Apple FS, Galvani M, et al. Universal definition of myocardial infarction. *Circulation* 2007; **116**: 2634–2653.

3 Roberts R, Sobel BE. Editorial: Isoenzymes of creatine phosphokinase and diagnosis of myocardial infarction. *Annals of internal medicine* 1973; **79**: 741–743.

4 Adams JE, 3rd, Bodor GS, Davila-Roman VG, Delmez JA, Apple FS, Ladenson JH, et al. Cardiac troponin I. A marker with high specificity for cardiac injury. *Circulation* 1993; **88**: 101–106.

5 Takeda S, Yamashita A, Maeda K, Maeda Y. Structure of the core domain of human cardiac troponin in the Ca(2+)-saturated form. *Nature* 2003; **424**: 35–41.

6 Katus HA, Remppis A, Neumann FJ, Scheffold T, Diederich KW, Vinar G, et al. Diagnostic efficiency of troponin T measurements in acute myocardial infarction. *Circulation* 1991; **83**: 902 912.

7 Bodor GS, Porter S, Landt Y, Ladenson JH. Development of monoclonal antibodies for an assay of cardiac troponin-I and preliminary results in suspected cases of myocardial infarction. *Clinical chemistry* 1992; **38**: 2203–2214.

8 Adams JE, 3rd, Schechtman KB, Landt Y, Ladenson JH, Jaffe AS. Comparable detection of acute myocardial infarction by creatine kinase MB isoenzyme and cardiac troponin I. *Clinical chemistry* 1994; **40**: 1291–1295.

9 Katus HA, Remppis A, Scheffold T, Diederich KW, Kuebler W. Intracellular compartmentation of cardiac troponin T and its release kinetics in patients with reperfused and nonreperfused myocardial infarction. *The American journal of cardiology* 1991; **67**: 1360–1367.

10 Hamm CW, Ravkilde J, Gerhardt W, Jorgensen P, Peheim E, Ljungdahl L, et al. The prognostic value of serum troponin T in unstable angina. *The New England journal of medicine* 1992; **327**: 146–150.

11 Heidenreich PA, Alloggiamento T, Melsop K, McDonald KM, Go AS, Hlatky MA. The prognostic value of troponin in patients with non-ST elevation acute coronary syndromes: a meta-analysis. *Journal of the American College of Cardiology* 2001; **38**: 478–485.

12 Newby LK, Alpert JS, Ohman EM, Thygesen K, Califf RM. Changing the diagnosis of acute myocardial infarction: implications for practice and clinical investigations. *American heart journal* 2002; **144**: 957–980.

13 Kontos MC, Fritz LM, Anderson FP, Tatum JL, Ornato JP, Jesse RL. Impact of the troponin standard on the prevalence of acute myocardial infarction. *American heart journal* 2003; **146**: 446–452.

14 Adams JE, 3rd, Sicard GA, Allen BT, Bridwell KH, Lenke LG, Davila-Roman VG, et al. Diagnosis of perioperative myocardial infarction with measurement of cardiac troponin I. *The New England journal of medicine* 1994; **330**: 670–674.

15 McCullough PA, Nowak RM, Foreback C, Tokarski G, Tomlanovich MC, Khoury NE, et al. Performance of multiple cardiac biomarkers measured in the emergency department in patients with chronic kidney disease and chest pain. *Acad Emerg Med* 2002; **9**: 1389–1396.

16 Jaffe AS. Elevations in cardiac troponin measurements: false false-positives: the real truth. *Cardiovascular toxicology* 2001; **1**: 87–92.

17 Wallace TW, Abdullah SM, Drazner MH, Das SR, Khera A, McGuire DK, et al. Prevalence and determinants of troponin T elevation in the general population. *Circulation* 2006; **113**: 1958–1965.

18 Brogan GX, Jr., Friedman S, McCuskey C, Cooling DS, Berrutti L, Thode HC, Jr., et al. Evaluation of a new rapid quantitative immunoassay for serum myoglobin versus CK-MB for ruling out acute myocardial infarction in the emergency department. *Annals of emergency medicine* 1994; **24**: 665–671.

19 de Winter RJ, Koster RW, Sturk A, Sanders GT. Value of myoglobin, troponin T, and CK-MBmass in ruling out an acute myocardial infarction in the emergency room. *Circulation* 1995; **92**: 3401–3407.

20 Gilkeson G, Stone MJ, Waterman M, Ting R, Gomez-Sanchez CE, I Iull A, et al. Detection of myoglobin by radioimmunoassay in human sera: its usefulness and limitations as an emergency room screening test for acute myocardial infarction. *American heart journal* 1978; **95**: 70–77.

21 Apple FS, Christenson RH, Valdes R, Jr., Andriak AJ, Berg A, Duh SH, et al. Simultaneous rapid measurement of whole blood myoglobin, creatine kinase MB, and cardiac troponin I by the triage cardiac panel for detection of myocardial infarction. *Clinical chemistry* 1999; **45**: 199–205.

22 Wu AH, Smith A, Christenson RH, Murakami MM, Apple FS. Evaluation of a point-of-care assay for cardiac markers for patients suspected of acute myocardial infarction. *Clinica chimica acta; international journal of clinical chemistry* 2004; **346**: 211–219.

23 Apple FS, Anderson FP, Collinson P, Jesse RL, Kontos MC, Levitt MA, et al. Clinical evaluation of the first medical whole blood, point-of-care testing device for detection of myocardial infarction. *Clinical chemistry* 2000; **46**: 1604–1609.

24 Apple FS, Murakami MM, Christenson RH, Campbell JL, Miller CJ, Hock KG, et al. Analytical performance of the i-STAT cardiac troponin I assay. *Clinica chimica acta; international journal of clinical chemistry* 2004; **345**: 123–127.

25 Heeschen C, Goldmann BU, Langenbrink L, Matschuck G, Hamm CW. Evaluation of a rapid whole blood ELISA for quantification of troponin I in patients with acute chest pain. *Clinical chemistry* 1999; **45**: 1789–1796.

26 Collinson PO, Jorgensen B, Sylven C, Haass M, Chwallek F, Katus HA, et al. Recalibration of the point-of-care test for CARDIAC T Quantitative with Elecsys Troponin T 3rd generation. *Clinica chimica acta; international journal of clinical chemistry* 2001; **307**: 197–203.

27 Goldmann BU, Langenbrink L, Matschuck G, Heeschen C, Kolbe-Busch S, Niederau C, et al. Quantitative bedside testing of troponin T: is it equal to laboratory testing? The Cardiac Reader Troponin T (CARE T) study. *Clinical laboratory* 2004; **50**: 1–10.

28 James SK, Lindahl B, Armstrong P, Califf R, Simoons ML, Venge P, et al. A rapid troponin I assay is not optimal for determination of troponin status and prediction of subsequent cardiac events at suspicion of unstable coronary syndromes. *International journal of cardiology* 2004; **93**: 113–120.

29 Wu AH, Apple FS, Gibler WB, Jesse RL, Warshaw MM, Valdes R, Jr. National Academy of Clinical Biochemistry Standards of Laboratory Practice: recommendations for the use of cardiac markers in coronary artery diseases. *Clinical chemistry* 1999; **45**: 1104–1121.

30 Panteghini M, Apple FS, Christenson RH, Dati F, Mair J, Wu AH. Use of biochemical markers in acute coronary syndromes. IFCC Scientific Division, Committee on Standardization of Markers of Cardiac Damage. International Federation of Clinical Chemistry. *Clin Chem Lab Med* 1999; **37**: 687–693.

31 Braunwald E, Antman EM, Beasley JW, Califf RM, Cheitlin MD, Hochman JS, et al. ACC/AHA guidelines for the management of patients with unstable angina and non-ST-segment elevation myocardial infarction: executive summary and recommendations. A report of the American College of Cardiology/American Heart Association task force on practice guidelines (committee on the management of patients with unstable angina). *Circulation* 2000; **102**: 1193–1209.

32 Caragher TE, Fernandez BB, Jacobs FL, Barr LA. Evaluation of quantitative cardiac biomarker point-of-care testing in the emergency department. *The Journal of emergency medicine* 2002; **22**: 1–7.

33 Hsu LF, Koh TH, Lim YL. Cardiac marker point-of-care testing: evaluation of rapid on-site biochemical marker analysis for diagnosis of acute myocardial infarction. *Annals of the Academy of Medicine, Singapore* 2000; **29**: 421–427.

34 Gaze D. The Use of a Quantitative Point-of-Care System Greatly Reduces the Turnaround Time of Cardiac Marker Determination. *Point of Care* 2004; **3**: 156–158.

35 Lee-Lewandrowski E, Corboy D, Lewandrowski K, Sinclair J, McDermot S, Benzer TI. Implementation of a point-of-care satellite laboratory in the emergency department of an academic medical center. Impact on test turnaround time and patient emergency department length of stay. *Archives of pathology & laboratory medicine* 2003; **127**: 456–460.

36 Collinson PO, John C, Lynch S, Rao A, Canepa-Anson R, Carson E, et al. A prospective randomized controlled trial of point-of-care testing on the coronary care unit. *Annals of clinical biochemistry* 2004; **41**: 397–404.

37 McCord J, Nowak RM, McCullough PA, Foreback C, Borzak S, Tokarski G, et al. Ninety-minute exclusion of acute myocardial infarction by use of quantitative point-of-care testing of myoglobin and troponin I. *Circulation* 2001; **104**: 1483–1488.

38 Altinier S, Zaninotto M, Mion M, Carraro P, Rocco S, Tosato F, et al. Point-of-care testing of cardiac markers: results from an experience in an Emergency Department. *Clinica chimica acta; international journal of clinical chemistry* 2001; **311**: 67–72.

39 Sieck S. The Evolution of a New Standard of Hospital Care: Paradigm Shift to the Emergency Department and the Role of Point-of-Care Testing. *Point of Care* 2006; **5**: 2–5.

40 Singer AJ, Ardise J, Gulla J, Cangro J. Point-of-care testing reduces length of stay in emergency department chest pain patients. *Annals of emergency medicine* 2005; **45**: 587–591.

41 Murray RP, Leroux M, Sabga E, Palatnick W, Ludwig L. Effect of point of care testing on length of stay in an adult emergency department. *The Journal of emergency medicine* 1999; **17**: 811–814.

42 Svensson L, Axelsson C, Nordlander R, Herlitz J. Prehospital identification of acute coronary syndrome/myocardial infarction in relation to ST elevation. *International journal of cardiology* 2005; **98**: 237–244.

43 Cawdery M, Burg MD. Emergency medicine career paths less traveled: cruise ship medicine, Indian health, and critical care medicine. *Annals of emergency medicine* 2004; **44**: 79–83.

44 Roth A, Malov N, Golovner M, Sander J, Shapira I, Kaplinsky E, et al. The "SHAHAL" experience in Israel for improving diagnosis of acute coronary syndromes in the prehospital setting. *The American journal of cardiology* 2001; **88**: 608–610.

45 Schuchert A, Hamm C, Scholz J, Klimmeck S, Goldmann B, Meinertz T. Prehospital testing for troponin T in patients with suspected acute myocardial infarction. *American heart journal* 1999; **138**: 45–48.

46 De Luca G, Suryapranata II, Ottervanger JP, Antman EM. Time delay to treatment and mortality in primary angioplasty for acute myocardial infarction: every minute of delay counts. *Circulation* 2004; **109**: 1223–1225.

47 Cohen M, Demers C, Gurfinkel EP, Turpie AG, Fromell GJ, Goodman S, et al. A comparison of low-molecular-weight heparin with unfractionated heparin for unstable coronary artery disease. Efficacy and Safety of Subcutaneous Enoxaparin in Non-Q-Wave Coronary Events Study Group. *The New England journal of medicine* 1997; **337**: 447–452.

48 A comparison of aspirin plus tirofiban with aspirin plus heparin for unstable angina. Platelet Receptor Inhibition in Ischemic Syndrome Management (PRISM) Study Investigators. *The New England journal of medicine* 1998; **338**: 1498–1505.

49 Inhibition of platelet glycoprotein IIb/IIIa with eptifibatide in patients with acute coronary syndromes. The PURSUIT Trial Investigators. Platelet Glycoprotein IIb/IIIa in Unstable Angina: Receptor Suppression Using Integrilin Therapy. *The New England journal of medicine* 1998; **339**: 436–443.

50 Mehta SR, Cannon CP, Fox KA, Wallentin L, Boden WE, Spacek R, et al. Routine vs selective invasive strategies in patients with acute coronary syndromes: a collaborative meta-analysis of randomized trials. *Jama* 2005; **293**: 2908–2917.

51 Luepker RV, Apple FS, Christenson RH, Crow RS, Fortmann SP, Goff D, et al. Case definitions for acute coronary heart disease in epidemiology and clinical research studies: a statement from the AHA Council on Epidemiology and Prevention; AHA Statistics Committee; World Heart Federation Council on Epidemiology and Prevention; the European Society of Cardiology Working Group on Epidemiology and Prevention; Centers for Disease Control and Prevention; and the National Heart, Lung, and Blood Institute. *Circulation* 2003; **108**: 2543–2549.

52 Braunwald E, Antman EM, Beasley JW, Califf RM, Cheitlin MD, Hochman JS, et al. ACC/AHA 2002 guideline update for the management of patients with unstable angina and non-ST-segment elevation myocardial infarction–summary article: a report of the American College of Cardiology/American Heart Association task force on practice guidelines (Committee on the Management of Patients With Unstable Angina). *Journal of the American College of Cardiology* 2002; **40**: 1366–1374.

53 Morrow DA, Cannon CP, Jesse RL, Newby LK, Ravkilde J, Storrow AB, et al. National Academy of Clinical Biochemistry Laboratory Medicine Practice Guidelines: clinical characteristics and utilization of biochemical markers in acute coronary syndromes. *Clinical chemistry* 2007; **53**: 552–574.

54 Bassand JP, Hamm CW, Ardissino D, Boersma E, Budaj A, Fernandez-Aviles F, et al. Guidelines for the diagnosis and treatment of non-ST-segment elevation acute coronary syndromes: The Task Force for the Diagnosis and Treatment of Non-ST-Segment Elevation Acute Coronary Syndromes of the European Society of Cardiology. *Eur Heart J* 2007; **28**: 1598–1660.

55 Newby LK, Kaplan AL, Granger BB, Sedor F, Califf RM, Ohman EM. Comparison of cardiac troponin T versus creatine kinase-MB for risk stratification in a chest pain evaluation unit. *The American journal of cardiology* 2000; **85**: 801–805.

56 Hamm CW, Goldmann BU, Heeschen C, Kreymann G, Berger J, Meinertz T. Emergency room triage of patients with acute chest pain by means of rapid testing for

cardiac troponin T or troponin I. *The New England journal of medicine* 1997; **337**: 1648–1653.

57 Ierren KR, Mackway-Jones K, Richards CR, Seneviratne CJ, France MW, Cotter L. Is it possible to exclude a diagnosis of myocardial damage within six hours of admission to an emergency department? Diagnostic cohort study. *BMJ* (Clinical research ed. 2001; **323**: 372.

58 Kontos MC, Anderson FP, Hanbury CM, Roberts CS, Miller WG, Jesse RL. Use of the combination of myoglobin and CK-MB mass for the rapid diagnosis of acute myocardial infarction. *The American journal of emergency medicine* 1997; **15**: 14–19.

59 Ng SM, Krishnaswamy P, Morissey R, Clopton P, Fitzgerald R, Maisel AS. Ninety-minute accelerated critical pathway for chest pain evaluation. *The American journal of cardiology* 2001; **88**: 611–617.

60 Kontos MC, Anderson FP, Schmidt KA, Ornato JP, Tatum JL, Jesse RL. Early diagnosis of acute myocardial infarction in patients without ST-segment elevation. *The American journal of cardiology* 1999; **83**: 155–158.

61 Fesmire FM, Percy RF, Bardoner JB, Wharton DR, Calhoun FB. Serial creatinine kinase (CK) MB testing during the emergency department evaluation of chest pain: utility of a 2-hour deltaCK-MB of +1.6ng/ml. *American heart journal* 1998; **136**: 237–244.

62 Sallach SM, Nowak R, Hudson MP, Tokarski G, Khoury N, Tomlanovich MC, et al. A change in serum myoglobin to detect acute myocardial infarction in patients with normal troponin I levels. *The American journal of cardiology* 2004; **94**: 864–867.

63 Fesmire FM, Christenson RH, Fody EP, Feintuch TA. Delta creatine kinase-MB outperforms myoglobin at two hours during the emergency department identification and exclusion of troponin positive non-ST-segment elevation acute coronary syndromes. *Annals of emergency medicine* 2004; **44**: 12–19.

64 Macrae AR, Kavsak PA, Lustig V, Bhargava R, Vandersluis R, Palomaki GE, et al. Assessing the requirement for the 6-hour interval between specimens in the American Heart Association Classification of Myocardial Infarction in Epidemiology and Clinical Research Studies. *Clinical chemistry* 2006; **52**: 812–818.

65 Eggers KM, Oldgren J, Nordenskjold A, Lindahl B. Diagnostic value of serial measurement of cardiac markers in patients with chest pain: limited value of adding myoglobin to troponin I for exclusion of myocardial infarction. *American heart journal* 2004; **148**: 574–581.

66 Apple FS, Wu AH, Jaffe AS. European Society of Cardiology and American College of Cardiology guidelines for redefinition of myocardial infarction: how to use existing assays clinically and for clinical trials. *American heart journal* 2002; **144**: 981–986.

67 Panteghini M, Pagani F, Yeo KT, Apple FS, Christenson RH, Dati F, et al. Evaluation of imprecision for cardiac troponin assays at low-range concentrations. *Clinical chemistry* 2004; **50**: 327–332.

68 Amodio G, Antonelli G, Varraso L, Ruggieri V, Di Serio F. Clinical impact of the troponin 99th percentile cut-off and clinical utility of myoglobin measurement in the early management of chest pain patients admitted to the Emergency Cardiology Department. *Coronary artery disease* 2007; **18**: 181–186.

69 Kavsak PA, MacRae AR, Newman AM, Lustig V, Palomaki GE, Ko DT, et al. Effects of contemporary troponin assay sensitivity on the utility of the early markers myoglobin and CKMB isoforms in evaluating patients with possible acute myocardial infarction. *Clinica chimica acta; international journal of clinical chemistry* 2007; **380**: 213–216.

Chapter 2

Troponin and other markers of necrosis for risk stratification in patients with acute coronary syndromes

Thomas E. Noel and Michael C. Kontos

Introduction

The assessment of patients with chest pain or symptoms consistent with myocardial ischemia typically begins in the emergency department (ED) with a history, physical, and electrocardiogram (ECG). In the absence of ischemic ST-segment elevation, the ECG lacks sensitivity as well as specificity, necessitating serial assessment of biomarkers to exclude myocardial infarction (MI), with further diagnostic testing to identify ischemia in those in whom MI is excluded. Although a wide variety of biomarkers have been used routinely for diagnosis, currently three—myoglobin, CK-MB, and troponin—are most commonly used for diagnosing MI. Additionally, these three markers have prognostic power for identifying patients at risk for short- and long-term cardiac events.

Myoglobin

Myoglobin is a relatively small heme protein (18.8 kD) that is present in both cardiac and skeletal muscle. It was one of the first cardiac markers used for the rapid identification of MI in ED chest pain patients because of its early detection in the serum (1–3 hours) after infarction. Because it is renally excreted and is found in all striated muscle, it has low cardiac specificity in the presence of skeletal muscle damage or renal failure. This lower specificity dramatically affects its diagnostic value when applied to low-risk chest pain patients, as the number of false positives can markedly exceed that of the true positives [1]. Although prior studies demonstrated a utility for early diagnosis of MI, more recent studies have questioned its usefulness when compared to newer, more sensitive CK-MB (1) and troponin assays [2].

Biomarkers in Heart Disease, 1st edition. Edited by James A. de Lemos.
© 2008 American Heart Association, ISBN: 978-1-4051-7571-5

The ability to predict cardiac events for myoglobin has varied across studies. Differences in study design, patient inclusion criteria, and choice of end-points likely contribute to this inconsistency. Studies in which both death and MI were used as end-points frequently found that troponin was the best predictor of this combination [3], as myoglobin did not predict recurrent MI [6]. However, when only mortality was assessed, myoglobin was a powerful predictor of short- and long-term mortality [3–7]. In a study by de Lemos et al. using the pooled data from the Thrombolysis in Myocardial Infarction (TIMI) 11B and TIMI 18 trials, myoglobin was an independent predictor of 6-month mortality, even after taking into account clinical variables and TnI [5]. Mortality was approximately 3-fold higher in patients with elevated myoglobin compared to those without, for both TnI positive and negative patients. Because TnI was sampled at only one time point, one possibility was that myoglobin identified patients who had undetectable TnI at presentation. However, in an analysis of 3461 patients admitted for exclusion of MI who underwent serial sampling with myoglobin, CK-MB, and TnI, myoglobin was the cardiac marker most predictive of 30-day and 1-year mortality [7].

Why myoglobin elevations predict mortality is unclear. Because it is eliminated primarily through the kidneys, one possible explanation is that myoglobin elevations are a surrogate for renal insufficiency. However, Kontos et al. found that variables that predicted mortality in the subgroup of patients with renal insufficiency were similar to those when all patients were included [7]. In addition, myoglobin remained the most important independent predictor of mortality in the renal dysfunction subgroup. The fact that myoglobin-associated mortality remained high in TnI-negative patients suggests that myoglobin predicts mortality through mechanisms distinct from myocardial ischemia. For example, hypotension and reduced renal perfusion can cause skeletal muscle release of myoglobin [8] and could contribute to mortality. Consistent with this hypothesis, in a small study of patients who had sepsis or hypovolemic shock, myoglobin was more commonly elevated (97%) than TnI (74%) [9].

Although myoglobin is a strong predictor of short- and long-term mortality in chest pain patients, it appears to be primarily identifying those at risk for death from mechanisms other than myocardial ischemia.

CK-MB

Creatine kinase (CK) is a dimer comprised of two subunits types, M and B, which are 39–42 kD. The MB form comprises 20–30% of cardiac muscle, while skeletal muscle is predominantly MM with only small amounts of MB, and the BB dimer primarily in the brain and kidney. Measurement traditionally was performed by assaying enzymatic activity with the relative amounts of the different isoenzymes being separated by electrophoresis, and then quantitated.

In contrast, mass assays measure the actual protein concentration, allowing quantitation of lower amounts with higher accuracy. Smaller elevations, even when total CK levels are normal, have been associated with increased cardiac events [10]. These elevations, previously considered a "micro-infarct," result from minimal amounts of myocardial damage, which are now typically identified by using troponin.

Increased levels of CK-MB correlate with the extent of necrosis, and can be used to indirectly estimate MI size [11]. Data from the PURSUIT trial revealed an incremental increase in mortality in non–ST-elevation acute coronary syndrome (NSTEACS) based on CK-MB. Patients who had a normal CK-MB had a 30-day mortality of 1.8%, compared to 3.3% in those with 1- to 2-fold increase and 8.3% in those with >10-fold elevation [12].

Although relatively cardiac specific, CK-MB is found in skeletal muscle; hence, significant skeletal muscle injury will result in elevations making detection of myocardial injury difficult. For example, in one study, although CK-MB elevations were detectable in the majority of patients with acute skeletal muscle injury and chronic skeletal muscle disease, elevated TnI was found in only six patients, all of whom were ultimately diagnosed with acute myocardial injury [13].

CK-MB is a more specific cardiac marker than myoglobin. Increased levels predict mortality in a step-wise fashion. Despite improved accuracy, CK-MB remains suboptimal for identifying patients with minimal myocardial necrosis. Although it may play a role in early diagnosis of MI, the additional prognostic value over cardiac troponins is less; therefore routine CK-MB measurement for risk assessment is not recommended.

Troponin

Among patients with possible MI, TnI and TnT have a number of advantages compared to other biomarkers, of which the most important is its cardiac specificity [14], allowing accurate detection of small amounts of myocardial necrosis [15]. Much of the early data demonstrating the prognostic value of troponins were derived from substudies of clinical trials, and therefore were limited by the trial-specific inclusion and exclusion criteria. In addition, in most cases markers were sampled at only one time point, which varied from the time of true enrollment. Nevertheless, these studies were critical in demonstrating the strong predictive value of troponins.

In one of the first large prognostic studies, Lindahl et al. evaluated TnT in 996 patients with NSTEACS in a substudy of the Fragmin in Unstable Coronary Artery Disease (FRISC) Trial (16). The 5-month death/MI rate was 16.1% for the highest tertile (TnT > 0.18 ng/mL), 10.5% for the second tertile (TnT 0.06 to 0.18 ng/mL), compared to 4.3% in the lowest tertile (TnT < 0.06 ng/mL). TnT remained an independent predictor of death and MI at 5 months, even after adjusting for age, gender, diabetes, hypertension, prior MI, and ST-segment depression [16].

In a subsequent study, Ohman and colleagues evaluated TnT in 755 patients enrolled in the Global Utilization of Strategies To Open occluded arteries (GUSTO) IIa trial who had STEMI (56%), non-STEMI (NSTEMI), or unstable angina (UA). Thirty-day mortality was more than 2-fold higher among patients with TnT elevation for all three ACS categories (13% vs. 4.7% for STEMI, 7.6% vs. 1.2% for NSTEMI, and 12.3% vs. 4.1% for UA, all p < 0.001). When combined, increased TnT was associated with 30-day mortality in a linear fashion [17]. Subsequent studies have confirmed this increased risk. A meta-analysis of 21 studies involving 18,982 patients found troponin elevations were associated with a 3.4-fold increased risk of death and MI at 30 days [18].

In contrast to substudies from clinical trials, studies from single institutions have a number of advantages. Most performed serial sampling, which can better delineate the role of marker timing. In addition, the absence of specific enrollment criteria results in inclusion of patients who have a broader range of clinical risk. This broader range of clinical risk enhances the prognostic power of troponin. For example, in a meta-analysis that included only patients with NSTEACS, Heidenreich et al. found that in 11,963 patients, the risk of death increased from 1.6% to 5.2% (OR 3.1) among patients with troponin elevation. Risk associated with troponin elevation was greater in cohort studies (OR 8.5 for TnI and 5.1 for TnT) than in clinical trials (OR 2.6 for TnI and 3.0 for TnT), indicating that clinical trial data may underestimate the prognostic value for troponin [19].

Despite the development of other biomarkers, most studies have continued to demonstrate that troponin remains an important predictor of adverse events, including mortality and subsequent MI [20,21]. Although the ability to predict mortality is not superior to other markers [21], troponin is a much stronger predictor of recurrent MI, and therefore identifies patients in whom risk can be reduced by appropriate treatment. For example, in the GUSTO IV trial, biomarkers that predicted 1-year mortality included TnT, NT-proBNP, C-reactive protein (CRP), and creatinine clearance. Of these, only TnT was an independent marker of recurrent MI at 30 days [21]. Similarly, in a single site study that enrolled 457 patients admitted for MI exclusion, the independent predictive value of multiple markers including myeloperoxidase, CRP, NT-proBNP, soluble CD40 ligand, placental growth factor, metalloproteinase-9, and TnT was assessed. Of these, only TnI and NT-proBNP were independent predictors of the combination of MI, revascularization, and mortality [20].

Mechanisms associated with the increased risk associated with troponin elevation

An obvious explanation for the increased risk associated with elevated troponin is that higher values indicate more extensive necrosis. Peak troponin value is highly correlated with infarct size [22,23]. However, this does not explain the

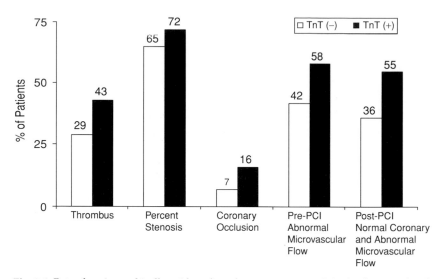

Fig. 2.1 Rate of angiographically evident thrombus, percent stenosis in the disease related epicardial artery, rate of suboptimal TIMI 0/1 epicardial flow prior to PCI (percutaneous coronary intervention), pre-PCI abnormal microvascular flow, and abnormal microvascular flow after successful PCI stratified by troponin T status. Adapted from [26].

higher risk associated with lower values not meeting prior CK-MB criteria for MI, which would be unlikely to cause systolic dysfunction.

An important finding is that even minor troponin elevations have been associated with higher risk angiographic findings such as more extensive atherosclerosis [24], higher rates of visible thrombus [25–28], more complex lesions [26–29], a higher likelihood of having an occluded vessel, and slower coronary blood flow in patients who have a patent vessel [28–29]. In addition, microvascular flow is more likely to be abnormal despite successful percutaneous coronary intervention (PCI), even when patients are treated with a glycoprotein (GP) IIb/IIIa antagonist (Fig. 2.1) [26], suggesting that troponin elevations are secondary to distal thrombus embolization from the site of plaque rupture to the microcirculation.

In a study that further explored the relationship between troponin elevations and outcomes, the FRISC II investigators reported the interesting finding that mortality was relatively stable for the three tertiles of patients with an elevated TnT. In contrast, later MI showed an inverted U-shaped relationship, with the lowest rate in those without TnT elevations and those in the upper tertile, compared to significantly higher rates in the two intermediate TnT groups [28] (Fig. 2.2). It was hypothesized that lower TnT values identified patients who had unstable plaque with a significant amount of myocardium at risk, who were at high risk for recurrent ischemic events. In contrast, patients with higher

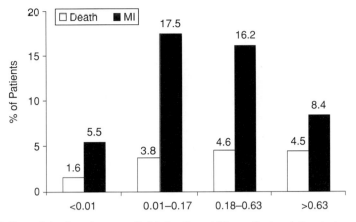

Fig. 2.2 Rate of death and myocardial infarction at 12 months in relation to troponin T status. White bars: death; dark bars: myocardial infarction. Adapted from [28].

TnT values were more likely to have larger infarcts, and therefore less viable myocardium at ischemic risk [30].

ST-Segment elevation myocardial infarction

Although the majority of ACS studies using troponin to predict risk focused on patients with non-STEMI, troponin elevations are also predictive in patients with STEMI. Detectable troponin at the time of presentation was associated with a worse prognosis, whether treated with fibrinolytics [31] or primary PCI [32,33]. In a GUSTO III substudy involving 12,666 patients [31], patients who had an initially positive TnT were more likely to present later than those who were TnT negative (3.5 vs. 2.3 hours), and had a significantly higher mortality at all subsequent time points (24 hours, 6.7 vs. 2.2%, and at 30 days, 15.7 vs. 6.2%, all p < 0.001). Symptom duration did not appear to completely explain these results as mortality was significantly higher at each time point for the TnT-positive patients (Fig. 2.3) [31]. Therefore, detectable troponin at the time of presentation may more accurately reflect infarction duration than symptoms [31]. Data from patients undergoing primary PCI have demonstrated similar results, with consistently worse outcomes in patients who were troponin positive at the time of presentation [32,33]. Tn-positive patients also had a lower likelihood of achieving normal TIMI grade 3 blood flow post-intervention [32,33], despite similar coronary flow prior to PCI and use of GP IIb/IIIa antagonists during the procedure [32].

Difference between TnI and TnT

Although meta-analyses indicated that the predictive ability of TnT and TnI appeared similar, the more appropriate way to compare the two is to measure

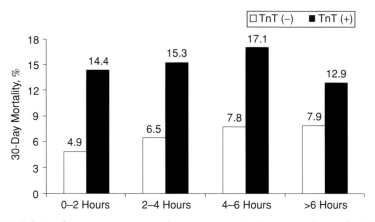

Fig. 2.3 Relationship among symptom duration, troponin T status, and mortality. White bars: TnT (+); black bars: TnT (−). Adapted from [31].

both assays simultaneously in the same patients. Despite the frequent poor standardization of different TnI assays, most studies that used appropriate diagnostic values reported similar prognostic ability between TnI and TnT. Luscher and colleagues compared the incidence of MI and death at 30 days in 491 patients with NSTEACS [34]. Outcomes were similar when comparing elevated TnT (11% vs. 4%) to elevated TnI (11% vs. 5%). Other ACS trials also have reported similar outcomes between TnT and TnI [35]. Further, in the TIMI-18 study, angiographic findings did not differ between patients with elevations in either TnT or TnI [26], and the benefit of an invasive approach was similar whether TnT or TnI was used to define troponin status [36]. Therefore, other than in patients with renal disease [37], as long as appropriate diagnostic values are used, both TnT and TnI appear to predict outcomes in ACS patients with comparable accuracy.

Implications of the troponin as the diagnostic standard for myocardial infarction

In 2000 a consensus conference recommended using troponin as the diagnostic standard for MI [17]. The clinical and research implications of this change are significant. In most studies, MI is used as a "hard" outcome event. Currently, the majority of U.S. hospitals use TnI [38]. Because different TnI assays can have up to a 20-fold difference in values for the same absolute TnI concentration [39], comparing results from one hospital to another is difficult. Even if the same assay is used, using a different diagnostic value would result in different rates of MI.

The variation in diagnostic values has important implications for comparing outcomes between physicians and institutions, particularly in the era of "scorecard medicine." For example, Kontos et al. compared mortality using a

CK-MB versus a TnI standard for MI [40]. Patients who met CK-MB criteria for MI had the highest mortality (7.1%), whereas those who were TnI negative had the lowest (1.9%). Patients with TnI elevation but normal CK-MB levels had an intermediate morality (5.4%). Using a TnI standard for MI would decrease overall mortality in both the unstable angina patients (to 1.6%) and MI patients (to 5.9%), giving the impression of improved outcomes in both cohorts.

Treatment strategies for patients with troponin elevation

Although critical for diagnosis as well as for prognosis, the ability to identify specific treatments based an elevated biomarker is an important benefit. Troponin fulfills this role, as elevations define a subgroup of ACS patients who benefit from aggressive pharmacologic treatment, as well as those in whom early coronary angiography and revascularization may be more appropriate. [41]

Low molecular weight heparins

Unfractionated heparin (UFH) was previously the anti-thrombotic of choice for treating NSTEACS. Low molecular weight heparins (LMWH) offer a convenient alternative and appear to modestly reduce recurrent ischemic events in this patient population [42,43]. Two trials—the FRISC trial, which compared the LMWH dalteparin with UFH, and the TIMI 11B trial, which used enoxaparin—presented results based on troponin status. In the FRISC TnT substudy, patients who were TnT negative had a nonsignificant reduction in the incidence of death and MI at 6 days when treated with dalteparin instead of UFH (2.4 vs. 0%; p = 0.12) (32). In contrast, the incidence of death and MI was higher in TnT-positive patients, which was significantly reduced when treated with dalteparin. Similarly, in the TIMI 11B TnI substudy, the primary end-point of death, MI, or urgent revascularization was reduced with enoxaparin in patients with TnI elevations, whereas rates of these events were low and not significantly different in patients without TnI elevations whether UFH or enoxaparin was used [44].

Glycoprotein IIb/IIIa antagonists

GP IIb/IIIa antagonists are potent parenteral antiplatelet agents that have been associated with a modest 9% reduction in death or MI at 30 days among patients with NSTEACS in a recent meta-analysis [45]. However, troponin elevations appear to identify patients who receive preferential treatment benefit from these agents. As discussed earlier, angiographic studies have shown that patients who are troponin positive are more likely to have visible thrombus and suboptimal coronary flow [25,27], both of which are improved by treatment with GP IIb/IIIa antagonists [27].

The first trial to report an interaction between troponin levels and GP IIb/IIIa inhibitor benefit was the Chimeric c7E3 Antiplatelet Therapy in Unstable Angina Refractory to Standard Treatment (CAPTURE) trial [46]. Inclusion

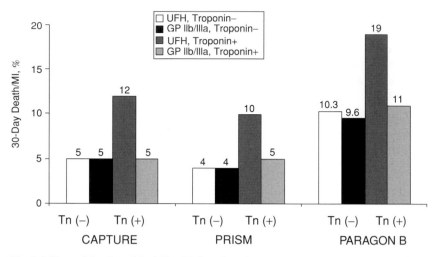

Fig. 2.4 Rate of death and/or MI at 30 days based on troponin positivity and use of GP IIb/IIIa antagonists. White bars, troponin negative, no GP IIb/IIIa antagonist; black bars, troponin negative, GP IIb/IIIa antagonist given; dark gray bars, troponin positive, no GP IIb/IIIa antagonist; light gray bars, troponin positive, GP IIb/IIIa antagonist given.

criteria required patients to have symptoms requiring intravenous nitroglycerin and who were scheduled to undergo PCI the next day. Troponin-negative patients had a low pre-PCI cardiac event rate of 0.7%, which increased to 4.5% 72 hours post-PCI. Treatment with abciximab in these patients had no effect on outcomes. In contrast, abciximab in patients with a TnT level > 0.1 ng/mL significantly reduced cardiac events pre-PCI (6.6% vs. 0.7% p = 0.02) as well as 72 hours post-PCI (17.4% vs. 3.6% p = 0.007) and at 30 days (Fig. 2.4).

Similarly, efficacy of the small molecule GP IIb/IIIa antagonist tirofiban was demonstrated in the Tn-positive subgroup of 2222 patients enrolled in the Platelet Receptor Inhibition in Ischemic Syndrome Management (PRISM) trial. Treatment with tirofiban in patients who had a TnI > 1.0 ng/mL significantly reduced death and MI at 48 hours (2.8% vs. 0.3% p < 0.001), an effect that persisted at 30 days (12% vs. 4.3% p < 0.001). In patients with a TnI < 1.0 ng/mL or TnT < 0.1 ng/mL, the overall cardiac event rate was low at 48 hours and not significantly different with and without GP IIb/IIIa treatment. Finally, data from the PARAGON B TnT substudy, using the small molecule GP IIb/IIIa lamifiban, found improvement in outcomes in the TnT-positive but not the TnT-negative patients [6].

In summary, troponin elevations in these 3 trials approximately doubled the risk of 30-day death/MI. Treatment with a GP IIb/IIIa antagonist significantly reduced risk in the troponin-positive patients (combined results, OR 0.33, 95% CI 0.19 to 0.57) [6], with treatment effectively converting the risk to that of troponin-negative patients (Fig. 2.4). By contrast, there was no significant treat-ment effect in troponin-negative patients (OR, 1.06; 95% CI, 0.78–1.43).

In contrast to the 3 prior studies, the GUSTO IV ACS study failed to demon-strate benefit of abciximab, when given as a 24- or 48-hour infusion, either in the trial as a whole, or in the troponin subgroup [47]. One potential explanation for the lack of efficacy was the very low rate of revascularization, especially in the first 48 hours (only 2%).

In a prospective trial designed to clarify the role of GP IIb/IIIa antagonists in troponin-positive patients in the setting of a high clopidogrel loading dose, the Intracoronary Stenting and Antithrombotic Regimen: Rapid Early Action for Coronary Treatment 2 (ISAR-REACT 2) trial was performed [48]. ACS patients undergoing PCI were pretreated with 600 mg of clopidogrel at least 2 hours before the procedure, and patients were randomized to treatment with abcix-imab during PCI. Abciximab had no significant effect in the troponin-negative patients. In contrast, there was a significant 30% reduction in the combination of death, MI, and urgent target vessel revascularization in the troponin-positive subgroup.

Thus, data from retrospective [6,35,46] as well as prospective [48] trials in patients who were managed medically [35], invasively [46,48], or both [6,35] demonstrated that troponin elevations define a group of patients who bene-fit preferentially when treated with GP IIb/IIIa antagonists, with little to no treatment benefit in troponin-negative patients.

Other agents

In contrast to LMWH and GP IIb/IIIa antagonists, treatment with clopidogrel in high-risk ACS patients was beneficial across most subgroups and not dependent on troponin status [49]. Another intravenous agent, the direct thrombin inhibitor bivalirudin, was tested in the Acute Catheterization and Urgent Intervention Triage Strategy (ACUITY) trial. This trial compared bivalirudin to treatment with the combination of GP IIb/IIIa antagonists and either UFH or LMWH in patients with NSTEACS. There was a nonsignificant trend toward more ischemic end-points in the troponin positive patients who were treated with bivalirudin, although bleeding events were significantly less [50].

Invasive vs. conservative therapy

In the last 10 years, a number of trials have investigated the role of a routine invasive compared to a medical management strategy in NSTEACS patients. In general, the routine invasive strategy has a higher short-term adverse event rate (primarily related to procedural complications) that was more than offset by a reduction in long-term events [51]. Two trials have reported outcomes based on troponin.

The FRISC II trial was the first early invasive trial in the stent era. A total of 2457 patients who had symptoms consistent with ischemia along with either ST-segment depression or elevated cardiac markers were enrolled. There was a significant 22% relative and 2.7% absolute risk reduction in death/MI in the early invasive group compared to the non-invasive group at 6 months [52]. Although there was no significant benefit in those who had TnT $\geq$ 0.1 ng/mL at 6 months (13.4% vs. 10.2%, p = ns), by 1 year the difference had become significant (16.6% vs. 11.6%, p = 0.005) [53].

The TACTICS-TIMI 18 trial found a benefit of early invasive treatment, particularly in patients who were troponin positive. This trial enrolled 2220 NSTEACS patients using enrollment criteria similar to the FRISC II trial. All patients received aspirin, heparin, and the GP IIb/IIIa antagonist tirofiban. Patients in the invasive arm underwent coronary angiography within 48 hours, while those in the conservative arm underwent stress testing prior to discharge, with subsequent coronary angiography for those who had high-risk, non-invasive findings. The primary end-point of death, MI, and/or rehospitalization at 6 months was significantly lower with the invasive strategy (15.9 vs. 19.4%, p = 0.025). Subanalysis revealed the importance of troponin elevations for risk-stratifying patients. Patients who had elevated troponin (defined as a TnT > 0.01 ng/mL, or TnI > 0.1 ng/mL) had a significant reduction of death and MI with the early invasive approach (24.5% vs. 16.4% p < 0.001), while no benefit was seen in patients without troponin elevations [36].

More recently, the Early Invasive versus Selectively Invasive Management for Acute Coronary Syndromes (ICTUS) reported no difference in outcomes between an early invasive or conservative strategy [54]. In contrast to the prior two studies, evidence of myocyte necrosis, based on an elevated TnT > 0.03 ng/mL (along with ECG changes or history of coronary disease) was required for trial enrollment. Patients were randomized to either coronary angiography within 48 hours or aggressive medical therapy that included aspirin, clopidogrel, LMWH, and statins. There was no difference in the primary end-point of death, MI, or readmission for ACS at 1 year between the two arms (23% vs. 21% p = 0.3). An important difference in this study compared to prior ones was the high rate of crossover among conservatively managed patients; by 1 year 54% had undergone revascularization (compared to 79% of patients in the early invasive group [54].

The ACC/AHA guidelines provide a class I recommendation for an early invasive approach in patients with UA/NSTEMI who have high-risk features such as ST-segment depression or elevated TnT or TnI [55]. However, the results of the ICTUS trial indicate that selected troponin-positive patients can undergo noninvasive risk stratification, in conjunction with appropriate follow-up and intensive medical treatment. At a minimum, these data would indicate that further risk stratification should be considered for patients who have troponin elevations and symptoms suggestive of ACS [55].

Pitfalls

Despite the large amount of data currently demonstrating the prognostic implications of troponin elevations, a number of points of controversy remain. These
include the significance of low-level troponin elevations, elevations in patients
without obvious ACS, and elevations in other non-ACS conditions, such as
renal failure, heart failure, sepsis, and neurologic conditions. Because troponin
is cardiac specific, not ACS specific, any condition that causes myocyte necrosis
will result in detectable troponin. Therefore, troponin elevations should not be
considered synonymous with ACS or MI, although risk is usually increased.

Another important consideration is recognizing that the absence of troponin
elevations in potential ACS patients identifies a group who is at lower risk,
but not necessarily low risk, in whom further evaluation is often warranted to
exclude ischemia as a cause for their symptoms.

Low troponin values

Low-level troponin elevations are often a source of considerable diagnostic confusion even in the modern era where assay-related issues are less likely to contribute to false-positive test results. ACS trials using modern high-precision
assays have demonstrated that even small elevations in troponin are clinically meaningful. For example, James et al. [56] using a third-generation TnT
assay performed a prospective evaluation of three cut-off levels (0.1 ng/mL,
0.03 ng/mL, and 0.01 ng/mL) in 7115 patients with NSTEACS from the GUSTO-
IV trial. Patients with TnT levels > 0.1 ng/mL had a 30-day mortality of 5.5%. A
cut-off value of 0.03 ng/mL provided better discrimination between high and
low risk: 5.1% versus 1.6%. However, a cut-off value at the lower limit of detection, 0.01 ng/mL, provided the best discrimination: 5.0% versus 1.1% (p < 0.001).

In contrast to ACS trials, studies performed during the same time frame in
lower risk patients failed to find a difference in outcomes [36,57]. This can be
attributed to two factors: risk and number of patients evaluated. In contrast to
patients included in ACS trials, most ED patients are at lower risk. Thus, the
number of patients included would be insufficient to demonstrate a significant
difference in outcomes in those with low troponin values.

In a study of 4123 consecutive patients admitted from the ED, Kontos et al.
separated patients into 4 groups based on peak TnI values [58]. Similar to studies
in high-risk ACS patients, there was a stepwise increase in events when using
death, MI, revascularization, or a combination of these at 30 days, and when
mortality alone was analyzed at 6 months (p < 0.0001). However, non-ischemic
outcomes showed an inverse relationship to peak TnI values, decreasing as
peak TnI values increased (Fig. 2.5). In fact, over 40% of the patients who had
low peak TnI values had a non-ischemic evaluation. The results of this study
are consistent with the ICTUS trial [54], indicating that although low troponin
values are associated with increased risk, further evaluation should be based

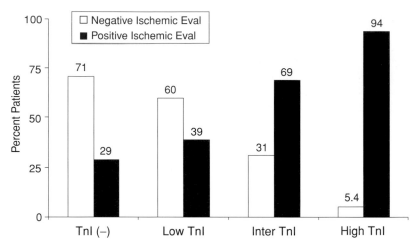

Fig. 2.5 Outcomes based on peak troponin I (TnI) values. Groups were defined as follows: Negative: no detectable TnI; Low: peak TnI values ≥ lower limit of detectability and < optimal diagnostic value; Intermediate: peak TnI values ≥ optimal diagnostic value < upper reference limit; High: peak TnI values ≥ upper reference limit. The incidence of positive outcomes (either death, CK-MB MI, revascularization, significant disease on angiography, or abnormal rest myocardial perfusion imaging) increased significantly as peak TnI increased (black bars). The differences between outcomes in each TnI group was significant (p < 0.001 for the trend). Non-ischemic outcomes (no CK-MB MI, significant disease on revascularization, reversibility on stress imaging, or negative rest myocardial perfusion imaging) based on peak TnI values showed an inverse relationship (p < 0.001 for the trend). Adapted from [57].

on the clinical presentation, and that invasive management is not necessarily indicated in every patient [58].

Another point of controversy is patients who have symptoms suggestive of ACS and troponin elevations, but subsequent coronary angiography does not demonstrate significant coronary disease. Although the troponin elevations are usually considered false positive, it appears in some cases it is the angiogram that is "false negative." In the TIMI 18 trial, Dokainish et al. found that despite the absence of significant disease, troponin-positive patients had a rate of death, MI, or rehospitalization of 6.3%, compared to only 2.7% in those who were troponin negative [59].

Conclusions

The measurement of troponin has been shown to provide important diagnostic and prognostic information in patients with ACS. Troponin has also been extremely useful in defining a group of patients who benefit from more aggressive pharmacologic treatment, such as LMWH and GP IIb/IIIa antagonists, and who are likely to benefit from early invasive management. Just as importantly, the absence of troponin elevations identifies a group of patients who account for the majority of those treated for suspected ACS who are unlikely to benefit from these treatments. Although myoglobin and CK-MB appear to provide incremental prognostic value to cardiac troponins, their role in contemporary practice remains undefined, largely because the therapeutic implications are not clear.

References

1 Kontos MC, Anderson FP, Schmidt KA, Ornato JP, Tatum JL, Jesse RL. Early diagnosis of acute myocardial infarction in patients without ST-segment elevation. *Am J Cardiol* 1999; **83**: 155–158.

2 Eggers KM, Oldgren J, Nordenskjold A, Lindahl B. Diagnostic value of serial measurement of cardiac markers in patients with chest pain: limited value of adding myoglobin to troponin I for exclusion of myocardial infarction. *Am Heart J* 2004; **148**: 574–581.

3 McCord J, Nowak RM, Hudson MP, McCullough PA, Tomlanovich MC, Jacobsen G et al. The prognostic significance of serial myoglobin, troponin I, and creatine kinase-MB measurements in patients evaluated in the emergency department for acute coronary syndrome. *Ann Emerg Med* 2003; **42**: 343–350.

4 Newby LK, Storrow AB, Gibler WB, Garvey JL, Tucker JF, Kaplan AL et al. Bedside multimarker testing for risk stratification in chest pain units: The chest pain evaluation by creatine kinase-MB, myoglobin, and troponin I (CHECKMATE) study. *Circulation* 2001; **103**: 1832–1837.

5 de Lemos JA, Morrow DA, Gibson CM, Murphy SA, Sabatine MS, Rifai N et al. The prognostic value of serum myoglobin in patients with non-ST-segment elevation acute coronary syndromes. Results from the TIMI 11B and TACTICS-TIMI 18 studies. *J Am Coll Cardiol* 2002; **40**: 238–244.

6 Newby LK, Ohman EM, Christenson RH, Moliterno DJ, Harrington RA, White HD et al. Benefit of glycoprotein IIb/IIIa inhibition in patients with acute coronary syndromes and troponin T-positive status: the paragon-B troponin T substudy. *Circulation* 2001; **103**: 2891–2896.

7 Kontos MC, Garg R, Anderson P, Roberts C, Ornato JP, Tatum JL et al. Ability of myoglobin to predict mortality in patients admitted for exclusion of myocardial infarction. *Am J Emerg Med* 2007; **25**: 873–89.

8 Spangenthal EJ, Ellis AK. Cardiac and skeletal muscle myoglobin release after reperfusion of injured myocardium in dogs with systemic hypotension. *Circulation* 1995; **91**: 2635–2641.

9 Arlati S, Brenna S, Prencipe L, Marocchi A, Casella GP, Lanzani M et al. Myocardial necrosis in ICU patients with acute non-cardiac disease: a prospective study. *Intensive Care Med* 2000; **26**: 31–37.

10 Ravkilde J, Nissen H, Horder M, Thygesen K. Independent prognostic value of serum creatine kinase isoenzyme MB mass, cardiac troponin T and myosin light chain levels in suspected acute myocardial infarction. Analysis of 28 months of follow-up in 196 patients. *J Am Coll Cardiol* 1995; **25**: 574–581.

11 Roberts R, Henry PD, Sobel BE. An improved basis for enzymatic estimation of infarct size. *Circulation* 1975; **52**: 743–754.

12 Alexander JH, Sparapani RA, Mahaffey KW, Deckers JW, Newby LK, Ohman EM et al. Association between minor elevations of creatine kinase-MB level and mortality in patients with acute coronary syndromes without ST-segment elevation. *JAMA* 2000; **283**: 347–353.

13 Adams JE, 3rd, Bodor GS, Davila-Roman VG, Delmez JA, Apple FS, Ladenson JH et al. Cardiac troponin I. A marker with high specificity for cardiac injury. *Circulation* 1993; **88**: 101–106.

14 Potter JD. Preparation of troponin and its subunits. *Methods Enzymol* 1982; **85** Pt B: 241–263.

15 Alpert JS, Thygesen K, Antman E, Bassand JP. Myocardial infarction redefined—a consensus document of the Joint European Society of Cardiology/American College of Cardiology Committee for the redefinition of myocardial infarction. *J Am Coll Cardiol* 2000; **36**: 959–969.

16 Lindahl B, Venge P, Wallentin L. Troponin T identifies patients with unstable coronary artery disease who benefit from long-term antithrombotic protection. Fragmin in Unstable Coronary Artery Disease (FRISC) Study Group. *J Am Coll Cardiol* 1997; **29**: 43–48.

17 Ohman EM, Armstrong PW, Christenson RH, Granger CB, Katus HA, Hamm CW et al. Cardiac troponin T levels for risk stratification in acute myocardial ischemia. GUSTO IIA Investigators. *N Engl J Med* 1996; **335**: 1333–1341.

18 Ottani F, Galvani M, Nicolini FA, Ferrini D, Pozzati A, Di Pasquale G et al. Elevated cardiac troponin levels predict the risk of adverse outcome in patients with acute coronary syndromes. *Am Heart J* 2000; **140**: 917–927.

19 Heidenreich PA, Alloggiamento T, Melsop K, McDonald KM, Go AS, Hlatky MA. The prognostic value of troponin in patients with non-ST elevation acute coronary syndromes: a meta-analysis. *J Am Coll Cardiol* 2001; **38**: 478–485.

20 Apple FS, Pearce LA, Chung A, Ler R, Murakami MM. Multiple biomarker use for detection of adverse events in patients presenting with symptoms suggestive of acute coronary syndrome. *Clin Chem* 2007; **53**: 874–881.

21 James SK, Lindahl B, Siegbahn A, Stridsberg M, Venge P, Armstrong P et al. N-terminal pro-brain natriuretic peptide and other risk markers for the separate prediction of mortality and subsequent myocardial infarction in patients with unstable coronary artery disease: a Global Utilization of Strategies To Open occluded arteries (GUSTO)-IV substudy. *Circulation* 2003; **108**: 275–281.

22 Panteghini M, Cuccia C, Bonetti G, Giubbini R, Pagani F, Bonini E. Single-point cardiac troponin T at coronary care unit discharge after myocardial infarction correlates with infarct size and ejection fraction. *Clin Chem* 2002; **48**: 1432–1436.

23 Ingkanisorn WP, Rhoads KL, Aletras AH, Kellman P, Arai AE. Gadolinium delayed enhancement cardiovascular magnetic resonance correlates with clinical measures of myocardial infarction. *J Am Coll Cardiol* 2004; **43**: 2253–2259.

24 Jurlander B, Farhi ER, Banas JJ, Jr, Keany CM, Balu D, Grande P et al. Coronary angiographic findings and troponin T in patients with unstable angina pectoris. *Am J Cardiol* 2000; **85**: 810–814.

25 Benamer H, Steg PG, Benessiano J, Vicaut E, Gaultier CJ, Aubry P et al. Elevated cardiac troponin I predicts a high-risk angiographic anatomy of the culprit lesion in unstable angina. *Am Heart J* 1999; **13**: 815–820.

26 Wong GC, Morrow DA, Murphy S, Kraimer N, Pai R, James D et al. Elevations in troponin T and I are associated with abnormal tissue level perfusion: a TACTICS-TIMI 18 substudy. Treat Angina with Aggrastat and Determine Cost of Therapy with an Invasive or Conservative Strategy-Thrombolysis in Myocardial Infarction. *Circulation* 2002; **106**: 202–207.

27 Heeschen C, van Den Brand MJ, Hamm CW, Simoons ML. Angiographic findings in patients with refractory unstable angina according to troponin T status. *Circulation* 1999; **100**: 1509–1514.

28 Lindahl B, Diderholm E, Lagerqvist B, Venge P, Wallentin L, FRISC II (Fast Revascularization during InStability in CAD) Investigators. Mechanisms behind the prognostic value of troponin T in unstable coronary artery disease: a FRISC II substudy. *J Am Coll Cardiol* 2001; **38**: 979–986.

29 Benamer H, Steg PG, Benessiano J, Vicaut E, Gaultier CJ, Aubry P et al. Elevated cardiac troponin I predicts a high-risk angiographic anatomy of the culprit lesion in unstable angina. *Am Heart J* 1999; **137**: 815–820.

30 Antman EM. Troponin measurements in ischemic heart disease: more than just a black and white picture. *J Am Coll Cardiol* 2001; **38**: 987–990.

31 Ohman EM, Armstrong PW, White HD, Granger CB, Wilcox RG, Weaver WD et al. Risk stratification with a point-of-care cardiac troponin T test in acute myocardial infarction. GUSTO III Investigators. Global Use of Strategies To Open Occluded Coronary Arteries. *Am J Cardiol* 1999; **84**: 1281–1286.

32 Matetzky S, Sharir T, Domingo M, Noc M, Chyu KY, Kaul S et al. Elevated troponin I level on admission is associated with adverse outcome of primary angioplasty in acute myocardial infarction. *Circulation* 2000; **102**: 1611–1616.

33 Kurowski V, Hartmann F, Killermann DP, Giannitsis E, Wiegand UK, Frey N et al. Prognostic significance of admission cardiac troponin T in patients treated successfully with direct percutaneous interventions for acute ST-segment elevation myocardial infarction. *Crit Care Med* 2002; **30**: 2229–2235.

34 Luscher MS, Thygesen K, Ravkilde J, Heickendorff L. Applicability of cardiac troponin T and I for early risk stratification in unstable coronary artery disease. TRIM Study Group. Thrombin Inhibition in Myocardial Ischemia. *Circulation* 1997; **96**: 2578–2585.

35 Heeschen C, Hamm CW, Goldmann B, Deu A, Langenbrink L, White HD. Troponin concentrations for stratification of patients with acute coronary syndromes in relation to therapeutic efficacy of tirofiban. *Lancet* 1999; **354**: 1757–1762.

36 Morrow DA, Cannon CP, Rifai N, Frey MJ, Vicari R, Lakkis N et al. Ability of minor elevations of troponins I and T to predict benefit from an early invasive strategy in patients with unstable angina and non-ST elevation myocardial infarction: results from a randomized trial. *JAMA* 2001; **286**: 2405–2412.

37 Apple FS, Murakami MM, Pearce LA, Herzog CA. Predictive value of cardiac troponin I and T for subsequent death in end-stage renal disease. *Circulation* 2002; **106**: 2941–2945.

38 Apple FS, Murakami M, Panteghini M, Christenson RH, Dati F, Mair J et al. International survey on the use of cardiac markers. *Clin Chem* 2001; **47**: 587–588.

39 Wu AH, Feng YJ, Moore R, Apple FS, McPherson PH, Buechler KF et al. Characterization of cardiac troponin subunit release into serum after acute myocardial infarction and comparison of assays for troponin T and I. American Association for Clinical Chemistry Subcommittee on cTnI Standardization. *Clin Chem* 1998; **44**: 1198–1208.

40 Kontos MC, Fritz LM, Anderson FP, Tatum JL, Ornato JP, Jesse RL. Impact of the troponin standard on the prevalence of acute myocardial infarction. *Am Heart J* 2003; **146**: 446–452.

41 Panteghini M. The new definition of myocardial infarction and the impact of troponin determination on clinical practice. *Int J Cardiol* 2006; 106: 298–306.

42 Cohen M, Demers C, Gurfinkel EP, Turpie AG, Fromell GJ, Goodman S et al. A comparison of low-molecular-weight heparin with unfractionated heparin for unstable coronary artery disease. *N Engl J Med* 1997; **337**: 447–452.

43 Antman EM, McCabe CH, Gurfinkel EP, Turpie AG, Bernink PJ, Salein D et al. Enoxaparin prevents death and cardiac ischemic events in unstable angina/non-Q-wave myocardial infarction. Results of the Thrombolysis in Myocardial Infarction (TIMI) 11B Trial. *Circulation* 1999; **100**: 1593–1601.

44 Morrow DA, Antman EM, Tanasijevic M, Rifai N, de Lemos JA, McCabe CH et al. Cardiac troponin I for stratification of early outcomes and the efficacy of enoxaparin in unstable angina: a TIMI-11B substudy. *J Am Coll Cardiol* 2000; **36**: 1812–1817.

45 Boersma E, Harrington RA, Moliterno DJ, White H, Simoons ML. Platelet glycoprotein IIb/IIIa inhibitors in acute coronary syndromes. *Lancet* 2002; **360**: 342–343.

46 Hamm CW, Heeschen C, Goldmann B, Vahanian A, Adgey J, Miguel CM et al. Benefit of abciximab in patients with refractory unstable angina in relation to serum troponin T levels. *N Engl J Med* 1999; **340**: 1623–1629.

47 Simoons ML, GUSTO IV-ACS Investigators. Effect of glycoprotein IIb/IIIa receptor blocker abciximab on outcome in patients with acute coronary syndromes without early coronary revascularisation: the GUSTO IV-ACS randomised trial. *Lancet* 2001; **357**: 1915–1924.

48 Kastrati A, Mehilli J, Neumann FJ, Dotzer F, ten Berg J, Bollwein H et al. Abciximab in patients with acute coronary syndromes undergoing percutaneous coronary intervention after clopidogrel pretreatment: the ISAR-REACT 2 randomized trial. *JAMA* 2006; **295**: 1531–1538.

49 Yusuf S, Zhao F, Mehta SR, Chrolavicius S, Tognoni G, Fox KK et al. Effects of clopidogrel in addition to aspirin in patients with acute coronary syndromes without ST-segment elevation. *N Engl J Med* 2001; **345**: 494–502.

50 Stone GW, McLaurin BT, Cox DA, Bertrand ME, Lincoff AM, Moses JW et al. Bivalirudin for patients with acute coronary syndromes. *N Engl J Med* 2006; **355**: 2203–2216.

51 Mehta SR, Cannon CP, Fox KA, Wallentin L, Boden WE, Spacek R et al. Routine vs. selective invasive strategies in patients with acute coronary syndromes: a collaborative meta-analysis of randomized trials. *JAMA* 2005; **293**: 2908–2917.

52 Invasive compared with non-invasive treatment in unstable coronary artery disease: FRISC II prospective randomised multicentre study. FRagmin and Fast Revascularisation during InStability in Coronary artery disease Investigators. *Lancet* 1999; **354**: 708–715.

53 Wallentin L, Lagerqvist B, Husted ST, Kontny F, Stahle E, Swahn E et al. Outcome at 1 year after an invasive compared with a non-invasive strategy in unstable coronary-artery disease: the FRISC II invasive randomized trial. *Lancet* 2000; **356**: 9–16.

54 de Winter RJ, Windhausen F, Cornel JH, Dunselman PH, Janus CL, Bendermacher PE et al. Early invasive versus selectively invasive management for acute coronary syndromes. *N Engl J Med* 2005; **353**: 1095–1104.

55 Anderson JL, Adams CD, Antman EM, Bridges CR, Califf RM, Casey DE Jr, et al. ACC/AHA 2007 Guideline for the Management of Patients With Unstable Angina Non-ST Elevation Myocardial Infarction—summary article: a report of the American College of Cardiology/American Heart Association task force on practice guidelines (Committee on the Management of Patients With Unstable Angina). *J Am Coll Cardiol* 2007; **50**: 652–726.

56 James S, Armstrong P, Califf R, Simoons ML, Venge P, Wallentin L et al. Troponin T levels and risk of 30-day outcomes in patients with the acute coronary syndrome: prospective verification in the GUSTO-IV trial. *Am J Med* 2003; **115**: 178–184.

57 Johnson PA, Goldman L, Sacks DB, Garcia T, Albano M, Bezai M et al. Cardiac troponin T as a marker for myocardial ischemia in patients seen at the emergency department for acute chest pain. *Am Heart J* 1999; **137**: 1137–1144.

58 Kontos MC, Shah R, Fritz LM, Anderson FP, Tatum JL, Ornato JP et al. Implication of different cardiac troponin I levels for clinical outcomes and prognosis of acute chest pain patients. *J Am Coll Cardiol* 2004; **43**: 958–965.

59 Dokainish H, Pillai M, Murphy SA, DiBattiste PM, Schweiger MJ, Lotfi A et al. Prognostic implications of elevated troponin in patients with suspected acute coronary syndrome but no critical epicardial coronary disease: a TACTICS-TIMI-18 substudy. *J Am Coll Cardiol* 2005; **45**: 19–24.

Chapter 3

Challenges interpreting cardiac troponin values

Fred S. Apple

Introduction

The story describing the evolution of cardiac troponin T (cTnT, first introduced in 1995) and I (cTnI, first introduced in 1996) to become the gold standard biomarkers for the detection of myocardial injury is an educational one and is described in an article by Rosalki, Roberts, Katus, and Ladenson [1]. Guideline endorsement for cTn use in clinical practice initially came from the laboratory medicine group, National Academy of Clinical Biochemistry (NACB), in 1999 [2]. This was followed in 2000 by the consensus document for the redefinition of myocardial infarction (MI) jointly issued by the European Society of Cardiology (ESC) and American College of Cardiology (ACC) [3]. Support continued to grow with the publications of case definitions for acute coronary disease by the epidemiology community in 2003 [4] and emergency medicine and cardiology groups in 2005 [6]. Most recently practice guidelines for cTn addressing its clinical utilization and analytical, methodologic specifications and recommendations have been jointly published by the NACB and the International Federation of Clinical Chemistry (IFCC) Committee for Standardization of Marker of Cardiac Damage (C-SMCD) [5,6]. The Global Task Force of the Joint ESC-ACC-AHA-WHF for redefinition of MI recently issued a revised universal definition of MI in 2007, [7] which will serve as an update of the ESC-ACC consensus document [3].

The criteria for acute MI, supported by all the associations noted here, is predicated on an increased cardiac biomarker, preferably cTn, above the 99th percentile reference value, along with evidence of myocardial ischemia with at least: ischemic symptoms, electrocardiograph (EKG) changes indicative of new ischemia, or infarction or imaging evidence of regional myocardial dysfunction

Biomarkers in Heart Disease, 1st edition. Edited by James A. de Lemos.
© 2008 American Heart Association, ISBN: 978-1-4051-7571-5

consistent with ischemia. Yet, many clinicians and laboratorians remain confused on how to interpret cardiac troponin concentrations based on both a single result and from serial, timed results. The three areas addressed in this chapter regard: 1) the need for universal incorporation of the 99th percentile value as the accepted cutoff for myocardial injury; 2) how we should utilize and interpret serial, timed cTn values in patients presenting to rule in/out MI; and 3) non-ischemic mechanisms that may be responsible for increased cTn, recognizing that while increased cTn concentrations do imply myocardial injury, these should not be confused with the concept that all cTn increases define an MI.

Universal acceptance of the 99th percentile value as the accepted cut-off

Lowering the biomarker cutoff of cardiac troponin to the 99th percentile value has been a challenge for clinicians who see the >5 million patients who present to emergency departments with chest discomfort and related symptoms [6]. Of the >1 million patients who are hospitalized, an accurate diagnosis and appropriate treatment is critical for optimal short- and long-term outcomes. With improvements in the analytical aspects of cardiac troponin assays [9–14], the 99th percentile reference values have become lower and lower (Table 3.1). The challenge to clinicians involves the substantially greater number of positive cTn values that are now being observed compared to when higher cardiac troponin cutoffs were used that were either based on a) the WHO-ROC curved derived values or b) CK-MB as the gold-standard diagnostic biomarker [5,15–20]. Historically, CK-MB was used as the primary biomarker to aid in the diagnosis of MI and cutoffs were defined to optimize clinical sensitivity (>90%) and clinical specificity (>90%) [1,18–20]. It has been recognized that CK-MB is not 100% cardiac tissue specific [21].

When biomarker superiority shifted to cTn from CK-MB, the initial cTn cut-off values were optimized based on ROC curves to maintain high clinical specificity. However, multiple studies performed over the past 10 years have clearly shown that when improved analytical cTn assays are used, any increase above the 99th percentile reference (normal) value is both diagnostic and implicates greater risk of adverse outcomes for patients presenting with symptoms suggestive of ACS [22–26]. Consequently, the decreased cut-off concentrations from the older WHO-ROC curve values to the current 99th percentile values demonstrates a 2- to 25-fold decrease in reference ranges as shown in Table 3.1. Over the past several years, clinical and epidemiology studies have translated the decreased cTn cutoffs to an increased number of patients diagnosed with MI. Numerous studies have provided the evidence demonstrating the increased rates of MI when biomarker use has shifted from a) total CK or CK-MB to cTn or b) from using cTn WHO-ROC cutoffs to the lower cTn 99th percentile cutoffs. In this author's personal experiences at Hennepin County Medical Center, an increased

Table 3.1 Characteristics of FDA-cleared cTn assays from manufacturer package inserts.

Assay	LLD	99th	WHO-ROC	Ratio[†]
Abbott Architect	0.009	0.012	0.3	25
Abbott AxSYM ADV	0.02	0.04	0.4	10
Abbott i-STAT	0.02	0.08 (WB)	ND	–
Beckman Accu	0.01	0.04	0.5	12.5
Biosite Triage*	0.05	<0.05	0.4	8
bioMerieux Vidas	0.001	0.01	0.16	16
MKl Pathfast	0.006	0.01	0.06	6
Ortho Vitros ES	0.012	0.032	0.12	3.25
Response Biomedical	0.03	<0.03 (WB)	ND	–
Roche Elecsys	0.01	<0.01	0.03	3
Roche Reader*	0.05	<0.05 (WB)	0.1	2
Siemens (Bayer) Centaur*	0.02	0.1	1.0	10
Siemens (Bayer) Ultra	0.006	0.04	0.9	2.25
Siemens (Dade Behring) RxL	0.04	0.07	0.6–1.5	8.5
Siemens (Dade Behring) CS*	0.03	0.07	0.6–1.5	8.5
Siemens (DPC) Immulite*	0.1	0.2	1.0	5
Tosoh AIA	0.06	0.06	0.31–0.64	5.1

LLD, lower limit of detection; 99th percentile reference limit; ROC, receiver operator characteristics curve optimized cutoff; *older generation of assay; [†] Ratio of WHO-ROC/99th percentile

rate of MI detection from 11% to 24% was seen when transitioning from MI diagnosed by CK-MB values compared to cTnI values at the ROC-WHO cutoff [17]. In a second series of 1719 consecutive patients with cTn measured to rule out MI, we observed an increase from 13.1% using the WHO-ROC cutoff to 25% using the 99th percentile cutoff; an 85% increase [15].

Utilization and interpretation of serial, timed cTn values

Few data are available regarding the effective use of serial cTn or CK-MB results after the diagnosis of MI has been established. As noted earlier and in chapter 1, contemporary guidelines adequately address early serial biomarker measurement in patients with suspected ACS, with consensus that serial negative results over a minimum of 6–9 hours following presentation in a patient presenting with clinical symptoms suggestive of ACS rules out an MI. However, in this author's experience, serial biomarker measurement often continues for the duration of the hospital stay, even among patients with normal values at 6–9 hours. This cost-inefficient process may have adverse effects on revenue for hospitals under DRG reimbursement rules. It should be noted that there is no clinical evidence to support the need for serial Tn or CK-MB testing once the diagnosis has been established. A single daily measurement is sufficient in the days following an MI, to document a decreasing value; once values have started downtrending, measurement is typically no longer necessary. Additional measurements may be performed as necessary to detect reinfarction among patients with recurrent ischemic symptoms [27].

Another challenge regarding serial monitoring of cardiac troponin values is demonstrated in the patient who presents with a normal cTn at presentation (below the 99th percentile value) and the follow-up 6h cTn value is slightly increased above the 99th percentile. For example, consider a 48-year-old man with a history of coronary artery disease who presents with 12 hours of nausea, shortness of breath, and left shoulder discomfort. His EKG is normal. However, although his baseline cTnI was undetectable (at <0.3 ng/mL; by the assay used in this lab), his 4h value was normal but detectable (0.4 ng/mL), and his 8h value was above the 99th percentile (0.5 ng/mL) at 0.6 ng/mL. The challenge is how does one interpret this minor changing pattern in a low-risk patient? Fesmire has initially championed the approach for identifying myocardial necrosis by relying on changes in serum biomarkers over an abbreviated time interval, which he designates slope or delta values [28,29]. This is opposed to the traditional recommended approach of relying on a single value exceeding a threshold reference (normal) cutoff. Specifically, as assays become more analytically sensitive and precise, this approach has the potential for both identifying and excluding MI patients earlier than the 6h window as well as identifying patients at risk, without compromising clinical specificity.

Non-ischemic etiologies of cTn increases

Numerous pathologies causing both primary and secondary myocardial injury of a non-ischemic nature may potentially result in increased cTn concentrations in the circulation [30]. These pathologies (listed in Table 3.2) include heart failure, trauma, electrical cardioversion, pulmonary emboli, sepsis, critical illness myocarditis, stroke, noncardiac surgery, extreme exercise, drug-induced damage, end-stage renal disease, and others. The increased cTn values observed in patients who present to hospitals often confuse the clinical impression of the health care provider as the differential diagnosis often includes an MI. Therefore, clinicians must rely on their clinician skills, history, and physical, as well as the

Table 3.2 Diagnostic groups frequently associated with increased cardiac troponin concentrations in non-ischemic pathologies.

 1 Congestive heart failure*

 2 Trauma, cardiac contusion

 3 Cardioversion, electrical defibrillation

 4 Pulmonary embolism, edema*

 5 Sepsis, septic shock*

 6 Myocarditis

 7 Exercise, vital exhaustion

 8 Stroke*

 9 Non-cardiac, vascular surgery

10 End-stage renal disease*

11 Hypertension

12 Hypotension

13 Critically ill intensive care patients*

14 Aneurismal subarachnoid hemorrhage

15 Drugs of abuse toxicity, including ethanol

16 Chemotherapy

17 Heart surgery, transplantation

18 Polymyositis, dermatomyositis

19 Cardiomyopathy

20 Rhabdomyolysis, trauma (non-chest)

21 Hematologic malignances

22 Acute pericarditis

23 Amyloid cardiomyopathy

24 Idiopathic dilated cardiomyopathy

25 Neonates

26 Lung disease

* Evidence of role of cardiac troponin for risk stratification for short- or long-term outcomes.

role of cTn in their diagnostic pathway. Because of the specificity of cardiac troponin, which is only released from the heart following necrosis of myocytes, these findings are true positive results, and are rarely false-positive results due to analytical assay issues [11]. False-positive analytical results occur rarely, with the most common causes being heterophilic antibody interferences or fibrin clot interferences. Manufacturers have optimized their assays and laboratories have improved their sample handling techniques to minimize these issues.

Clinically however, the challenge remains that health care providers must understand that the clinical specificities of cTn, with the newer second-, third-, and fourth-generation assays (with correspondingly low 99th percentile values; Table 3.1) will be in the 75% to 80% range [31,32]. Thus, at least 2 out of every 10 positive cTn findings will be a result of a disorder other than MI. Importantly, rarely do these other etiologies demonstrate the classic rising and falling pattern experienced with an MI, highlighting the value of serial monitoring when the clinical scenario is confusing. In addition, numerous studies also now support that increases in cTn in conditions other than MI also imply risk of both short- and long-term adverse cardiac and all-cause death outcomes. Three clinical pathologies will be expanded upon which highlight the potential value of cTn for risk in non-ACS cases.

cTn in end-stage renal disease

One challenge confronting the nephrology community is to explore more aggressive treatment modalities for cardiovascular disease in end-stage renal disease (ESRD) patients. Cardiac disease is the major cause of death in patients with ESRD, accounting for approximately 45% of all deaths [33–56]. In dialysis patients, about 20% of cardiac deaths are attributed to acute MI. MI is a catastrophic clinical event in ESRD patients, with a 2-year mortality of 73%. Recent evidence demonstrates that cTnT and cTnI are important predictors of long-term, all-cause mortality and cardiovascular mortality in patients with ESRD. cTn elevation detected in outpatient dialysis patients is a powerful predictor of all-cause mortality as shown in Fig. 3.1 for cTnT and cTnI. Elevated versus normal cTnT defined by the 99th percentile cutoff was associated with a 2- to 4-fold increased risk of death over 2 to 3 years. The relative risk of death remained increased following adjustment for other risk factors. It is likely that other mechanisms beside ACS are responsible for the troponin increase and adverse outcome, as evidenced by concomitant increases c-reactive protein (CRP) and NT-proBNP. The clinical duality of cardiac troponin testing in dialysis patients must be acknowledged to avoid incorrect clinical judgments, that is, recognizing that while defining ACS may be challenging, prediction of mortality remains robust.

Several studies substantiate that cTnT is increased more frequently than cTnI among patients with ESRD, as well as noting differences between different cTnI assays. Speculation as to the possible causes for the difference in increases in cTnT compared to cTnI include the following. First, increased cTnT, but not cTnI,

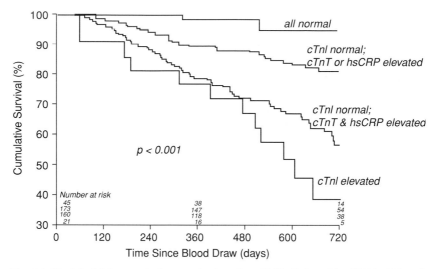

Fig. 3.1 Kaplain-Meier survival curves by baseline cTnT, cTnI, and hs-CRP in 399 end-stage renal disease patients (reproduced with permission from [55]).

reflects increased left ventricular mass in the ESRD population with a different release pattern of cTnT compared to cTnI. Second, cTnT released from injured myocardium may have a longer circulating half-life compared to cTnI due to advanced glycation end products known to accumulate in diabetic patients with renal disease. Third, cTnI may decrease postdialysis, either directly due to removal by dialysis or indirectly by degradation of the labile cTnI molecule. In contrast, cTnT concentrations trend toward increasing postdialysis. This would result in lower circulating cTnI levels compared to cTnT. Additional studies are needed to elucidate the mechanism responsible for the cTnI/cTnT differences found in ESRD patients. Regardless of the mechanisms of myocardial injury in ESRD patients, findings continue to substantiate the prognostic power of cardiac troponin testing for predicting mortality in ESRD patients. One plausible, cost-effective scenario is the developing role of outpatient cardiac troponin testing. Incorporation of quarterly or semi-annual cardiac troponin monitoring in ESRD patients may assist in initiating more aggressive treatment of underlying coronary artery disease (CAD), detection of subclinical myocardial injury, and assist in treatment therapies before renal transplantation.

Congestive heart failure

Congestive heart failure (CHF) is a dynamic process with spontaneous, progressive severity, and is structurally characterized by cellular degeneration and multiple foci of myocardial cell death. Increased concentrations of cTnI and cTnT have been found in patients with CHF [57–61]. The specific underlying mechanisms remain unclear. In the majority of heart failure (HF) patients studied, cTns were detected in patients with advanced CHF predominantly involving NYHA III and IV classifications [8]. Increased cTnI and cTnT values in patients with advanced HF also serve as an independent biomarker for a decline in left ventricular ejection fraction and higher mortality rates for both all-cause death and cardiac death. In addition, the prognostic power of cardiac troponin appears to be additive to other biomarker predictors of death in HF; with the combination of increased cTnI and increased B-type natriuretic peptide (BNP) identifying patients with HF who have a markedly (12-fold) increased risk of death. The future role of cardiac troponin testing in HF patients, alone or in combination with BNP monitoring, will need to be determined regarding aggressive treatment strategies.

Pulmonary embolism

Although the number of patients studied is small (<200), both cTnI and cTnT have demonstrated increases in one-third to one-half of patients clinically diagnosed with pulmonary embolism (PE) [62,63]. cTnI identified patients with right ventricular dysfunction who had a burden of lung perfusion abnormalities. cTnT, at concentrations >0.1 µg/L, was associated with poor long-term survival and provided an independent prediction of mortality in patients with acute PE (Fig. 3.2). Although these prognostic data are encouraging, clinicians need to be

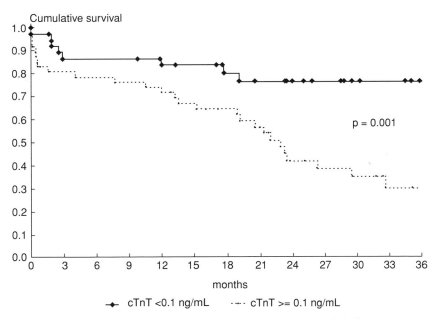

Fig. 3.2 Kaplain-Meier survival curves for patients with pulmonary embolism; cTnT <0.1 ng/mL (solid circles) and ≥ 0.1 ng/mL (open circles) (reproduced with permission from [62]).

aware that troponin elevation is common in PE, and this diagnosis must be considered in differential diagnosis of patients with chest symptoms and troponin elevation, as the diagnostic and therapeutic pathways diverge distinctly from ACS.

Conclusions

Improvements in the analytical sensitivity of cardiac troponin assays, with the introduction of newer generation assays, allow for the sensitive and precise detection of lower cardiac troponin concentrations. Further advances in this area are forthcoming. These more sensitive assays identify a greater number of patients with myocardial injury, reduce the time for detecting an increased cardiac troponin from the onset of clinical symptoms, improve the diagnosis of myocardial infarction, and enhance risk stratification for both ACS and non-ischemic syndromes. However, with these advances come new challenges: these new assays will also identify a larger number of patients with troponin elevation from causes other than ACS. Although the troponin elevation in such patients does represent myocardial injury and is associated with excess cardiovascular risk, additional research is needed to identify the best diagnostic and therapeutic strategies.

References

1 Rosalki S, Roberts R, Katus HA, Giannitsis E, Ladenson JH, Apple FS. Cardiac biomarkers for detection of myocardial infarction: perspectives from past to present. *Clin Chem* 2004; **50**: 2205–2213.

2 Wu AHB, Apple FS, Gibler WB, Jesse RL, Warshaw MM, Valdes Jr R. National academy of clinical biochemistry standards of laboratory practice: recommendations for use of cardiac markers in coronary artery diseases. *Clin Chem* 1999; **45**: 1104–1121.

3 Alpert JS, Thygesen K, for the Cardiology Committee for the Redefinition of Myocardial Infarction. Myocardial infarction redefined – a consensus document of the Joint European Society of Cardiology/American College of Cardiology Committee for the redefinition of myocardial infarction. *J Am Coll Cardiol* 2000; **21**: 1502–1513.

4 Luepker RV, Apple FS, Christenson RH, Crow RS, Fortmann SP, Goff D, Goldberg RJ, Hand MM, Jaffe AS, Julian DG, Levy D, Manolio T, Mendis S, Mensah G, Pajak A, Prineas RJ, Reddy KS, Roger VL, Rosamond WD, Shahar E, Sharrett AR, Sorlie P, Tunstall-Pedoe H. Case definitions for acute coronary heart disease in epidemiology and clinical research studies. *Circulation* 2003; **108**: 2543–2549.

5 Gibler WB, Cannon CP, Blomkalns AL, Drew BJ, Hollander JE, Jaffe AS, Newby LK, Ohman EM, Peterson ED, Pollack CV. Practical implementation of the guidelines for unstable angina/non-St-segment elevation myocardial infarction in the emergency department. *Ann Emerg Med* 2005; **46**: 185–197.

6 Morrow DA, Cannon CP, Jesse RL, Newby LK, Ravkilde J, Storrow AB, Wu AHB, Christenson RH. National Academy of Clinical Biochemistry Laboratory Medicine

practice guidelines: clinical characteristics and utilization of biochemical markers in acute coronary syndromes. *Clin Chem* 2007; **53**: 552–574.

7 Thygesen K., Alpert J. S., White H. D., Jaffe A. S., Apple F. S., Galvani M., Katus A., Newby K., *et al.* Universal definition of myocardial infarction. Eur. Heart J., October 2, 2007; **28**: 2525–2538.

8 Apple FS, Jesse RL, Newby LK, Wu AHB, Christenson RH. National Academy of Clinical Biochemistry and IFCC Committee for Standardization of Markers of Cardiac Damage Laboratory Medicine practice guidelines: analytical issues for biomarkers of acute coronary syndromes. *Clin Chem* 2007; **53**: 547–551.

9 Apple FS. Cardiac troponin monitoring for detection of myocardial infarction: newer generation assays are here to stay. *Clin Chim Acta* 2007; **380**: 1–3.

10 Apple FS, Wu AHB, Jaffe AS. European Society of Cardiology and American College of Cardiology guidelines for redefinition of myocardial infarction: how to use existing assays clinically and for clinical trials. *Am Heart J* 2002; **144**: 981–986.

11 Apple FS, Jaffe AS. Cardiac function. In: Burtis C, Ashwood E, & Bruns DE, eds. *Tietz' Textbook of Clinical Chemistry and Molecular Diagnostics*, 4th edn. WB Saunders, Philadelphia, 2005: 1619–1670.

12 Wu AHB, Fukushima N, Puskas R, Todd J, Goix P. Development and preliminary clinical validation of a high sensitivity assay for cardiac troponin using a capillary flow (single molecule) fluorescence detector. *Clin Chem* 2006; **52**: 2157–2159.

13 Panteghini M, Gerhardt W, Apple FS, Dati F, Ravkilde J, Wu AH. Quality specifications for cardiac troponin assays. *Clin Chem Lab Med* 2001; **39**: 175–179.

14 Apple FS, Murakami MM. Serum and plasma cardiac troponin I 99th percentile reference values for 3 2nd-generation assays. *Clin Chem* 2007; **53**: 1558–1560.

15 Lin JC, Apple FS, Murakami MM, Luepker RV. Rates of positive cardiac troponin I and creatine kinase MB among patients hospitalized for suspected acute coronary syndromes. *Clin Chem* 2004; **50**: 333–338.

16 Jaffe AS, Babuin L, Apple FS. Biomarkers in acute coronary disease: the present and the future. *J Am Coll Cardiol* 2006; **48**: 1–11.

17 Apple FS, Johari V, Hoybook KJ, Weber-Shrikant E, Davis GK, Murakami MM. Operationalizing cardiac troponin I testing along ESC/ACC consensus guidelines for defining myocardial infarction. *Clin Chim Acta* 2003; **331**: 165–166.

18 Apple FS, Falahati A, Paulson PR, Miller E, Sharkey SW. Improved detection of minor ischemic myocardial injury with measurement of serum cardiac troponin I. *Clin Chem* 1997; **43**: 2047–2051.

19 Tucker JF, Collins RA, Anderson AJ, Hauser J, Kalas J, Apple FS. Early diagnostic efficiency of cardiac troponin I and cardiac troponin T for acute myocardial infarction. *Acad Emerg Med* 1997; **4**: 13–21.

20 Kavsak PA, MacRae AR, Lustig V, Bhargava R, Vandersluis R, Palomaki GE et al. The impact of the ESC/ACC redefinition of myocardial infarction and new sensitive troponin assays on the frequency of acute myocardial infarction. *Am Heart J* 2006; **152**: 118–125.

21 Apple FS. Tissue specificity of cardiac troponin I, cardiac troponin T, and creatine kinase MB. *Clin Chim Acta* 1999; **284**: 151–159.

22 Apple FS, Pearce LA, Doyle PJ, Otto AP, Murakami MM. Cardiac troponin risk stratification based on 99th percentile reference cutoffs in patients with ischemic symptoms

suggestive of acute coronary syndrome: influence of estimated glomerular filtration rates. *Am J Clin Path* 2007; **127**: 598–603.

23 Apple FS, Pearce LA, Chung A, Ler R, Murakami MM. Multiple biomarker use for detection of adverse events in patients presenting with symptoms suggestive of acute coronary syndrome. *Clin Chem* 2007; **53**: 874–881.

24 Ottani F, Galvani M, Nicolini FA, Ferrini D, Pozzati A, Di Pasquele G, Jaffe AS. Elevated cardiac troponin levels predict the risk of adverse outcome in patients with acute coronary syndromes. *Am Heart J* 2000; **140**: 917–927.

25 Morrow DA, Cannon CP, Rifai N, Frey MJ, Vican R, Lakkis N et al. Ability of minor elevations of troponins I and T to predict benefit from an early invasive strategy in patients with unstable angina and non-ST-elevation myocardial infarction: results from a randomized trial. *JAMA* 2001; **286**: 2405–2412.

26 Heidenreich PA, Alloggiamento T, Melsop K, McDonald KM, Go AS, Tllatky MA. The prognostic value of troponin in patients with non-ST elevation acute coronary syndromes: a meta-analysis. *J Am Coll Cardiol* 2001; **38**: 478–485.

27 Apple FS, Murakami MM. Cardiac troponin and creatine kinase MB monitoring during in-hospital myocardial reinfarction. *Clin Chem* 2005; **51**: 460–463.

28 Fesmire FM, Percy RF, Bardoner JB, Wharton DR, Calhoun FB. Serial creatine kinase (CK) MB testing during emergency department evaluation of chest pain: utility of a 2-hour delta CKMB of +1.6 ng/mL. *Am Heart J* 1998; **136**: 237–244.

29 Fesmire FM. Improved identification of acute coronary syndromes with delta cardiac serum marker measurements during the emergency department evaluation of chest pain patients. *Cardiovasc Tox* 2001; **1**: 117–123.

30 Apple FS, Morrow DA. Cardiac troponin in conditions other than acute coronary syndromes. In: Morrow DA, ed. *Cardiovascular Biomarkers: Pathophysiology and Disease Management*. Humana, Totowa, NJ, 2006, 139–160.

31 Apple FS, Chung AY, Kogut ME, Bubany S, Murakami MM. Decreased patient charges following implementation of point-of-care cardiac troponin monitoring in acute coronary syndrome patients in a community hospital cardiology unity. *Clin Chim Acta* 2006; **370**: 191–195.

32 Apple FS, Smith SW, Pearce LA, Kaczmarek JM, Murakami MM, Vlaminck J, Meyers J, Kilburn BJ, DeSantis T, Uettwiller-Geiger D. Clinical and analytical validation of the Ortho-Clinical Diagnostics second generation VITROS troponin I ES assay for the diagnosis of myocardial infarction and detection of adverse events in patients presenting with symptoms suggestive of acute coronary syndrome. *Clin Chem* 2007; **53**: A9 (abstract).

33 McLaurin MD, Apple FS, Falahati A, Murakami MA, Miller EA, Sharkey SW. Cardiac troponin I and creatine kinase MB mass to rule out myocardial injury in hospitalized patients with renal insufficiency. *Am J Cardiol* 1998; **82**: 973–975.

34 Apple FS. The role of cardiac troponin testing in renal disease. In: Apple FS, Adams III, Wu AHB, & Jaffe AS, eds. *Markers in Cardiology: Current and Future Clinical Applications*. Futura, Armonk, NY, 2001: 203–209.

35 Herzog CA, Ma JZ, Collings AJ. Poor long-term survival after acute myocardial infarction among patients on long-term dialysis. *N Engl J Med* 1998; **339**: 779–805.

36 Bleyer AJ, Russell GB, Satko SG. Sudden and cardiac death rates in hemodialysis patients. *Kid Internal* 1999; **55**: 1553–1559.

37 Ooi D, Zimmerman D, Graham J, Wells G. Cardiac troponin T predicts long-term outcomes in hemodialysis patients. *Clin Chem* 2001; **47**: 412–417.

38 McCullough P, Nowak R, Foreback C, Tokarski G, Tomlanovich M et al. Performance of multiple cardiac biomarkers measured in the emergency department in patients with chronic kidney disease and chest pain. *Acad Emerg Med* 2002; **9**: 1389–1396.

39 Iliou M, Fumeron C, Benoit M, Tuppin P, Courvoisier C et al. Factors associated with increased serum levels of cardiac troponins T and I in chronic haemodialysis patients: chronic haemodialysis and new cardiac markers evaluation (CHANCE) study. *Nephrol Dial Transplant* 2001; **16**: 1452–1458.

40 Dierkes J, Domrose U, Westphal D, Ambrosch A, Bosselmann H et al. Cardiac troponin T predicts mortality in patients with end-stage renal disease. *J Am Coll Cardiol* 2000; **102**: 1964–1969.

41 Aviles R, Askari A, Lindahl B, Wallentin L, Jia G et al. Troponin T levels in patients with acute coronary syndromes, with or without renal dysfunction. *N Engl J Med* 2002; **346**: 2047–2052, 2079–2082.

42 Lowbeer C, Ottosson-Seeberger A, Gustafsson S, Norrman R, Hulting J et al. Increased cardiac troponin T and endothelin-1 concentrations in dialysis patients may indicate heart disease. *Nephrol Dial Transplant* 1999; **14**: 1948–1955.

43 Roppolo L, Fitzgerald R, Dillow J, Ziegler T, Rice M et al. A comparison of troponin T and troponin I as predictors of cardiac events in patients undergoing chronic dialysis at a veteran's hospital: a pilot study. *J Am Coll Cardiol* 1999; **34**: 448–454.

44 Khan I, Wattanasuwan N, Mehta N, Tun S, Singh N et al. Prognostic value of serum cardiac troponin I in ambulatory patients with chronic renal failure undergoing long-term hemodialysis. *J Am Coll Cardiol* 2001; **38**: 991–998.

45 Jaffe S. Editorial comment: Testing the wrong hypothesis: the failure to recognize the limitations of troponin assays. *J Am Coll Cardiol* 2001; **38**: 999–1001.

46 Mockel M, Schindler R, Knorr L, Muller C, Heller Jr G et al. Prognostic value of cardiac troponin T and I elevations in renal disease patients without acute coronary syndromes: a 9-month outcome analysis. *Nephrol Dial Transplant* 1999; **14**: 1489–1495.

47 Apple FS, Sharkey S, Hoeft P, Skeate R, Voss E et al. Prognostic value of serum cardiac troponin I and T in chronic dialysis patients: a 1-year outcomes analysis. *Am J Kid Dis* 1997; **29**: 399–403.

48 McLaurin M, Apple FS, Voss E, Herzog C, Sharkey S. Cardiac troponin I, cardiac troponin T, and creatine kinase MB in dialysis patients without ischemic heart disease: evidence of cardiac troponin T expression in skeletal muscle. *Clin Chem* 1997; **43**: 976–982.

49 Frankel W, Herold D, Ziegler T, Fitzgerald R. Cardiac troponin T is elevated in asymptomatic patients with chronic renal failure. *Clin Chem* 1995; **106**: 118–123.

50 Apple FS, Murakami MA, Pearce L, Herzog C. Predictive value of cardiac troponin I and T for subsequent death in end-stage renal disease. *Circulation* 2002; **61**: 2941–2945.

51 Hamm C, Giannitsis E, Katus H. Cardiac troponin elevations in patients without acute coronary syndrome. *Circulation* 2002; **106**: 2871–2872.

52 Roberts MA, Fernando D, Macmillan N, Proimos G, Bach LA et al. Single and serial measurements of cardiac troponin I in asymptomatic patients of chronic hemodialysis. *Clin Nephrol* 2004; **61**: 40–46.

53 Diris J, Hackeng C, Kooman J, Pinto Y, Hermens W et al. Impaired renal clearance explains elevated troponin T fragments in hemodialysis patients. *Circulation* 2004; **109**: 23–25.

54 Donnino M, Karriem-Norwood V, Rivers E, Gupta A, Nguyen B et al. Prevalence of elevated troponin I in end-stage renal disease patients receiving hemodialysis. *Acad Emerg Med* 2004; **11**: 979–981.

55 Apple FS, Murakami MA, Pearce L, Herzog C. Multi-biomarker risk stratification on N-terminal pro-B-type natriuretic peptide, high-sensitivity C-reactive protein, and cardiac troponin T and I in end-stage renal disease for all-cause death. *Clin Chem* 2004; **50**: 1–7.

56 deFilippi C, Wasserman S, Rosanio S, Tiblier E, Sperger H et al. Cardiac troponin T and C-reactive protein for predicting prognosis, coronary atherosclerosis, and cardiomyopathy in patients undergoing long-term hemodialysis. *JAMA* 2003; **290**: 353–359.

57 Setsuta K, Seino Y, Takahashi N, Ogawa T, Sasaki K, et al. Clinical significance of elevated levels of cardiac troponin T in patients with chronic heart failure. *Am J Cardiol* 1999; **84**: 608–611.

58 Horwich T, Patel J, MacLellan R, Fonarow G. Cardiac troponin I is associated with impaired hemodynamics, progressive left ventricular dysfunction, and increased mortality rates in advanced heart failure. *Circulation* 2003; **108**: 833–838.

59 Del Carlo C, O'Connor C. Cardiac troponins in congestive heart failure. *Am Heart J* 1999; **138**: 646–653.

60 Vecchia L, Mezzena G, Ometto R, Finocchi G, Bedogni F et al. Detectable serum troponin I in patients with heart failure of non-myocardial ischemic origin. *Am J Cardiol* 1997; **80**: 88–90.

61 Missov E, Mair J. A novel biochemical approach to congestive heart failure: cardiac troponin T. *Am Heart J* 1999; **138**: 95–99.

62 Perna E, Macin S, Parras J, Pantich R, Farias E et al. Cardiac troponin T levels are associated with poor short- and long-term prognosis in patients with acute cardiogenic pulmonary edema. *Am Heart J* 2002; **143**: 814–820.

63 Meyer T, Binder L, Hruska N, Luthe H, Buchwald A. Cardiac troponin I elevation in acute pulmonary embolism is associated with right ventricular dysfunction. *J Am Coll Cardiol* 2000; **36**: 1632–1636.

Chapter 4

Natriuretic peptides and inflammatory markers for risk stratification in patients with ischemic heart disease

Torbjørn Omland and Torgun Wæhre

Introduction

Acute coronary syndromes (ACS) encompass a range of clinical manifestations caused by the rupture or erosion of a coronary atherosclerotic plaque [1]. The clinical presentation may vary from unstable angina pectoris to non–ST-elevation myocardial infarction (MI) or ST-elevation MI, depending on whether the acute plaque rupture results in subtotal, or transient, or permanent total occlusion of the diseased vessel. Major progress has been made in the management of patients with ACS during recent years. Commensurate with advances in medical therapy and increasing use of an early invasive strategy, the concept of using circulating biomarkers for early risk stratification and targeting of therapy has gained widespread attention [2,3]. Currently, measurement of cardiac-specific troponins is routinely performed in patients with ACS, both for diagnostic and prognostic purposes (see chapters 1 and 2). Moreover, troponins have convincingly been shown to identify subsets of patients at high risk who benefit from aggressive medical intervention and early coronary interventions, resulting in reduced extent of myocardial injury. Multiple other circulating biomarkers have also been shown to be independently related to outcome [3]. Among a number of candidate biomarkers, the strongest and most consistent evidence supporting a role in prognostic assessment in both ACS and in stable ischemic heart disease (IHD) appears to be for B-type natriuretic peptides (BNPs) [4,5] and high sensitivity C-reactive protein (hs-CRP) [4,6]. Accordingly, this chapter will review data concerning the prognostic value of BNPs and hs-CRP in IHD and discuss strengths and limitations of these biomarkers as tools for risk stratification in clinical practice.

Biomarkers in Heart Disease, 1st edition. Edited by James A. de Lemos.
© 2008 American Heart Association, ISBN: 978-1-4051-7571-5

B-type natriuretic peptides

Biology of B-type natriuretic peptide (BNP)

Originally identified in porcine brain and termed brain natriuretic peptide [7], BNP was soon detected in ventricular cardiomyocytes and found circulating in human plasma. The ventricular myocardium is now recognized as the major source of circulating BNP [8], but BNP is also produced in considerable amounts in human atrial tissue [9]. BNP is formed by cleavage of its prohormone (proBNP) by the enzyme corin into the 32 amino-acid, biologically active C-terminal fragment, BNP, and an inactive N-terminal fragment, NT-proBNP. ProBNP is only partially stored in granules, and regulation of BNP synthesis and secretion occurs mainly at the level of gene expression.

Increments in wall stress represent a potent stimulus for BNP and NT-proBNP release from cardiomyocytes. High circulating levels of BNP and NT-proBNP may also be observed in critically ill patients despite normal or near normal cardiac function [10], suggesting that neurohormonal and immune activation may also be important determinants of circulating BNP and NT-proBNP levels in some circumstances.

Although the N- and C-terminal fragments of proBNP are believed to be secreted in a 1:1 fashion, circulating levels of BNP and NT-proBNP differ considerably due to different clearance characteristics. In humans, the in vivo plasma half-life of BNP has been estimated to be approximately 21 minutes. Concerning NT-proBNP, investigations in sheep indicate that the half-life of NT-proBNP in the circulation is approximately 70 minutes. Binding to clearance receptors and the enzyme neutral endopeptidase both contribute to clearance of BNP. Clearance mechanisms for NT-proBNP are less understood. Impaired renal function is associated with increased circulating levels of both BNP and NT-proBNP. Properties of BNP and NT-proBNP are summarized in Table 4.1.

BNPs and myocardial ischemia

Acute ischemic injury is a potent stimulus for activation of the cardiac natriuretic peptide system [11–13]. A variety of factors may cause increased production of BNPs following acute ischemia and their relative contributions are difficult to assess. Left ventricular systolic and diastolic dysfunction, induced by myocardial ischemia, are major stimuli for BNP production. Notably, impaired ventricular relaxation, an early consequence of ischemia that precedes anginal pain and electrocardiographic changes, may enhance the production and release of BNP and NT-proBNP. During the process of ventricular remodeling following acute MI, both increased intra-ventricular pressure and an increase in chamber diameter may contribute to elevation of circulating BNPs. Other factors, including hypoxia, increased heart rate, and a variety of pro-inflammatory cytokines and neurohormones with vasoconstrictory, antidiuretic, hypertrophic, and cytoproliferative effects, may also contribute to increased BNP production.

Table 4.1 Properties of BNP and NT-proBNP.

Property	BNP	NT-proBNP
Molecular weight	3.5 kd	8.5 kd
Physiological activity	Active	Probably inactive
Plasma half-life	21 min	70 min
FDA approved cut-off values for heart failure diagnosis	<100 pg/mL	Age <75 y: 125 pg/mL Age >75 y: 450 pg/mL
Clearance mechanisms	Clearance receptors (NPR-C) Neutral endopeptidase (NEP)	Unclear, possibly renal clearance
Analyzed in	Whole blood and EDTA plasma (plastic tubes)	Serum and plasma
In vitro stability	4–24 h at room temperature	>3 days at room temperature

FDA = Food and Drug Administration
NPR-C = Natriuretic peptide receptor-C

Atherosclerotic lesions may represent an additional source of circulating BNPs.

Clinical observations also suggest that ischemia per se is a stimulus for BNP and NT-proBNP release. Unstable angina is associated with increased circulating levels of BNPs [14,15], which decrease following successful percutaneous coronary intervention. Post-ischemic elevation of both BNP and NT-proBNP appear to be associated with the magnitude of the ischemic territory as assessed by nuclear imaging or stress echocardiography [16,17]. Not surprisingly, given differences in plasma half-lives and baseline levels, the acute changes in peptide concentrations during stress testing are somewhat more pronounced for BNP than for NT-proBNP [17].

BNPs in ACS
Plasma profile and determinants of BNP elevation
In patients with acute MI, the magnitude and duration of the increase in plasma concentrations of NT-proBNP are associated with the size of the infarcted area and subsequent left ventricular dysfunction [12]. Following transmural infarction, circulating levels of BNPs increase rapidly and peak after approximately 24 hours [12,18]. The pattern of BNP production following ACS may vary according

to the extent and the site of ischemia. Accordingly, a biphasic profile of BNP and NT-proBNP secretion may be more common in patients with large, anterior wall infarctions than in those with less extensive, inferior infarctions.

Prognostic value of BNPs in ACS

The first studies reporting an association between BNP levels and survival after MI were published in 1996 [13,19]. Currently, more than 15 studies have been published concerning the association between circulating levels of BNP and NT-proBNP in patients with ACS and the subsequent incidence of death and heart failure [13,19–31]. Early studies comprised mainly patients with ST-elevation MI, but based on studies showing that BNP and NT-proBNP were elevated in unstable angina and could be normalized following successful percutaneous coronary intervention [14], it was subsequently postulated that BNP and NT-proBNP would be predictive of outcome across the spectrum of ACS. In aggregate, these studies clearly demonstrate that both circulating BNP and NT-proBNP levels obtained acutely or in the subacute phase are strongly associated with both short-term and long-term cardiovascular mortality across the spectrum of ACS, independently of conventional risk factors, including older age, female gender, renal impairment, extent of myocardial necrosis and of coronary artery disease, clinical heart failure, and left ventricular systolic dysfunction (Figs. 4.1 and 4.2). Importantly, BNP and NT-proBNP identify patients without clinical signs of heart failure and with preserved ventricular function who are at high risk for death and heart failure events [27]. Given that recurrent ischemic events are a common cause of death in patients with ACS, it is somewhat surprising that the association between natriuretic peptides and recurrent MI is generally weak, and in most studies nonexistent after adjustment for potential confounders [22,25]. In contrast, BNPs are closely associated with the incidence of heart failure, suggesting that the ability of BNP and NT-proBNP to predict death in ACS is mainly explained by its ability to predict heart failure. Accordingly, BNPs provide complementary prognostic information to troponins: whereas troponins are superior to BNPs in predicting ischemic events, the converse is true for prediction of heart failure and death [25] (Fig. 4.3).

Timing of measurements of natriuretic peptides

The literature on the potential additional value of serial measurements of natriuretic peptides in patients with ACS is still relatively sparse. In a substudy of the A-Z trial, BNP levels were measured serially after ACS, during the hospital phase, and again at 4 and 8 months [24]. After adjustment for relevant confounders, a BNP concentration >80 pg/mL on study entry was associated with increased risk of death and heart failure. Interestingly, when the repeat measurement at 4 months was considered, patients with newly elevated levels of BNP (>80 pg/mL) had increased risk, whereas patients with elevated levels on study entry but with BNP levels <80 pg/mL at 4 months had

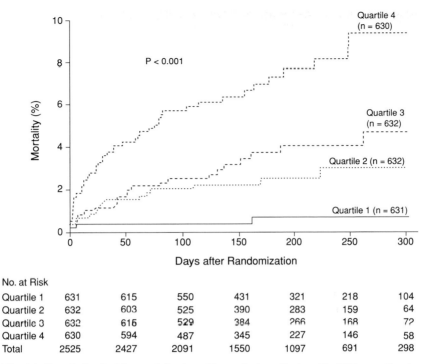

No. at Risk							
Quartile 1	631	615	550	431	321	218	104
Quartile 2	632	603	525	390	283	159	64
Quartile 3	632	616	529	384	266	168	72
Quartile 4	630	594	487	345	227	146	58
Total	2525	2427	2091	1550	1097	691	298

Fig. 4.1 Cumulative incidence of death at 10 months in patients with ACS according to the quartile of B-type natriuretic peptide at baseline (reproduced from [22]).

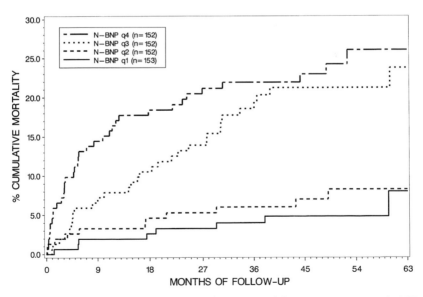

Fig. 4.2 Cumulative incidence of death during long-term follow-up in patients with ACS according to the quartile of N-terminal pro-B-type natriuretic peptide (reproduced from [27]).

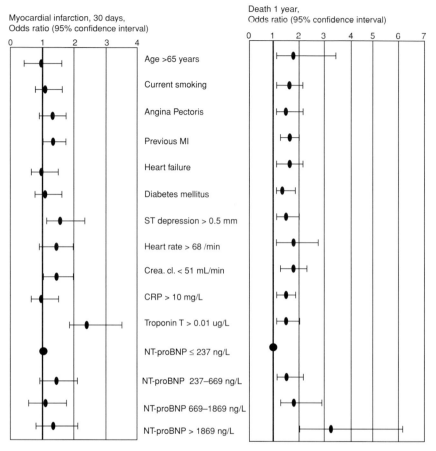

Myocardial infarction, 30 days,
Odds ratio (95% confidence interval)

Death 1 year,
Odds ratio (95% confidence interval)

Age >65 years

Current smoking

Angina Pectoris

Previous MI

Heart failure

Diabetes mellitus

ST depression > 0.5 mm

Heart rate > 68 /min

Crea. cl. < 51 mL/min

CRP > 10 mg/L

Troponin T > 0.01 ug/L

NT-proBNP ≤ 237 ng/L

NT-proBNP 237–669 ng/L

NT-proBNP 669–1869 ng/L

NT-proBNP > 1869 ng/L

Fig. 4.3 Potential risk markers and their association with the incidence of myocardial infarction at 30 days and death at 1 year in patients with ACS (reproduced from [25]).

only marginally increased risk compared to patients with BNP levels <80 pg/mL at both time points (Fig. 4.4).

As mentioned earlier, circulating concentrations of natriuretic peptides change markedly over time after presentation [12]. Accordingly, it seems reasonable to assume that the timing of measurement may affect the association with risk. Data from the FRISC-II trial show that NT-proBNP levels are highest on admission, decrease markedly the first 24 hours and then gradually over the following 6 months [32]. Interestingly, the predictive ability of NT-proBNP appears to increase with time, suggesting that persistent elevation is a particularly strong marker of adverse outcome. In a substudy of PRISM, the addition of a second NT-proBNP value 72 hours following admission appeared to improve risk prediction concerning the end-point of death or recurrent MI at 30 days [26].

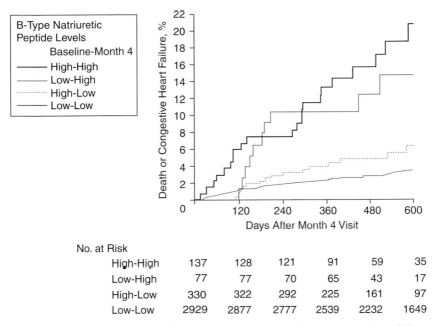

No. at Risk

High-High	137	128	121	91	59	35
Low-High	77	77	70	65	43	17
High-Low	330	322	292	225	161	97
Low-Low	2929	2877	2777	2539	2232	1649

Fig. 4.4 Cumulative incidence of death or new or worsening congestive heart failure according to the B-type natriuretic peptide levels at baseline and month 4 in patients with ACS (reproduced from [24]).

Regardless of the NT-proBNP value on admission, a NT-proBNP concentration >250 pg/mL at 72 hours indicated a markedly increased risk. However, the impact of this observation on contemporary clinical practice is unclear, as most patients presenting with ACS will be referred to coronary angiography within 72 hours of presentation. Although more data concerning the optimal timing of natriuretic peptide determination is warranted, at this point it seems reasonable to measure BNP or NT-proBNP on presentation for initial risk assessment and once during the subacute phase (either at hospital discharge or at an early postdischarge outpatient visit) for long-term risk assessment.

What BNP and NT-proBNP concentrations define increased risk?

The relationship between circulating concentrations of BNP and NT-proBNP in patients with ACS and the incidence of subsequent death and heart failure is largely monotonic and does not appear to allow definition of a specific threshold value. Accordingly, the absolute natriuretic peptide level carries clinically valuable information with regard to the magnitude of risk. For the clinician, however, identification of threshold concentrations of BNP and NT-proBNP that define increased risk would be helpful. The approved BNP cutoff for diagnosing heart failure (100 pg/mL) is derived from trials of acutely dyspneic patients and does not take into account the confounding effects of age and gender. As it is not based on healthy individuals it should not be regarded as a conventional upper normal value, and may be imperfect for defining risk in ACS patients. Nevertheless, a decision limit of 80 pg/mL has been validated in 2 ACS studies using different BNP assays [22,24]. Although the prognostic value of NT-proBNP has been examined in numerous studies, cut-off points have been study-specific and not prospectively defined. However, data from several NT-proBNP studies suggest that a cutoff of approximately 250 pg/mL discriminates well between patients with a poor and a favorable prognosis [25,26,32]. Unfortunately, both the 80 pg/mL decision limit for BNP and the 250 pg/mL decision limit for NT-proBNP are derived from clinical trials, which may imply a selection bias. Clearly, prospective studies in more unselected patient groups are warranted to define decision limits for BNP and NT-proBNP in ACS. Important questions that need to be addressed are whether thresholds should be age and/or gender adjusted and whether stratification in three strata (high-risk, intermediate risk, low-risk) is likely to be more helpful to the clinician than a conventional two-strata approach.

Impact on therapeutic decision making

Only limited retrospective data are currently available to elucidate whether the use of BNP or NT-proBNP in ACS is predictive of the effect of therapeutic intervention and should affect subsequent management. In contrast to troponins, natriuretic peptides are poor predictors of recurrent ischemic events but strong predictors of death [25]. Unfortunately, few contemporary clinical trials document a significant effect of intervention on mortality in ACS. Consequently, it is inherently difficult to demonstrate a significant interaction between natriuretic peptide levels and a specific therapeutic strategy. Three studies have evaluated whether natriuretic peptides can be used to identify patients who will benefit from routine early referral for coronary angiography and revascularization (early invasive strategy) following ACS [23,29,33]. Although all studies confirmed the association between BNP and NT-proBNP and outcome, discrepant results were obtained concerning the effect of routine invasive therapy in the high NT-proBNP or BNP subgroups.

In the TACTICS-TIMI 18 trial, the risk of death was not reduced significantly in the routine invasive arm and was similar regardless of whether the baseline BNP concentration was above or below the cutoff of 80 pg/mL [23]. Likewise, in the ICTUS trial an early invasive strategy for patients with higher NT-proBNP levels (above the 75th percentile) was not associated with mortality reduction [33]. In the FRISC-II trial, however, the mortality reduction in the routine invasive arm tended to be greater among patients in the highest NT-proBNP tertile than those in the lower two NT-proBNP tertiles [29]. Moreover, recent data based on a non-randomized, post hoc observational analysis from the GUSTO-IV trial suggest that patients with higher NT-proBNP levels may have a survival benefit from

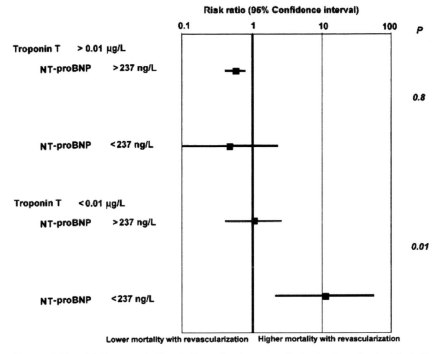

Risk ratio (95% Confidence interval)

Fig. 4.5 NT-proBNP, troponin T, and effect of early revascularization in patients with ACS (reproduced from [34]).

coronary revascularization [34]. Thirty-day survivors with elevated troponin and NT-proBNP levels undergoing early coronary revascularization had a significantly lower mortality rate at 1 year than those not revascularized. In contrast, patients without combined troponin and NT-proBNP elevations did not benefit from revascularization, and those with normal value of both biomarkers had a significant increase in mortality at 1 year following revascularization (Fig. 4.5).

BNPs in stable IHD

Myocardial ischemia can induce a reversible increase in regional wall stress that may lead to augmented production of natriuretic peptides, and both BNP and NT-proBNP concentrations are increased in patients with stable IHD after episodes of ischemia [16,17]. Several studies have reported a relationship between circulating levels of natriuretic peptides and long-term, all-cause mortality in patients with stable IHD, independently of left ventricular systolic dysfunction and other conventional risk factors [35,36]. An association between natriuretic peptide levels and specific cardiovascular end-points

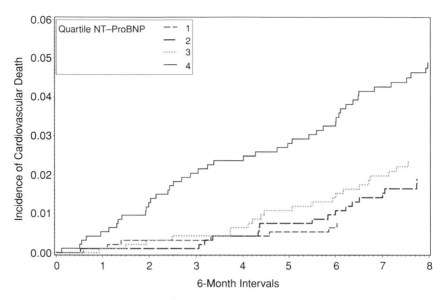

Fig. 4.6 Cumulative incidence of death due to a cardiovascular cause in patients with stable coronary artery disease and preserved ventricular function according to quartiles of plasma N-terminal B-type natriuretic peptide concentrations (reproduced from [38]).

(cardiovascular death, MI, stroke, heart failure) in patients with stable IHD has been reported in two separate studies [37,38] (Fig. 4.6).

In the Heart and Soul substudy, NT-proBNP provided prognostic information above and beyond that obtained from echocardiography and nuclear stress tests [37]. Furthermore, the addition of NT-proBNP to standard clinical assessment and echocardiographic indices improved the area under the receiver-operating characteristics curve for prediction of adverse cardiovascular events compared to clinical risk factors and echocardiographic indices alone. In the PEACE substudy, baseline plasma BNP and NT-proBNP concentrations were measured in 3761 patients with stable IHD and preserved left ventricular function. BNP and NT-proBNP levels were strongly related to the incidence of cardiovascular mortality, heart failure, and stroke, but not MI. BNP and NT-proBNP significantly improved the predictive accuracy of the best available model for incident heart failure, and NT-proBNP also improved the model for cardiovascular death (Table 4.2). However, the clincal implications of elevated BNPs in stable IHD are less clear. Lack of prediction of MI suggests that determination of BNPs may not be useful for selection of anti-ischemic therapies in low-risk patients. Moreover, BNP and NT-proBNP failed to identify stable IHD patients who will benefit from angiotensin converting enzyme (ACE)-inhibition. In conclusion, current data support measurement of BNPs in stable IHD for prognostic assessment,

Table 4.2 Incremental prognostic value of B-type natriuretic peptide and N-terminal-proB-type natriuretic peptide to the best available multivariable* model for cardiovascular end-points

Outcome	C-statistic Covariates	C-statistic Covariates & BNP	C-statistic Covariates & NT-proBNP
CV mortality	0.74 (0.70–0.79)	0.75 (0.71–0.80)	0.77 (0.73–0.81)*
CHF	0.82 (0.78–0.86)	0.84 (0.80–0.87)*	0.85 (0.81–0.88)*
Stroke	0.78 (0.73–0.83)	0.78 (0.73–0.83)	0.80 (0.76 to 0.85)

CV: cardiovascular; CHF: congestive heart failure
* $p < 0.05$
Covariates include treatment assignment, age, sex, body mass index, ejection fraction <50%, estimated glomerular filtration rate, current smoking, history of hypertension or measured hypertension, history of myocardial infarction, history of diabetes, history of stroke, history of percutaneous coronary intervention, history of coronary artery bypass grafting, total cholesterol, C-reactive protein, use of a beta blocker, use of a lipid-lowering drug, use of aspirin or an antiplatelet medication, and use of a diuretic. (reproduced from Omland T et al. *JACC* 2007; **50**: 205–14).

but do not provide a mandate for the use of these peptides for tailoring therapy in individual patients.

C-reactive protein (CRP)

Introduction

Inflammatory mechanisms play an important pathogenic role in atherogenesis—from early formation and progression of plaques to development of ACS and thrombotic complications [39]. The inflammatory activation in IHD is not isolated to the atherosclerotic plaques, as IHD is also characterized by systemic signs of inflammation, reflected as elevated plasma levels of CRP, soluble adhesion molecules, chemokines, and cytokines, including interleukin (IL)-6, soluble CD40 ligand, and tumor necrosis factor (TNF)-α [40]. Particularly high levels of inflammatory markers are found in patients with unstable IHD. CRP is the prototypical acute-phase reactant and the most extensively studied inflammatory marker in clinical studies, and hs-CRP has emerged as a robust predictor of cardiovascular risk at all stages, from healthy subjects to patients with ACS [41].

CRP as a potential mediator of inflammation and atherosclerosis

CRP is a nonspecific acute-phase reactant that serves as a pattern-recognition molecule in the innate immune systems. It is produced in hepatocytes in response to stimulation by inflammatory cytokines, primarily IL-6, TNF-α, and IL-1β. CRP levels may increase several 100-fold in response to infectious stimuli. In chronic inflammatory disorders such as rheumatoid arthritis and inflammatory bowel disease, variation in CRP levels reflects disease activity. A commonly assigned cut-off value of "conventional" CRP assays is <10 mg/L, with concentrations of 10–40 mg/L associated with mild inflammation and concentrations of 40–200 mg/L associated with acute inflammation and bacterial infections. To assess cardiovascular risk caused by atherosclerotic inflammation, particularly in the nonacute setting, the use of hs-CRP assays with accurate and reproducible CRP measurements down to 0.3 mg/L is required [42].

Whether CRP is merely a marker of vascular inflammation or plays a pathogenetic role in the inflammatory process is yet unclear; however, several lines of evidence support the latter theory. First, in endothelial cells, CRP attenuates nitric oxide production, promotes apoptosis, and induces expression of adhesion molecules [43,44]. Second, CRP stimulates release of inflammatory cytokines from monocytes and serves as an opsonin on low-density lipoprotein (LDL) particles mediating LDL uptake in macrophages. Third, CRP is localized in the early atherosclerotic lesions where it may precede and mediate monocyte recruitment. Finally, inflammatory cytokines have been shown to induce production of CRP in vascular smooth muscle cells and macrophages [45], suggesting that not only hepatic but also local vascular production of CRP may occur. However, in an atherosclerotic model using Apo E knockout mice, transgenic expression of human CRP did not accelerate atherosclerosis, suggesting that the in vitro observations of potential pro-inflammatory CRP effects do not necessarily reflect the in vivo situation [46].

hs-CRP as a predictor of risk in IHD

hs-CRP and short-term prognosis

Numerous studies have reported elevated levels of hs-CRP in patients with IHD, with particularly high levels in those with unstable disease. In a hallmark study, Liuzzo et al. reported that hs-CRP levels above 3 mg/L on admission in patients with unstable angina were associated with increased risk of recurrent ischemic events [47]. A similar observation was made in >1000 non–ST-elevation ACS patients undergoing early revascularization procedures, where an hs-CRP >10 mg/L predicted short-term mortality [48]. In the TIMI 11A substudy the 14-day mortality rate in non–ST-elevation ACS was as high as 5.6% in patients with hs-CRP >15.5 mg/L but only 0.3% in the patients with hs-CRP under this cut-off level [49]. In the GUSTO IV-ACS trial, hs-CRP levels >9.62 mg/L were associated with a significantly increased risk of death, but not recurrent ischemic events at 48 hours, 7 days, and 30 days [50]. However, other studies have not

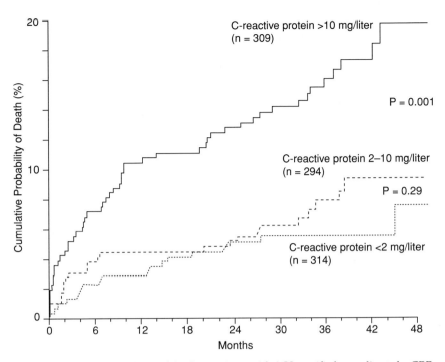

Fig. 4.7 Cumulative incidence of death in patients with ACS stratified according to hs-CRP levels at baseline (reproduced from [54]).

been able to confirm the same association between hs-CRP levels on admission and short-term prognosis [51,52].

hs-CRP and long-term prognosis

More consistent data exist concerning hs-CRP levels and long-term prognosis in non–ST-elevation ACS patients. Biasucci et al. found that unstable angina patients with hs-CRP >3 mg/L at discharge from hospital were more likely to have persistent hs-CRP elevation after 3 months, suggesting persistent inflammatory activation, and a significantly higher rate of new ischemic episodes the following year [53]. Confirming evidence has been provided by other investigators (Table 4.3), although controversy still exists whether hs-CRP is primarily predictive of mortality or whether it also predicts recurrent ischemic events [48,50,52,54] (Fig. 4.7).

Whether the worse outcome seen in patients with elevated hs-CRP after non–ST-elevation ACS is a consequence of persistent coronary inflammation or is related to myocardial injury during the ischemic episode has been evaluated in several large-scale studies. A consistent finding has been that troponins and hs-CRP are complementary predictors of adverse outcome: in the GUSTO-IV

Table 4.3 Selected studies examining the association between hs-CRP levels and moderate to long-term outcome in patients with acute coronary syndromes.

Author (Trial)	n	Mean Follow-up	CRP cut-off (mg/L)	End-point	OR or HR (95% CI)
Mueller [48]	1042	6 months	>10	Death	4.1 (2.3–7.2)
Lindahl [54]	917	37 months	>10	Death	2.5 (1.6–3.9)
Heeschen [51]	447	6 months	>10	Death+MI	2.0 (1.2–3.6)
James [50]	7108	12 months	>10	Death	1.5 (1.1–1.9)
Biasucci [53]	53	12 months	>3	Death+MI+RI	4.7 (1.8–12.0)
Ferreiros [52]	194	3 months	>1.5	Death+MI+RI	1.9 (1.2–8.3)

OR, odds ratio; HR, hazard ratio; MI, myocardial infarction; RI, recurrent ischemia

study, the FRISC II study, and the TIMI 11B study, hs-CRP and troponins were independently associated with mortality [49,50,54]. Indeed, increased risk was also observed in patients with normal troponin levels and elevated hs-CRP, suggesting that myocardial injury does not totally explain the unfavorable outcome associated with hs-CRP-elevation [49,54]. Moreover, patients with unstable angina have higher hs-CRP levels than patients with variant angina despite a higher ischemic burden in the latter group, suggesting a plaque-dependent inflammatory response [55].

Although there is evidence that myocardial necrosis is responsible for some of the inflammatory response and risk associated with hs-CRP elevation following non–ST-elevation ACS, hs-CRP also has been found to predict future coronary events in apparently healthy subjects [56–58], in patients with stable IHD [59], in subjects undergoing revascularization procedures [60,61], and in patients with chest pain but without evidence of non–ST-elevation ACS [62]. Interestingly, hs-CRP levels do not seem to be related to the total burden of atherosclerosis as assessed by number of stenoses at coronary angiography after adjustment for other risk factors [63]. The more pronounced hs-CRP elevation found in patients with ACS might indicate a process different from the more low-grade hs-CRP elevation in the chronic phase of the atherosclerotic disease.

Timing of hs-CRP measurements

The optimal timing for measurement of hs-CRP for risk assessment in ACS remains to be determined. hs-CRP appears to provide prognostic information regardless of whether samples are obtained on presentation, at discharge, or during the postdischarge convalescent phase. However, the inflammatory response to myocardial necrosis may affect hs-CRP levels in MI patients when measured late after presentation. Indeed, it is likely that hs-CRP concentrations obtained on admission and during the convalescent phase differ with respect to pathophysiologic determinants and association with subsequent risk.

What hs-CRP concentrations define increased risk?

Although most investigators agree that optimal decision limits for hs-CRP in ACS should be higher than for primary prevention, a wide range of limits have been evaluated in ACS. Receiver-operating characteristics analysis derived from one prospective study has suggested that a decision limit of 15 mg/L may be optimal in ACS [52]. However, a lower decision limit of 10 mg/L has also been evaluated, and currently, no generally accepted consensus value exists. In patients with stable IHD, or in the convalescent phase following ACS, the following thresholds have been recommended to stratify patients into high risk (>3 mg/L), intermediate risk (1–3 mg/L), and low risk (<1 mg/L). These cut-off values have recently been evaluated in a large cohort of patients with stable IHD included in the PEACE trial. During a median follow-up period of 4.8 years, an elevated hs-CRP concentration >1 mg/L was associated with moderately increased risk of a composite end-point of cardiovascular death, MI, or stroke [59] (Fig. 4.8). Similarly, elevated hs-CRP was associated with increased risk of new heart failure and new-onset diabetes [59]. Recognition of the potential impact of race and ethnicity on the distribution of hs-CRP may be of consequence for determining optimal cutoffs in different populations of patients.

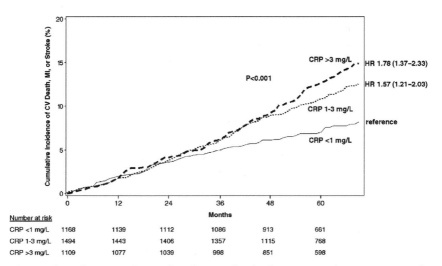

Fig. 4.8 Cumulative incidence of cardiovascular death, MI, or stroke in patients with stable coronary artery disease and preserved ventricular function according to quartiles of CRP concentrations (reproduced from [59]).

Impact on therapeutic decision making

Therapeutic strategies to reduce the recurrence of cardiovascular events in patients with established IHD include drugs from several classes, the most important being statins, platelet-inhibiting drugs such as aspirin and clopidogrel, β-adrenoreceptor blockers, and ACE-inhibitors. Of these, statins and aspirin have potential anti-inflammatory effects, and their relation with CRP and risk stratification will be briefly discussed.

Statins reduce circulating cholesterol levels and are shown to be useful in both primary and secondary prevention of IHD. Numerous in vitro animal and human studies have suggested potent anti-inflammatory effects of statins (reviewed in [64]). Statins lower hs-CRP levels in a manner largely independently of LDL-cholesterol levels, and several studies have suggested that statin therapy may have greater clinical benefit if hs-CRP levels are elevated [65]. In the PROVE-IT TIMI 22 study, the ACS patients who achieved low hs-CRP levels (<2 mg/L) after statin therapy had better clinical outcomes than those with higher hs-CRP levels, regardless of the degree of LDL-cholesterol lowering [66]. In the REVERSAL study the progression of coronary atherosclerosis, as assessed by intravascular ultrasound, was significantly reduced during intensive statin therapy, and particularly in those who achieved the lowest hs-CRP levels [67]. In both these intervention studies, the degree of reduction in LDL-cholesterol levels was a predictor of better outcome, but the correlation between hs-CRP and LDL-cholesterol levels was weak. In summary, these trials suggest a possible role for hs-CRP measurement as a guide to monitor the efficacy of statin therapy. However, no prospective data are as yet available testing different strategies for statin therapy among patients with higher versus lower hs-CRP levels.

Anti-platelet therapy with aspirin reduces the risk of death and MI in both stable and unstable IHD. Aspirin possesses anti-inflammatory properties, but these are probably modest at low daily doses (75–150 mg/day). Accordingly, although aspirin 300 mg has been shown to reduce hs-CRP levels in apparently healthy men and stable angina patients [56], more inconsistent effects have been seen with lower aspirin doses [68]. The clinical significance of any hs–CRP-lowering effect of aspirin in IHD patients remains uncertain, and is unlikely to affect treatment decisions as aspirin is routinely administered to all patients presenting with ACS. Finally, elevated hs-CRP concentrations do not appear to identify patients with stable IHD and preserved ejection fraction who benefit from ACE-inhibition [59].

Conclusions

Risk stratification of ACS patients is traditionally based on demographic data, presence of cardiovascular risk factors, medical history, clinical data, electrocardiographic findings, measures of left ventricular function, and evidence of myocardial necrosis as assessed by troponin measurements. Currently,

Table 4.4 National Academy of Clinical Biochemistry Laboratory Medicine (NACB) Practice Guidelines for Biomarkers in ACS: Recommendations for CRP and BNPs

Class IIa

1. Measurement of high-sensitivity C-reactive protein (hs-CRP) may be useful, in addition to cardiac troponin, for risk assessment in patients with a clinical syndrome consistent with ACS. The benefits of therapy based on this strategy remain uncertain.

2. Measurement of brain (B-type) natriuretic peptide (BNP) or N-terminal pro-BNP may be useful, in addition to cardiac troponin, for risk assessment in patients with a clinical syndrome consistent with ACS. The benefits of therapy based on this strategy remain uncertain.

(reproduced from [4]).

cardiac-specific troponins are routinely used for risk stratification and to decide the intensity of interventional and medical therapy in patients with non–ST-elevation ACS. There is ample evidence that the addition of both BNPs and CRP provide statistically independent prognostic information in both ACS and in stable IHD, and both BNPs and CRP have received Class IIa recommendations in the recently published National Academy of Clinical Biochemistry Laboratory Medicine Practice Guidelines [4] (Table 4.4). However, statistical independence does not necessarily imply better overall predictive performance of risk models including these markers [3]. Nevertheless, recent data from the HOPE and PEACE trials do suggest that BNPs, but not CRP, provide modest but statistically significant incremental prognostic information to the best available multivariable model based on conventional risk factors in stable patients (Table 4.2) [38,69]. For BNPs and CRP a number of practical issues of importance for the clinician, including the optimal time-points for sampling, appropriate decision limits, and potential usefulness of combinations with other biomarkers remain to be determined. Finally, the potential usefulness of BNPs and CRP for guiding treatment decisions in patients with ACS and stable IHD is still uncertain, but will be addressed in ongoing clinical trials.

References

1 Libby P. Current concepts of the pathogenesis of the acute coronary syndromes. *Circulation* 2001; **104**: 365–372.
2 Morrow DA, de Lemos JA. Benchmarks for the assessment of novel cardiovascular biomarkers. *Circulation* 2007; **115**: 949–952.
3 Vasan RS. Biomarkers of cardiovascular disease: molecular basis and practical considerations. *Circulation* 2006; **113**: 2335–2362.

4 Morrow DA, Cannon CP, Jesse RL et al. National Academy of Clinical Biochemistry Laboratory Medicine Practice Guidelines: clinical characteristics and utilization of biochemical markers in acute coronary syndromes. *Circulation* 2007; **115**: e356–e375.

5 de Lemos JA, McGuire DK, Drazner MH. B-type natriuretic peptide in cardiovascular disease. *Lancet* 2003; **362**: 316–322.

6 Biasucci LM. CDC/AHA Workshop on Markers of Inflammation and Cardiovascular Disease: Application to Clinical and Public Health Practice: clinical use of inflammatory markers in patients with cardiovascular diseases: a background paper. *Circulation* 2004; **110**: e560–e567.

7 Sudoh T, Kangawa K, Minamino N, Matsuo H. A new natriuretic peptide in porcine brain. *Nature* 1988; **332**: 78–81.

8 Mukoyama M, Nakao K, Hosoda K et al. Brain natriuretic peptide as a novel cardiac hormone in humans. Evidence for an exquisite dual natriuretic peptide system, atrial natriuretic peptide and brain natriuretic peptide. *J Clin Invest* 1991; **87**: 1402–1412.

9 Ruskoaho H. Cardiac hormones as diagnostic tools in heart failure. *Endocr Rev* 2003; **24**: 341–356.

10 Januzzi JL, Morss A, Tung R et al. Natriuretic peptide testing for the evaluation of critically ill patients with shock in the intensive care unit: a prospective cohort study. *Crit Care* 2006; **10**: R37.

11 Hama N, Itoh H, Shirakami G et al. Rapid ventricular induction of brain natriuretic peptide gene expression in experimental acute myocardial infarction. *Circulation* 1995; **92**: 1558–1564.

12 Morita E, Yasue H, Yoshimura M et al. Increased plasma levels of brain natriuretic peptide in patients with acute myocardial infarction. *Circulation* 1993; **88**: 82–91.

13 Omland T, Aakvaag A, Bonarjee VV et al. Plasma brain natriuretic peptide as an indicator of left ventricular systolic function and long-term survival after acute myocardial infarction. Comparison with plasma atrial natriuretic peptide and N-terminal proatrial natriuretic peptide. *Circulation* 1996; **93**: 1963–1969.

14 Kikuta K, Yasue H, Yoshimura M et al. Increased plasma levels of B-type natriuretic peptide in patients with unstable angina. *Am Heart J* 1996; **132**: 101–107.

15 Talwar S, Squire IB, Downie PF, Davies JE, Ng LL. Plasma N terminal pro-brain natriuretic peptide and cardiotrophin 1 are raised in unstable angina. *Heart* 2000; **84**: 421–424.

16 Bibbins-Domingo K, Ansari M, Schiller NB, Massie B, Whooley MA. B-type natriuretic peptide and ischemia in patients with stable coronary disease: data from the Heart and Soul study. *Circulation* 2003; **108**: 2987–2992.

17 Sabatine MS, Morrow DA, de Lemos JA et al. Acute changes in circulating natriuretic peptide levels in relation to myocardial ischemia. *J Am Coll Cardiol* 2004; **44**: 1988–1995.

18 Talwar S, Squire IB, Downie PF et al. Profile of plasma N-terminal proBNP following acute myocardial infarction; correlation with left ventricular systolic dysfunction. *Eur Heart J* 2000; **21**: 1514–1521.

19 Arakawa N, Nakamura M, Aoki H, Hiramori K. Plasma brain natriuretic peptide concentrations predict survival after acute myocardial infarction. *J Am Coll Cardiol* 1996; **27**: 1656–1661

20 Richards AM, Nicholls MG, Yandle TG et al. Plasma N-terminal pro-brain natriuretic peptide and adrenomedullin: new neurohormonal predictors of left ventricular function and prognosis after myocardial infarction. *Circulation* 1998; **97**: 1921–1929.

21 Richards AM, Nicholls MG, Espiner EA et al. B-type natriuretic peptides and ejection fraction for prognosis after myocardial infarction. *Circulation* 2003; **107**: 2786–2792.

22 de Lemos JA, Morrow DA, Bentley JH et al. The prognostic value of B-type natriuretic peptide in patients with acute coronary syndromes. *N Engl J Med* 2001; **345**: 1014–1021.

23 Morrow DA, de Lemos JA, Sabatine MS et al. Evaluation of B-type natriuretic peptide for risk assessment in unstable angina/non–ST-elevation myocardial infarction: B-type natriuretic peptide and prognosis in TACTICS-TIMI 18. *J Am Coll Cardiol* 2003; **41**: 1264–1272.

24 Morrow DA, de Lemos JA, Blazing MA et al. Prognostic value of serial B-type natriuretic peptide testing during follow-up of patients with unstable coronary artery disease. *JAMA* 2005; **294**: 2866–2871.

25 James SK, Lindahl B, Siegbahn A et al. N-terminal pro-brain natriuretic peptide and other risk markers for the separate prediction of mortality and subsequent myocardial infarction in patients with unstable coronary artery disease: a Global Utilization of Strategies To Open occluded arteries (GUSTO)-IV substudy. *Circulation* 2003; **108**: 275–281.

26 Heeschen C, Hamm CW, Mitrovic V, Lantelme NH, White HD. N-terminal pro-B-type natriuretic peptide levels for dynamic risk stratification of patients with acute coronary syndromes. *Circulation* 2004; **110**: 3206–3212.

27 Omland T, Persson A, Ng L et al. N-terminal pro-B-type natriuretic peptide and long-term mortality in acute coronary syndromes. *Circulation* 2002; **106**: 2913–2918.

28 Omland T, de Lemos JA, Morrow DA et al. Prognostic value of N-terminal pro-atrial and pro-brain natriuretic peptide in patients with acute coronary syndromes. *Am J Cardiol* 2002; **89**: 463–465.

29 Jernberg T, Lindahl B, Siegbahn A et al. N-terminal pro-brain natriuretic peptide in relation to inflammation, myocardial necrosis, and the effect of an invasive strategy in unstable coronary artery disease. *J Am Coll Cardiol* 2003; **42**: 1909–1916.

30 Sabatine MS, Morrow DA, de Lemos JA et al. Multimarker approach to risk stratification in non-ST elevation acute coronary syndromes: simultaneous assessment of troponin I, C-reactive protein, and B-type natriuretic peptide. *Circulation* 2002; **105**: 1760–1763.

31 Galvani M, Ottani F, Oltrona L et al. N-Terminal pro-brain natriuretic peptide on admission has prognostic value across the whole spectrum of acute coronary syndromes. *Circulation* 2004; **110**: 128–134.

32 Lindahl B, Lindback J, Jernberg T et al. Serial analyses of N-terminal pro-B-type natriuretic peptide in patients with non–ST-segment elevation acute coronary syndromes: a Fragmin and fast Revascularisation during In Stability in Coronary artery disease (FRISC)-II substudy. *J Am Coll Cardiol* 2005; **45**: 533–541.

33 Windhausen F, Hirsch A, Sanders GT et al. N-terminal pro-brain natriuretic peptide for additional risk stratification in patients with non–ST-elevation acute coronary syndrome and an elevated troponin T: an Invasive versus Conservative Treatment in Unstable coronary Syndromes (ICTUS) substudy. *Am Heart J* 2007; **153**: 485–492.

34 James SK, Lindback J, Tilly J et al. Troponin-T and N-terminal pro-B-type natriuretic peptide predict mortality benefit from coronary revascularization in acute coronary syndromes: a GUSTO-IV substudy. *J Am Coll Cardiol* 2006; **48**: 1146–1154.

35 Omland T, Richards AM, Wergeland R, Vik-Mo H. B-type natriuretic peptide and long-term survival in patients with stable coronary artery disease. *Am J Cardiol* 2005; **95**: 24–28.

36 Ndrepepa G, Braun S, Niemoller K et al. Prognostic value of N-terminal pro-brain natriuretic peptide in patients with chronic stable angina. *Circulation* 2005; **112**: 2102–2107.

37 Bibbins-Domingo K, Gupta R, Na B, Wu AH, Schiller NB, Whooley MA. N-terminal fragment of the prohormone brain-type natriuretic peptide (NT-proBNP), cardiovascular events, and mortality in patients with stable coronary heart disease. *JAMA* 2007; **297**: 169–176.

38 Omland T, Sabatine MS, Jablonski KA et al. Prognostic value of B-type natriuretic peptides in patients with stable coronary artery disease: the PEACE trial. *J Am Coll Cardiol* 2007; **50**: 205–214.

39 Libby P, Ridker PM, Maseri A. Inflammation and atherosclerosis. *Circulation* 2002; **105**: 1135–1143.

40 Armstrong EJ, Morrow DA, Sabatine MS. Inflammatory biomarkers in acute coronary syndromes: part I: introduction and cytokines. *Circulation* 2006; **113**: e72–e75.

41 Willerson JT, Ridker PM. Inflammation as a cardiovascular risk factor. *Circulation* 2004; **109**: II2–10.

42 Myers GL, Rifai N, Tracy RP et al. CDC/AHA workshop on markers of inflammation and cardiovascular disease: application to clinical and public health practice: report from the laboratory science discussion group. *Circulation* 2004; **110**: e545–e549.

43 Verma S, Wang CH, Li SH et al. A self-fulfilling prophecy: C-reactive protein attenuates nitric oxide production and inhibits angiogenesis. *Circulation* 2002; **106**: 913–919.

44 Pasceri V, Willerson JT, Yeh ET. Direct proinflammatory effect of C-reactive protein on human endothelial cells. *Circulation* 2000; **102**: 2165–2168.

45 Calabro P, Willerson JT, Yeh ET. Inflammatory cytokines stimulated C-reactive protein production by human coronary artery smooth muscle cells. *Circulation* 2003; **108**: 1930–1932.

46 Hirschfield GM, Gallimore JR, Kahan MC et al. Transgenic human C-reactive protein is not proatherogenic in apolipoprotein E-deficient mice. *Proc Natl Acad Sci USA* 2005; **102**: 8309–8314.

47 Liuzzo G, Biasucci LM, Gallimore JR et al. The prognostic value of C-reactive protein and serum amyloid a protein in severe unstable angina. *N Engl J Med* 1994; **331**: 417–424.

48 Mueller C, Buettner HJ, Hodgson JM et al. Inflammation and long-term mortality after non-ST elevation acute coronary syndrome treated with a very early invasive strategy in 1042 consecutive patients. *Circulation* 2002; **105**: 1412–1415.

49 Morrow DA, Rifai N, Antman EM et al. C-reactive protein is a potent predictor of mortality independently of and in combination with troponin T in acute coronary syndromes: a TIMI 11A substudy. thrombolysis in myocardial infarction. *J Am Coll Cardiol* 1998; **31**: 1460–1465.

50 James SK, Armstrong P, Barnathan E et al. Troponin and C-reactive protein have different relations to subsequent mortality and myocardial infarction after acute coronary syndrome: a GUSTO-IV substudy. *J Am Coll Cardiol* 2003; **41**: 916–924.

51 Heeschen C, Hamm CW, Bruemmer J, Simoons MI. Predictive value of C-reactive protein and troponin T in patients with unstable angina: a comparative analysis. CAP-TURE Investigators. Chimeric c7E3 AntiPlatelet Therapy in Unstable angina REfractory to standard treatment trial. *J Am Coll Cardiol* 2000; **35**: 1535–1542.

52 Ferreiros ER, Boissonnet CP, Pizarro R et al. Independent prognostic value of elevated C-reactive protein in unstable angina. *Circulation* 1999; **100**: 1958–1963.

53 Biasucci LM, Liuzzo G, Grillo RL et al. Elevated levels of C-reactive protein at discharge in patients with unstable angina predict recurrent instability. *Circulation* 1999; **99**: 855–860.

54 Lindahl B, Toss H, Siegbahn A, Venge P, Wallentin L. Markers of myocardial damage and inflammation in relation to long-term mortality in unstable coronary artery disease. FRISC Study Group. Fragmin during Instability in Coronary Artery Disease. *N Engl J Med* 2000; **343**: 1139–1147.

55 Liuzzo G, Biasucci LM, Rebuzzi AG et al. Plasma protein acute-phase response in unstable angina is not induced by ischemic injury. *Circulation* 1996; **94**: 2373–2380.

56 Ridker PM, Cushman M, Stampfer MJ, Tracy RP, Hennekens CH. Inflammation, aspirin, and the risk of cardiovascular disease in apparently healthy men. *N Engl J Med* 1997; **336**: 973–979.

57 Ridker PM, Hennekens CH, Buring JE, Rifai N. C-reactive protein and other markers of inflammation in the prediction of cardiovascular disease in women. *N Engl J Med* 2000; **342**: 836–843.

58 Koenig W, Sund M, Frohlich M et al. C-reactive protein, a sensitive marker of inflammation, predicts future risk of coronary heart disease in initially healthy middle-aged men: results from the MONICA (Monitoring Trends and Determinants in Cardiovascular Disease) Augsburg Cohort Study, 1984 to 1992. *Circulation* 1999; **99**: 237–242.

59 Sabatine MS, Morrow DA, Jablonski KA et al. Prognostic significance of the Centers for Disease Control/American Heart Association high-sensitivity C-reactive protein cut points for cardiovascular and other outcomes in patients with stable coronary artery disease. *Circulation* 2007; **115**: 1528–1536.

60 Buffon A, Liuzzo G, Biasucci LM et al. Preprocedural serum levels of C-reactive protein predict early complications and late restenosis after coronary angioplasty. *J Am Coll Cardiol* 1999; **34**: 1512–1521.

61 Chew DP, Bhatt DL, Robbins MA et al. Incremental prognostic value of elevated baseline C-reactive protein among established markers of risk in percutaneous coronary intervention. *Circulation* 2001; **104**: 992–997.

62 Bholasingh R, Cornel JH, Kamp O et al. The prognostic value of markers of inflammation in patients with troponin T-negative chest pain before discharge from the emergency department. *Am J Med* 2003; **115**: 521–528.

63 Sukhija R, Fahdi I, Garza L et al. Inflammatory markers, angiographic severity of coronary artery disease, and patient outcome. *Am J Cardiol* 2007; **99**: 879–884.

64 Balk EM, Lau J, Goudas LC et al. Effects of statins on nonlipid serum markers associated with cardiovascular disease: a systematic review. *Ann Intern Med* 2003; **139**: 670–682.

65 Ridker PM, Rifai N, Clearfield M et al. Measurement of C-reactive protein for the targeting of statin therapy in the primary prevention of acute coronary events. *N Engl J Med* 2001; **344**: 1959–1965.

66 Ridker PM, Cannon CP, Morrow D et al. C-reactive protein levels and outcomes after statin therapy. *N Engl J Med* 2005; **352**: 20–28.

67 Nissen SE, Tuzcu EM, Schoenhagen P et al. Statin therapy, LDL cholesterol, C-reactive protein, and coronary artery disease. *N Engl J Med* 2005; **352**: 29–38.

68 Feldman M, Jialal I, Devaraj S, Cryer B. Effects of low-dose aspirin on serum C-reactive protein and thromboxane B2 concentrations: a placebo-controlled study using a highly sensitive C-reactive protein assay. *J Am Coll Cardiol* 2001; **37**: 2036–2041.

69 Blankenberg S, McQueen MJ, Smieja M et al. Comparative impact of multiple biomarkers and N-Terminal pro-brain natriuretic peptide in the context of conventional risk factors for the prediction of recurrent cardiovascular events in the Heart Outcomes Prevention Evaluation (HOPE) Study. *Circulation* 2006; **114**: 201–208.

Chapter 5

Novel markers in patients with suspected acute coronary syndromes

Renato D. Lópes, Mark Chan, and L. Kristin Newby

Introduction

The acute coronary syndromes (ACS) comprise a continuum of biological events progressing from plaque instability to plaque rupture, coronary thrombosis, reduced coronary blood flow, myocardial ischemia, and, ultimately, myocardial necrosis [1,2]. Because the majority of these biological events are clinically unrecognizable and biochemically undetectable until the late stages of myocardial necrosis [3], there is a critical need to define biomarkers that provide information early in the continuum. If successful, such biomarkers will allow appropriate therapies to be instituted in a more timely fashion before the onset of irreversible myocardial damage, ultimately improving patient outcomes. In addition, if sufficiently sensitive, these markers should help to exclude ACS as a cause of chest pain and thereby decrease unnecessary admissions to the hospital.

Presently, troponin I or T, used alone or in combination with creatine kinase MB (CK-MB) or myoglobin, are the only markers accepted as part of the standard evaluation for ACS [4]. Unfortunately, these biomarkers are elevated only after irreversible myocardial damage has occurred. Biomarkers that provide real-time assessment of the early inflammatory, ischemic, and thrombotic processes occurring at the molecular and cellular level are preferable. In this context, three new biomarkers have shown potential for development as bedside tests of global atherosclerotic plaque vulnerability and atherothrombosis: myeloperoxidase (MPO), ischemia modified albumin (IMA), and growth differentiation factor-15 (GDF-15). In this chapter we review the available information supporting their potential role in identification of patients prior to or in the early stages of acute coronary events.

Biomarkers in Heart Disease, 1st edition. Edited by James A. de Lemos.
© 2008 American Heart Association, ISBN: 978-1-4051-7571-5

Myeloperoxidase (MPO)

Inflammation plays a principal role in atherosclerosis and atherothrombosis [5]. An ACS occurs when an atherosclerotic plaque ruptures, leading to thrombus formation and total or partial occlusion of an epicardial coronary artery. The leukocyte is intimately involved in this process, and the role of leukocyte-derived enzymes has been investigated recently [6]. Studies suggest numerous mechanisms through which leukocytes affect plaque stability in ACS. Evidence of leukocyte activation and degranulation has been found in patients with unstable angina [7,8], while extensive monocyte and neutrophil infiltration has been noted in fissured and thrombotic plaques in patients with ACS [9].

MPO is an enzyme that promotes the formation of potent oxidative products, and is released by activated neutrophils and monocytes [10]. Circulating MPO levels are elevated in individuals with angiographically documented coronary artery disease [11], and MPO is frequently found in infarcted myocardium [12]. MPO synthesis occurs during myeloid differentiation in bone marrow and is completed within granulocytes prior to their entry into the circulation [10,13]. The enzyme is stored within the primary granules of neutrophils and monocytes, and is not released until leukocyte activation and degranulation. MPO forms free radicals and diffusible oxidants with antimicrobial activity. However, MPO also promotes oxidative damage of host tissues at sites of inflammation, including atherosclerotic lesions. Immunohistochemical studies have demonstrated the presence of MPO in atheromatous plaque [14], and mass spectrometry studies have shown that oxidative products generated by MPO are enriched in human atheroma and in low-density lipoprotein (LDL) recovered from diseased arterial tissue [11].

MPO has been further implicated as an enzymatic catalyst of LDL oxidation in vivo, converting the lipoprotein into a high-uptake form for macrophages, leading to cholesterol deposition and foam cell formation [15]. The activation of leukocytes prompts the secretion of MPO and the generation of oxidants important in host defense [16]. MPO has been linked to the development of lipid-laden soft plaque, and the activation of protease cascades affecting the stability and thrombogenicity of plaque [17]. Moreover, hypochlorous acid (HOCl), a primary oxidant generated by MPO, may promote extracellular matrix degradation in vivo. MPO-generated HOCl both activates latent matrix metalloproteinases and inactivates their physiological inhibitors (tissue inhibitor of metalloproteinase 1 [TIMP1], for example), promoting destabilization and rupture of the atherosclerotic plaque surface [11]. Furthermore, MPO catalytically consumes endothelium-derived nitric oxide, reducing nitric oxide bioavailability and leading to vasoconstriction and endothelial dysfunction [18]. Following from this pathophysiology, it stands to reason that MPO would emerge as a useful marker for diagnosis and prognosis in a variety of clinical settings. However, there have been a few clinical studies examining the role of MPO as a marker of risk for ACS.

In a study published in 2003, MPO was shown to have prognostic value among 604 patients presenting with chest pain to the emergency department [17], among whom the final diagnosis was determined to be myocardial infarction (MI) in 23.5%, unstable angina in 17.1%, suspected ACS in 37.6%, and noncardiac chest pain in 21.5%. In this study, plasma MPO levels predicted cardiovascular risk independently of the levels of other markers of inflammation, such as C-reactive protein (CRP). A progressive increase of odds ratio (OR) for major adverse events (death, MI, or need for revascularization) at 30 days and 6 months was associated with each quartile increase in MPO levels. At 6 months the risk (OR [95% CI]) of adverse events associated with increasing quartiles (compared with quartile 1) of MPO were: 1.6 (1.0–2.7); 3.6 (2.2–5.8); and 4.7 (2.9–7.7), respectively. Similar results were observed at 30 days. Importantly, although elevated plasma MPO levels correlated with troponin T levels, MPO remained strongly associated with risk among patients who had persistently normal troponin levels, suggesting that MPO may identify high-risk patients who would not have been detected with standard troponin-based laboratory testing. Moreover, whereas 3–6 hours is required to detect a rise in troponins after ischemic myocardial injury, MPO levels were elevated at baseline among patients who were initially troponin-negative, but subsequently troponin-positive, even when fewer than 3 hours had elapsed since the onset the symptoms.

In this same study, four markers were compared for both the diagnosis of ACS and major adverse events to 30 days: CK-MB, CRP, troponin T, and MPO. The ability of these markers to discriminate between those with and without the outcome was compared using the area under the receiver operating characteristic (ROC) curves. MPO provided similar discrimination to that of the other two highest markers (troponin T and CK-MB). However, in the cohort who were negative for troponin T, MPO had significantly greater discrimination than any of the other markers for both outcomes (Fig. 5.1). These findings suggested that measurement of MPO levels might be useful in triage in the emergency department, and that elevated MPO values might be a marker of unstable angina preceding myocardial necrosis; therefore, a predictor of vulnerable plaque. Whereas elevated MPO levels were a predictor of cardiovascular risk among patients who had negative troponin T, CRP was not.

In a substudy of the CAPTURE (c7E3 Fab Antiplatelet Therapy in Unstable Refractory Angina) trial, MPO plasma levels were measured in 1090 patients with ACS [19]. The combined end-points of death and nonfatal MI were determined at 6-month follow-up. For a cutoff of 350 µg/L for baseline MPO plasma levels, the adjusted hazard ratio (HR) for death or MI among patients with elevated levels compared with those with levels below 350 µg/L was 2.25 (95% CI, 1.32–3.82) as shown in Figure 5.2. Interestingly, MPO plasma levels identified patients at risk who had admission troponin T levels below 0.01 µg/L (adjusted HR 7.48 [95% CI, 1.98–28.29]). Moreover, MPO levels were not correlated with

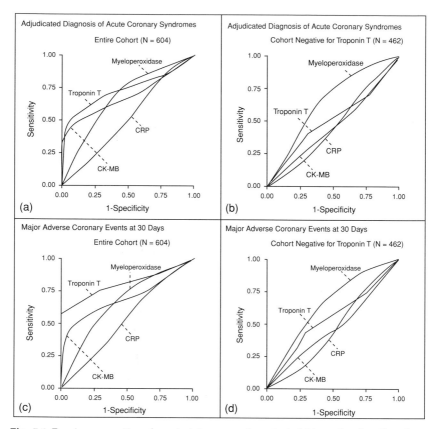

Fig. 5.1 Receiver operating characteristic curves for selected biomarker for all patients (panels a and c) and those with persistently negative troponin T (panels b and d) for the diagnosis of acute coronary syndrome (ACS; panels a and b) and 30-day major adverse cardiac events (MACE; panels c and d). Reproduced with permission from Brennan et al. [17].

troponin T, soluble CD40 ligand, CRP, or ST-segment changes, and in multivariable modeling remained significantly associated with 6-month death or MI in the context of other plasma biomarkers of risk (Table 5.1).

Recently, another study assessed the utility of MPO and N-terminal pro-B-type natriuretic peptide (NT-proBNP) in determining prognosis after acute MI [6]. In this study of 384 patients, there was a weak correlation between MPO and peak troponin T. MPO was elevated very early after acute MI, and levels fell rapidly during the first 24 hours, suggesting that neutrophil activation plays a role very early in acute MI and may even precede the onset of myocardial necrosis. Previous studies of multimarker strategies have used various combinations of markers including inflammatory markers, myocardial necrosis markers, and

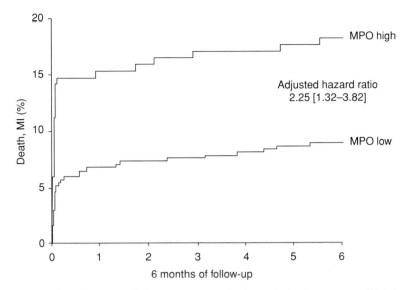

Fig. 5.2 Kaplan-Meier cumulative event curves for 6-month death or myocardial infarction (MI) according to baseline MPO level (diagnostic threshold 350 μg/L). Reproduced with permission from Baldus et al. [19].

markers of left ventricular systolic dysfunction in formulating a risk assessment profile in non–ST-segment elevation MI patients [20]. However, this was the first study to report the utility of MPO in combination with NT-proBNP among patients with ST-segment elevation MI. MPO levels above versus below the

Table 5.1 Multivariable Cox proportional-hazards regression model of multiple biomarkers for prediction of death and nonfatal myocardial infarction during 6 months of follow-up.

Variable	Adjusted Hazard Ratio	95% CI	P
Troponin T > 0.01 μg/L	1.99	1.16 to 3.64	0.023
C-reactive protein tertiles	1.25	1.02 to 1.68	0.044
Vascular endothelial growth factor >300 μg/L	1.87	1.03 to 3.51	0.041
sCD40L >5 μg/L	2.78	1.57 to 4.91	<0.001
MPO > 350 μg/L	2.11	1.21 to 3.67	0.008

Adapted with permission from Baldus et al. [19].

median were associated with higher rates of death or nonfatal MI (p = 0.0004) and also provided incremental prognostic information when combined in a multimarker approach with NT-proBNP (HR [hazard ratio] 6.91, 95% CI: 1.79–26.73 for MPO, and HR 4.21, 95% CI: 1.53–11.58 for NT-proBNP). Similar findings were shown more recently in a study that involved 512 patients with acute MI and 156 control subjects over a 5-year follow-up period for mortality [21]. In this study, MPO levels above the median (55 ng/mL) were independently predictive of mortality (OR 1.8, 95% CI: 1.0–3.0, p = 0.034). Moreover, patients with elevated MPO levels in combination with elevated NT-proBNP or low left ventricular ejection fraction had significantly higher long-term mortality.

Although MPO is an enzyme with an important pathophysiological role in ACS, neutrophil activation is apparently not induced by ischemia [22]; thus, MPO is more a marker of plaque instability than a marker of oxidative stress and myocardial damage [23]. The low specificity of elevated MPO levels (activation of neutrophils and macrophages can occur in any infectious, inflammatory, or infiltrative disease process) [23] for ACS mandates that it be interpreted in the context of associated clinical findings and other laboratory data.

Although a Food and Drug Administration (FDA)-approved assay is available for this promising biomarker, before it is ready for introduction into widespread clinical use additional studies of MPO alone and/or in combination with other biomarkers of cardiac events or subsequent risk will be needed to determine the appropriate role of this biomarker in clinical practice. As a first step, prospective large-scale studies of the relationship of MPO with clinical outcomes in general chest pain populations would provide reassurance of its diagnostic and prognostic utility and help to refine population-useful reference limits. Ultimately, the greatest value of a biomarker is its ability to guide patient management decisions. Therefore, ideally, the final step in its clinical development would include randomized trials designed to assess the incremental utility of incorporating MPO into routine testing strategies used to guide triage and treatment decisions.

Ischemia modified albumin (IMA)

Human serum albumin is a high-abundance protein with an N-terminus that binds free metals such as cobalt. During ischemic events, free radicals are released, resulting in acetylation of the N-terminus and alteration of the cobalt-binding site. Ischemia-modified albumin (IMA) has a reduced ability to bind cobalt, and the remaining free cobalt can then be detected with special assays [24]. This observation that myocardial ischemia produced a lower metal-binding capacity for cobalt to albumin led to the development of the now FDA-approved albumin cobalt binding (ACB) test [25]. The ACB test quantitatively measures IMA in human serum; cobalt added to serum does not bind to the amino terminus of IMA, leaving more free cobalt to react with dithiothreitol and form a darker color in samples from patients with ischemia [23]. The range of reference values in healthy individuals is from 52 to 116 kilounits/L [26].

IMA becomes rapidly positive (within a few minutes) after the onset of ischemia as demonstrated in a human angioplasty model of transient myocardial ischemia [27]. In this study, the investigators compared the concentration-time profiles of 2 markers of ischemia, IMA, and 8-iso prostaglandin F2-A, in 19 patients experiencing chest pain and/or ischemic electrocardiographic (ECG) changes after balloon inflation during elective percutaneous coronary intervention. Eleven patients undergoing diagnostic angiography served only as the control group. Both IMA and prostaglandin F2-A increased from baseline after balloon inflation in the group undergoing coronary intervention, but IMA levels were increased at much earlier time points compared with prostaglandin F2-A. Rapid hepatic clearance (6 hours) [28] allows further temporal specificity of IMA for acute ischemic events, with IMA levels returning to baseline at approximately 12 hours after resolution of ischemia [27]. In contrast, in an exercise model of ischemia, among 40 consecutive patients with coronary artery disease who underwent exercise stress testing, there was no difference in IMA levels relative to key time points in testing between groups with positive (n = 25) and negative (n = 14) stress tests [29]. Levels were decreased from baseline at peak stress in both positive and negative groups, and at 60-minutes poststress, levels were increased in both groups relative to peak stress levels. This response to exercise may suggest that IMA measures more than just coronary ischemia per se.

Several clinical studies have evaluated the performance of the ACB assay in detecting acute ischemia in a clinical setting, three of which warrant description in some detail. Christenson and colleagues conducted a case-control study of 224 patients enrolled within 3 hours after onset of symptoms of possible coronary ischemia to examine the ability of ACB to predict a subsequent increase in troponin I among patients with negative troponin I at baseline [30]. The sensitivity and specificity of ACB in predicting the troponin response were 70% and 80%, respectively, with a negative predictive value of 96%. Notably, the study yielded a very low positive predictive value of only 33% for the ACB test in predicting troponin results. An important shortcoming in this study was that troponin I alone was used as the outcome measure; ECG status at presentation was not considered.

Sinha and colleagues evaluated the utility of IMA for diagnosing cardiac ischemia in patients who presented to the emergency department with symptoms suggestive of ACS [31]. The study combined IMA (using a cutoff of >85 kilounits/L) with ECG results and troponin T concentrations in 208 patients presenting within 3 hours of acute chest pain. Baseline blood samples were taken for IMA and troponin T measurements, which were then correlated with the final diagnosis of ischemia based on the history, clinical examination, serial troponin T results, and data from medical records. In the overall study population, sensitivity of IMA for an ischemic cause of chest pain was 82%, specificity was 46%, the negative predictive value was 59%, and the positive predictive value was 72%. Despite these rather modest diagnostic indices for IMA alone, the combination of IMA, ECG, and troponin T identified 95% of patients whose chest pain was subsequently attributed to cardiac ischemia.

The ACB test performed better in a study by Bhagavan and colleagues, in which ACB results were correlated with final discharge diagnoses in 75 emergency department patients with myocardial ischemia, and 92 controls without ischemia [32]. The sensitivity and specificity for myocardial ischemia were 88% and 94%, respectively, and the positive and negative predictive values were 92% and 91%. However, the ACB test was not able to discriminate between ischemic patients with and without MI.

The same general principle applies to IMA and other serum biomarkers with a high negative predictive value, that their greatest value lies in "ruling out" or excluding ACS. In order to maximize their diagnostic potential, such biomarkers must be interpreted in the context of other clinical and biochemical data. In a meta-analysis of IMA used in the risk stratification patients presenting to the emergency department with suspected ACS (n = 1800), Peacock and colleagues demonstrated the clinical utility of a negative triple prediction test, defined as a nondiagnostic ECG, negative troponin, and negative IMA (Figs. 5.3 and 5.4) [33–36]. The triple prediction test sensitivity and NPV for acute coronary syndromes

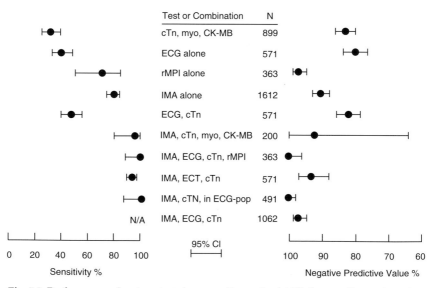

Fig. 5.3 Performance of various tests for acute diagnosis of ACS alone and in combination. cTn: Cardiac troponin; myo: myoglobin; rMPI, rest MPI. With permission from Peacock et al. [33].

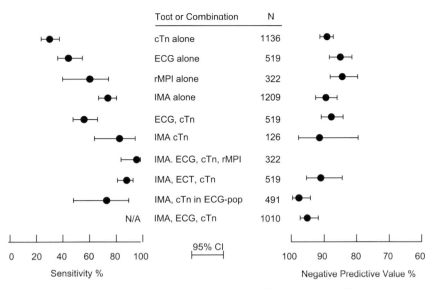

Fig. 5.4 Performance of various tests alone and in combination for predicting post-acute presentation events. With permission from Peacock et al. [33].

were 94.4% and 97.1%, respectively, and for longer-term outcomes, were 89.2% and 94.5%, respectively.

The positive predictive value of the ACB assay seems too low for "ruling in" ischemia. At present, whether patients with a negative ECG and troponin, but a positive IMA result might benefit from early treatment according to stratified pretest probabilities is unknown [23]. There is still a need for reference distributions by gender and ethnicity and an optimum diagnostic cut-off value for ACS patients. How IMA concentrations vary in common disease states with or without accompanying cardiac disease is yet unknown, but is important because IMA is known to be elevated in other conditions unrelated to cardiac ischemia (false positives) such as cancer, acute infections, cirrhosis, and end-stage renal disease [26,37]. Furthermore, the implications of an elevated IMA in the presence of common conditions that coexist with cardiac ischemia, such as congestive heart failure, diabetes mellitus, chronic renal failure, and hypertension, are still unknown. There are presently no published data on how these comorbid illnesses modify the IMA response, making it difficult to recommend appropriate cut-off values in these patients. Finally, IMA levels can be suppressed in the presence of elevated lactate levels, as seen in an experiment in which IMA levels were measured in a human model of forearm ischemia [38]. The same study also reported replication of the results in vitro when IMA was measured in the presence of blood spiked with exogenous lactate. Thus, the significance of a negative IMA result in patients with poorly controlled diabetes, sepsis, and/or renal failure is in question as all of these are situations in which increased lactate may exist (false negatives). Finally, the ACB test results should be interpreted with caution when serum albumin concentrations are <20 g/L or >55 g/L or in the presence of increased ammonia concentrations [23].

In summary, the greatest expected benefit of the ACB test is to rule out ACS in low to moderate pretest probability conditions with negative troponin and a negative ECG. The test seems to have limited specificity with a high false-positive rate. At present the assay is approved for use in combination with the ECG and troponin result to "rule-out" a suspected ACS, but not as a stand-alone test. However, an ongoing study (IMAGINE) is examining the relationship between an elevated IMA result and subsequent clinical outcomes, and may provide new insights into its independent prognostic value.

Growth differentiation factor-15 (GDF-15)

Macrophages play a key secretory role in the immune and inflammatory response, and participate in many normal biological processes, including wound healing and the elimination of tumors and infections. These cells are also important mediators of a range of chronic inflammatory and fibrotic diseases such as atherosclerosis and pulmonary fibrosis [39].

One of the first macrophage-secreted cytokines identified was macrophage-inhibitory cytokine-1 (MIC-1), which is a divergent member of the transforming grown factor-B (TGF-B) cytokine superfamily [40]. The TGF-B superfamily consists of several dimeric proteins having a conserved cysteine knot structure. These cytokines are involved in embryogenesis, regulation of growth and inflammation, and wound and fracture healing. This superfamily contains proteins such as TGF-B, bone morphogenetic proteins, inhibins, and glial-derived neurotrophic factors. TGF-B also constitutes a superfamily of cytokines that exert prominent functions in adult tissue homeostasis and adaptation by regulating cell survival, proliferation, and differentiation. Increases or decreases in the production of TGF-B have been linked to a number of disease states, including neurodegenerative disorders and atherosclerosis [41].

GDF-15 has been described in the literature as MIC-1 [39], placental bone morphogenetic protein (PLAB) [42], placental transforming grown factor-B (PTGF-B) [43], prostate-derived factor (PDF) [44], and nonsteroidal anti-inflammatory drug-activated gene-1 (NAG-1) [45], reflecting the different functions that have been implied for this protein [46]. However, biological functions of this protein are still uncertain. So, GDF-15 is considered a distant member of the TGF-B superfamily that is produced as a 40 kD pro-peptide monomer, which is processed to a mature 30 kD secreted peptide. Cell culture experiments suggest that GDF-15 can act as a neuronal survival factor and conversely can promote cell death in a number of tumor cell lines [39].

In a study by Kempf and colleagues, GDF-15 was strongly induced in the myocardium after ischemic injury, and was believed to provide endogenous protection against ischemia-reperfusion-induced cardiomyocyte apoptosis, possibly via PI3K-Akt-dependent signaling pathways [47], potentially promoting anti-apoptotic effects in cardiomyocytes. Together with the report of Xu et al. [48], this study showed that GDF-15 had a functional role in the cardiovascular system, and was the first study that assigned an in vivo function to GDF-15. This study showed that GDF-15 levels correlated with simulated ischemia and reperfusion, and it was observed in this mouse model of cardiac ischemia and reperfusion injury that GDF-15 expression levels rapidly increased in the ischemic area after coronary ligation. Expression remained elevated in the myocardium for several days after reperfusion. Additionally, studies in mice have shown that GDF-15 expression levels increase to a similar extent in the ischemic myocardium after transient coronary ligation (limited damage) or permanent coronary ligation (extensive necrosis), and that GDF-15 levels remain elevated in the heart for at least 1 week after the ischemic insult [47]. In cultured cardiomyocytes, GDF-15 expression is also strongly upregulated by several stressors such as nitric oxide, nitrosative stress, and inflammatory cytokines, all of which are putative signaling mediators in the ischemic and reperfused heart.

Atherosclerotic lesions progress through various stages, from a simple structure of the fatty streak, with accumulation of modified lipids, to the stable or sometimes unstable plaques of advanced atherosclerosis [49]. Evolution of these lesions revolves around a complex interplay among vascular endothelium, vascular smooth muscle, and the immune system, in which macrophage activation is determinant. This activation has been shown to lead to increased production of GDF-15 [40]. Although resting macrophages produce little GDF-15, macrophages within atherosclerotic lesions synthesize GDF-15. Based on that pathophysiology, it was hypothesized that GDF-15 may reflect macrophage activation and plaque evolution and be associated with cardiovascular events.

In 2002, data from a nested case-control study within the Women's Health Study showed that GDF-15 levels were associated with cardiovascular clinical outcomes, including stroke and acute MI [40]. In this study, median GDF-15 concentrations were higher at baseline among 257 women who developed cardiovascular events (cardiovascular death, MI, or thromboembolic stroke) than among 257 controls matched for age and smoking status who did not have these events (618 pg/mL vs. 538 pg/mL, p = 0.0002). GDF-15 concentrations above the 90th percentile (>856 pg/mL) were associated with an almost 3-fold higher adjusted risk compared for cardiovascular events compared with lower concentrations (OR: 2.7, 95% CI 1.6–4.9, p = 0.0001), and among participants with concentrations of both GDF-15 and CRP above the study median the OR for death, MI, or stroke of 4.32 (95% CI 2.0–9.1, p = 0.001). This risk estimate was greater than that associated with increases of either GDF-15 or CRP alone

Table 5.2 Odds ratio of developing cardiovascular events according to baseline concentrations of macrophage-inhibitory cytokine (MIC)-1 (a.k.a. GDF-15) and C-reactive protein (CRP).

MIC-1	CRP	Odd ratio (95% CI)	p
–	–	1.00 (reference)	…
+	–	1.30 (0.56–3.11)	0.5
–	+	2.32 (1.04–5.33)	0.04
+	+	4.32 (2.05–9.09)	0.001

+ = about study median; – = below study median.
Adapted from Brown et al. with permission [40].

(Table 5.2). These findings suggest that GDF-15 could be a novel target for cardiovascular disease risk stratification, and also could be an important factor in plaque evolution.

Recently, clinical studies in humans have shown that GDF-15 may provide prognostic information among patients with non–ST-segment elevation ACS. In a study that included 2081 patients from Global Utilization of Strategies to Open Occluded Arteries (GUSTO-IV) ACS trial, circulating GDF-15 levels were elevated above the upper limit of normal in two-thirds of patients. Increasing tertiles of GDF-15 were associated with a lower probability of 1-year survival (Fig. 5.5), and in a multivariable model that accounted for clinical factors that were significantly associated with GDF-15 levels and other biomarkers, including troponin T, NT-proBNP, creatinine clearance, and CRP, the HR for 1-year mortality per 1 standard deviation increase in GDF-15 was 1.49, CI 95% 1.21–1.85, p < 0.001 [50]. There was no incremental predictive utility for MI. ROC analyses showed that the best discriminatory level of this biomarker for predicting 1-year mortality was 1808 ng/L (AUC = 0.757; sensitivity, 68.5%; specificity, 68.8%). GDF-15 (AUC = 0.757), NT-proBNP (AUC = 0.735), and creatinine clearance (AUC = 0.728) were each superior to troponin T (AUC = 0.620) and CRP (AUC = 0.629) in discriminating risk for 1-year mortality (Fig. 5.6).

The levels of GDF-15 remained stable within each patient during serial testing over 72 hours, suggesting that a single measurement of GDF-15, obtained at any time point during the first 24 hours, and possibly even out to 72 hours after admission, could provide important prognostic information in patients with NSTE-ACS.

Eggers and colleagues [51] assessed the use of GDF-15 for risk stratification among 416 patients who were admitted to a coronary care unit with acute chest pain and no ST-segment elevation. They observed that higher GDF-15 levels were associated with increased risk of 6-month death or MI. Although

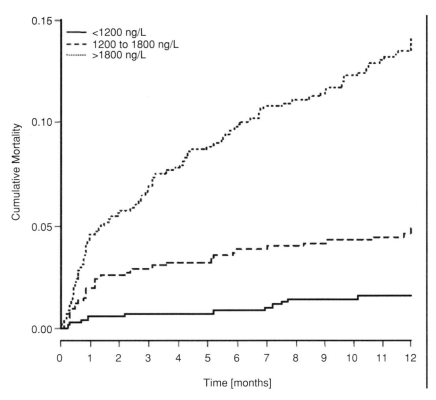

Fig. 5.5 Cumulative probability of death during 1 year according to tertiles of GDF-15 levels on admission in 2081 patients with NSTE-ACS enrolled in the GUSTO-IV trial (p < 0.001). Reproduced with permission from Wollert et al. [50].

this study had only 10 deaths and 19 MIs, the findings were consistent with the GUSTO-IV substudy observations.

GDF-15 is a novel biomarker that provides prognostic information beyond traditional clinical and biochemical markers among patients with NSTEACS. However, at present, there is no commercially available assay for clinical use, which would require completion of a number of remaining requisite steps in development of this novel biomarker (Fig. 5.7) [52].

Conclusion

Making an accurate diagnosis of ACS remains a major challenge to health care workers involved in the triage and care of patients suspected of having an ACS. Early diagnosis and treatment of myocardial ischemia should lead to improved triage and efficiency of patient care, the ability to target therapeutic options to

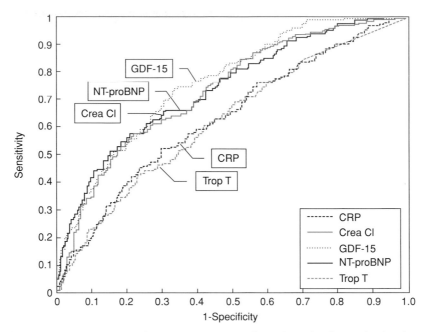

Fig. 5.6 Receiver operating characteristic curve analyses that relate biomarker levels to 1-year mortality risk in 2081 patients with NSTE-ACS enrolled in the GUSTO-IV trial. Crea Cl indicates creatinine clearance; Trop T, troponin T. Reproduced with permission from Wollert et al. [50].

Phases:	Phase 1 Preclinical Exploratory	Phase 2 Clinical Characterization & Assay Validation	Phase 3 Clinical Association: Retrospective Repository studies	Phase 4 Clinical Association: Prospective Screening studies	Phase 5 Disease control
Objective	Target Biomarker Identification, Feasibility	Study assay in people with & without disease	Case-control studies using repository specimens	Longitudinal studies to predict disease	Clinical use
Site	Biomarker Development Lab	Biomarker Validation Lab	Clinical Epidemiologic Centers	Cohort Studies	Community
Design	Cross-sectional	Cross-sectional	Case-control	Prospective	RCT
Sample Size	Small	Small	Modest	Medium	Large
Validity	Content & construct validity	Criterion validity	Predictive validity	Efficacy of strategy	Effectiveness
Result	Assay precision reliability, sensitivity	Reference limits, intra-individual variation	Screening characteristics, true & false+ rates	ROC analyses	No.-needed-to screen/treat

Fig. 5.7 Five phases of biomarker development: from discovery to delivery. Content validity refers to the degree to which the biomarker represents the biological phenomenon studied; construct validity refers to establishing that the biomarker is measuring the aspect of disease that we want to measure; and criterion validity refers to how well the biomarker identifies disease state when compared with a gold standard. Reproduced from Vasan [52].

those at greatest likelihood of benefit, and ultimately to better patient outcomes. Traditional biomarkers of diagnosis and risk are frequently not helpful early after presentation or provide an incomplete description of risk. Novel biomarkers such as MPO, IMA, and GDF-15 offer promise as adjuncts to conventional biomarker testing for diagnosis, risk stratification, and/or prognosis. Consideration of GDF-15 in clinical practice awaits additional data in larger populations as well as development of clinically useful and available assays that are FDA approved. Although MPO and IMA are now available commercially, at best, these novel tests must be interpreted together with other parts of the larger diagnostic landscape, which includes clinical findings, ECG changes, and troponin results. Importantly, both tests have limitations as outlined earlier, and neither is ready for widespread clinical application until additional prospective studies are completed to define their utility in refining diagnosis, defining prognosis, and most importantly providing incremental utility for clinical decision making in broad general clinical practice populations.

References

1 Fuster V, Badimon L, Badimon JJ et al. The pathogenesis of coronary artery disease and the acute coronary syndromes. *N Engl J Med* 1992; **326**: 242–250.

2 Fuster V, Badimon L, Badimon JJ et al. The pathogenesis of coronary artery disease and the acute coronary syndromes. *N Engl J Med* 1992; **326**: 310–318.

3 Lippi G, Montagnana M, Salvagno GL, Guidi GC. Potential value for new diagnostic markers in the early recognition of acute coronary syndromes. *CJEM* 2006; **8**: 27–31.

4 Morrow DA, Cannon CP, Jesse RL, Newby LK, Ravkilde J, Storrow AB, Wu AH, Christenson RH; National Academy of Clinical Biochemistry. National Academy of Clinical Biochemistry Laboratory Medicine Practice Guidelines: Clinical characteristics and utilization of biochemical markers in acute coronary syndromes. *Circulation* 2007; **115**: e356–375.

5 Ross R. Atherosclerosis—an inflammatory disease. *N Engl J Med* 1999; **340**: 115–126.

6 Khan SQ, Kelly D, Quinn P, Davies JE, Ng LL. Myeloperoxidase aids prognostication together with NT-BNP in high-risk patients with acute ST elevation myocardial infarction. *Heart* 2007; **93**: 826-831.

7 De Servi S, Mazzone A, Ricevute G et al. Expression of neutrophil and monocyte CD11B/CD18 adhesion molecules at different sites of the coronary tree in unstable angina pectoris. *Am J Cardiol* 1996; **78**: 564–568.

8 Buffon A, Biasucci LM, Liuzzo G, D'Onofrio G, Crea F, Maseri A. Widespread coronary inflammation in unstable angina. *N Engl J Med* 2002; **347**: 5–12.

9 Naruko T, Ueda M, Haze K, van der Wal AC, van der Loos CM, Itoh A, Komatsu R, Ikura Y, Ogami M, Shimada Y, Ehara S, Yoshiyama M, Takeuchi K, Yoshikawa J, Becker AE. Neutrophil infiltration of culprit lesions in acute coronary syndromes. *Circulation* 2002; **106**: 2894–2900.

10 Malech HL, Naussef WM. Primary inherited defects in neutrophil function: etiology and treatment. *Semin Hematol* 1997; **34**: 279–290.

11 Zhang R, Brennan ML, Fu X, Aviles RJ, Pearce GL, Penn MS, Topol EJ, Sprecher DL, Hazen SL. Association between myeloperoxidase levels and risk of coronary artery disease. *JAMA* 2001; **286**: 2136–2142.

12 Vasilyev N, Williams T, Brennan ML, Unzek S, Zhou X, Heinecke JW, Spitz DR, Topol EJ, Hazen SL, Penn MS. Myeloperoxidase-generated oxidants modulate left ventricular remodeling but not infarct size after myocardial infarction. *Circulation* 2005; **112**: 2812–2820.

13 Nauseef WM. Myeloperoxidase deficiency. *Hematol Oncol Clin North Am* 1988; **2**: 135–158.

14 Daugherty A, Dunn JL, Rateri DL, Heinecke JW. Myeloperoxidase, a catalyst for lipoprotein oxidation, is expressed in human atherosclerotic lesions. *J Clin Invest* 1994; **94**: 437–444.

15 Blake GJ, Ridker PM. C-reactive protein and other inflammatory risk markers in acute coronary syndromes. *J Am Coll Cardiol* 2003; **41**: 37S–42S.

16 Klebanoff SJ, Watersdorph AM, Rosen H. Antimicrobial activity of myeloperoxidase. *Methods Enzymol* 1984; **105**: 399–403.

17 Brennan ML, Penn MS, Van Lente F, Nambi V, Shishehbor MH, Aviles RJ, Goormastic M, Pepoy ML, McErlean ES, Topol EJ, Nissen SE, Hazen SL. Prognostic value of myeloperoxidase in patients with chest pain. *N Engl J Med* 2003; **349**: 1595–1604.

18 Vita JA, Brennan ML, Gokce N, Mann SA, Goormastic M, Shishehbor MH, Penn MS, Keaney JF, Jr., Hazen SL. Serum myeloperoxidase levels independently predict endothelial dysfunction in humans. *Circulation* 2004; **110**: 1134–1139.

19 Baldus S, Heeschen C, Meinertz T, Zeiher AM, Eiserich JP, Munzel T, Simoons ML, Hamm CW; CAPTURE Investigators. Myeloperoxidase serum levels predict risk in patients with acute coronary syndromes. *Circulation* 2003; **108**: 1440–1445.

20 Sabatine MS, Morrow DA, de Lemos JA, Gibson CM, Murphy SA, Rifai N, McCabe, Antman EM, Cannon CP, Braunwald E. Multimarker approach to risk stratification in non-ST elevation acute coronary syndromes: simultaneous assessment of troponin I, C-reactive protein, and B-type natriuretic peptide. *Circulation* 2002; **105**: 1760–1763.

21 Mocatta TJ, Pilbrow AP, Cameron VA, Senthilmohan R, Frampton CM, Richards AM, Winterbourn CC. Plasma concentrations of myeloperoxidase predict mortality after myocardial infarction. *J Am Coll Cardiol* 2007; **49**: 1993–2000.

22 Biasucci LM, D'Onofrio G, Liuzzo G, Zini G, Monaco C, Caligiuri G, Tommasi M, Rebuzzi AG, Maseri A. Intracellular neutrophil myeloperoxidase is reduced in unstable angina and acute myocardial infarction, but its reduction is not related to ischemia. *J Am Coll Cardiol* 1996; **27**: 611–616.

23 Apple FS, Wu AH, Mair J, Ravkilde J, Panteghini M, Tate J, Pagani F, Christenson RH, Mockel M, Danne O, Jaffe AS; Committee on Standardization of Markers of Cardiac Damage of the IFCC. Future biomarkers for detection of ischemia and risk stratification in acute coronary syndrome. *Clin Chem* 2005; **51**: 810–824.

24 Bar-Or D, Lau E, Winkler JV. Novel assay for cobalt-albumin binding and its potential as a marker for myocardial ischemia—a preliminary report. *J Emerg Med* 2000; **19**: 311–315.

25 Bar-Or D, Curtis G, Rao N, Bampos N, Lau E. Characterization of the Co_2 and Ni_2 binding amino-acid residues of the N-terminus of human albumin. *Eur J Biochem* 2001; **268**: 42–47.

26 Wu AHB. The ischemia-modified albumin biomarker for myocardial ischemia. *MLO Med Lab Obs* 2003; **6**: 36–40.

27 Sinha MK, Gaze DC, Tippins JR, Collinson PO, Kaski JC. Ischemia modified albumin is a sensitive marker of myocardial ischemia after percutaneous coronary intervention. *Circulation* 2003; **107**: 2403–2405.

28 Kontos MC, Schorer S, Kirk JD. Ischemia modified albumin, a new biomarker of myocardial ischemia, for the emergency diagnosis of acute coronary syndrome. *J Am Coll Cardiol* 2003; **41**: 340A.

29 Sbarouni E, Georgiadou P, Theodorakis GN, Kremastinos DT. Ischemia-modified albumin in relation to exercise stress testing. *JACC* 2006; **48**: 2482–2484.

30 Christenson RH, Duh SH, Sanhai WR, Wu AHB, Holtman V, Painter P et al. Characteristics of an albumin cobalt binding test for assessment of acute coronary syndrome patients: a multicentric study. *Clin Chem* 2001; **47**: 464–470.

31 Sinha MK, Roy D, Gaze DC, Collinson PO, Kaski J-C. Role of ischemia modified albumin a new biochemical marker of myocardial ischemia, in the early diagnosis of acute coronary syndromes. *Emerg Med J* 2004; **21**: 29–34.

32 Bhagavan NV, Lai EM, Rios PA, Yang J, Ortega-Lopez AM, Shinoda H et al. Evaluation of human serum albumin cobalt binding assay for the assessment of myocardial ischemia and myocardial infarction. *Clin Chem* 2003; **49**: 581–585.

33 Peacock F, Morris DL, Anwaruddin S, Christenson RH, Collinson PO, Goodacre SW, Januzzi JL, Jesse RL, Kaski JC, Kontos MC, Lefevre G, Mutrie D, Sinha MK, Uettwiller-Geiger D, Pollack CV. Meta-analysis of ischemia-modified albumin to rule out acute coronary syndromes in the emergency department. *Am Heart J* 2006; **152**: 253–262.

34 Goodacre SW, Morris FM, Campbell S et al. A prospective, observational study of a chest pain observation unit in a British hospital. *Emerg Med J* 2002; **19**: 117–121.

35 Lefevre G, Lefranc A, Garbarz E et al. Prognostic indications of a novel biological marker of cardiac ischemia in patients presenting with chest pain in an emergency setting. *J Am Coll Cardiol* 2004; **43**: 244A.

36 Anwaruddin S, Januzzi Jr JL, Baggish AL et al. Ischemia-modified albumin improves the usefulness of standard cardiac biomarkers for the diagnosis of myocardial ischemia in the emergency department setting. *Am J Clin Pathol* 2005; **123**: 140–145.

37 Aslan D, Apple FS. Ischemia modified albumin: clinical and analytical update. *Lab Med* 2004; **35**: 1–5.

38 Zapico-Muniz E, Santalo-Bel M, Merce'-Muntanola J, Montiel JA, Martinez-Rubio A, Ordonez-Llanos J. Ischemia-modified albumin during skeletal muscle ischemia. *Clin Chem* 2004; **50**: 1063–1065.

39 Bootcov MR, Bauskin AR, Valenzuela SM, Moore AG, Bansal M, He XY, Zhang HP, Donnellan M, Mahler S, Pryor K, Walsh BJ, Nicholson RC, Fairlie WD, Por SB, Robbins JM, Brett SN. MIC-1, a novel macrophage inhibitory cytokine, is a divergent member of the TGF-beta superfamily. *Proc Natl Acad Sci U S A* 1997; **94**: 11514–11519.

40 Brown DA, Breit SN, Buring J, Fairlie WD, Bauskin AR, Liu T, Ridker PM. Concentration in plasma of macrophage inhibitory cytokine-1 and risk of cardiovascular events in women: a nested case-control study. *Lancet* 2002; **359**: 2159–2163.

41 Blobe GC, Schiemann WP, Lodish HF. Role of transforming growth factor beta in human disease. *N Engl J Med* 2000; **342**: 1350–1358.

42 Hromas R, Hufford M, Sutton J, Xu D, Li Y, Lu L. PLAB, a novel placental bone morphogenetic protein. *Biochim Biophys Acta* 1997; **1354**: 40–44.

43 Yokoyama-Kobayashi M, Saeki M, Sekine S, Kato S. Human cDNA encoding a novel TGF-beta superfamily protein highly expressed in placenta. *J Biochem (Tokyo)* 1997; **122**: 622–626.

44 Paralkar VM, Vail AL, Grasser WA, Brown TA, Xu H, Vukicevic S, Ke HZ, Qi H, Owen TA, Thompson DD. Cloning and characterization of a novel member of the transforming growth factor-beta/bone morphogenetic protein family. *J Biol Chem* 1998; **273**: 13760–13767.

45 Baek SJ, Horowitz JM, Eling TE. Molecular cloning and characterization of human nonsteroidal anti-inflammatory drug-activated gene promoter. Basal transcription is mediated by Sp1 and Sp3. *J Biol Chem* 2001; **276**: 33384–33392.

46 Noorali S, Kurita T, Woolcock B, de Algara TR, Lo M, Paralkar V, Hoodless P, Vielkind J. Dynamics of expression of growth differentiation factor 15 in normal and PIN development in the mouse. *Differentiation* 2007; **75**: 325–336.

47 Kempf T, Eden M, Strelau J, Naguib M, Willenbockel C, Tongers J, Heineke J, Kotlars D, Xu J, Molkentin JD, Niessen HW, Drexler H, Wollert KC. The transforming growth factor-beta superfamily member growth-differentiation factor-15 protects the heart from ischemia/reperfusion injury. *Circ Res* 2006; **98**: 351–360.

48 Xu J, Kimball TR, Lorenz JN, Brown DA, Bauskin AR, Klevitsky R, Hewett TE, Breit SN, Molkentin JD. GDF15/MIC-1 functions as a protective and antihypertrophic factor released from the myocardium in association with SMAD protein activation. *Circ Res* 2006; **98**: 342–350.

49 Tegos TJ, Kalodiki E, Sabetai MM, Nicolaides AN. The genesis of atherosclerosis and risk factors: a review. *Angiology* 2001; **52**: 89–98.

50 Wollert KC, Kempf T, Peter T, Olofsson S, James S, Johnston N, Lindahl B, Horn-Wichmann R, Brabant G, Simoons ML, Armstrong PW, Califf RM, Drexler H, Wallentin L. Prognostic value of growth-differentiation factor-15 in patients with non–ST-elevation acute coronary syndrome. *Circulation* 2007; **115**: 962–971.

51 Eggers KM, Kempf T, Lindahl B, Wallentin L, Wollert KC. Growth-Differentiation Factor-15 for Early Risk Stratification in Patients with Acute Chest Pain. *J Am Coll Cardiol* 2007; **49**: 200A.

52 Vasan RS. Biomarkers of cardiovascular disease: molecular basis and practical considerations. *Circulation* 2006; **113**: 2335–2362.

PART II

Biomarkers for Evaluation of Patients Heart Failure

Chapter 6

Use of natriuretic peptides in the diagnosis of heart failure

Abelardo Martinez-Rumayor and James L. Januzzi

Biology of the natriuretic peptide system

The first important insights into the physiologic function of natriuretic peptides came in 1981, when de Bold and colleagues experimented by injecting atrial muscle cell extracts into rats and noted a marked increase in sodium and water excretion along with a drop in blood pressure [1]; the active hormone was named "atrial natriuretic factor" and subsequent studies later characterized the molecular structure unique to the cardiac natriuretic peptide family, which is composed of atrial natriuretic peptide (ANP), brain natriuretic peptide (BNP), and C-type natriuretic peptide (CNP), among others. The system is believed to have evolved for the common mechanism of sodium and volume homeostasis, but the molecules are encoded by separate genes, have distinct mechanisms of regulation, different main sites of synthesis, and are stored as three different precursor pro-hormone molecules with variable amino acid lengths [2,3].

Both ANP and BNP activate the same transmembrane guanylate cyclase receptor (natriuretic peptide receptor, NPR-A) on target organs for common physiologic effects, which include promotion of renal excretion of sodium and water, vasodilation by relaxation of vascular smooth muscle cells, improved diastolic relaxation, inhibition of the renin-angiotensin system, and prevention of myocardial fibrosis. ANP is stored and constitutively released during both normal and abnormal physiologic conditions; this particular biological characteristic—together with the fact that measurement of ANP is fraught with difficulties related to its short half-life—made BNP the more logical choice of the two molecules for clinical application; BNP and related compounds have

Biomarkers in Heart Disease, 1st edition. Edited by James A. de Lemos.
© 2008 American Heart Association, ISBN: 978-1-4051-7571-5

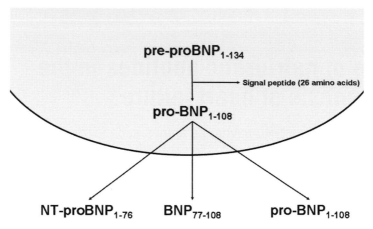

Fig. 6.1 Biochemical structure of pro-BNP, BNP, and NT-proBNP.

therefore become the most widely studied biomarkers of left ventricular (LV) systolic and diastolic dysfunction [4,5].

Although BNP was originally isolated from porcine brain (and hence its original name, "brain" natriuretic peptide), it is believed that the majority of BNP gene products are synthesized and released by the myocardium of the heart [2]. There are two related BNP-type markers, derived from a common intracellular 108-amino acid precursor peptide, proBNP$_{108}$, which is synthesized mainly in the atrial and ventricular cardiomyocytes in response to myocyte stretch. During its release from the cardiomyocyte, proBNP$_{108}$ is cleaved to release two portions in equimolar amounts: the biologically inert amino-terminal portion, NT-proBNP, and the carboxy-terminal portion, BNP, which represents the bioactive portion of the molecule, with a characteristic 17-amino acid ring formed by disulfide-linked cysteines, essential for biological activity [6] (see Fig. 6.1).

Among patients with heart failure, measurable concentrations of NT-proBNP, BNP, and proBNP$_{108}$ are found. It is well established at present that the currently available assays for detection of "NT-proBNP" or "BNP" in fact measure a mixture of each peptide *plus* a significant amount of proBNP$_{108}$ as well; this is important, as proBNP$_{108}$ demonstrates markedly reduced (or absent) biologic activity, relative to bioactive BNP, and raises the question as to whether different relative proportions of circulating proBNP$_{108}$ correlate with worsening states of heart failure [7,8].

After release, BNP is quickly cleared by several mechanisms, which include enzymatic degradation by the neutral endopeptidase (NEP) 24.11 and receptor-mediated endocytosis by the NPR-C receptor, both of which complement passive renal excretion; bioactive BNP has a half-life of about 20 minutes [6]. As for NT-proBNP, it is estimated that 20–25% is cleared by passive renal excretion, with the rest being removed through other, less well-understood

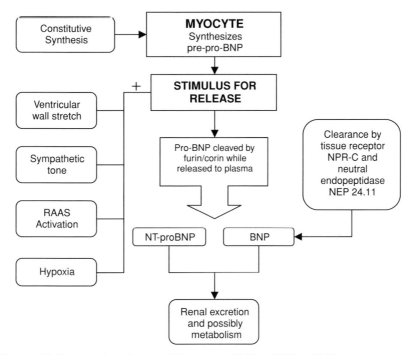

Fig. 6.2 Mechanisms for release and clearance of BNP and NT-proBNP.

mechanisms such as reticulo-endothelial system processing or passive removal by organs with high degrees of blood flow such as the liver. The half-life of NT-proBNP has been measured at around 60 to 120 minutes [6]. Figure 6.2 provides an overview of the mechanisms of release and clearance of BNP and NT-proBNP.

Major studies and operating characteristics

Four major fields of study have been established for natriuretic peptides in relation to heart failure, which include: 1) diagnosis and triage in the acute setting, 2) evaluation and diagnosis of heart failure in the primary care setting, 3) population screening for LV dysfunction, and 4) guiding therapy of heart failure (see also chapter 8). Table 6.1 summarizes the largest trials in the current areas of research in natriuretic peptide (NP) testing for heart failure. We will focus the major portion of the discussion on the utility of natriuretic peptides for diagnosis and triage in the acute setting.

The first clinical studies performed in the mid-1990s were small proof in principal studies that showed higher levels of BNP among dyspneic patients with versus without heart failure, and also showed a correlation of BNP with LV

Table 6.1 Summary of the major trials in the four areas of NP testing for heart failure.

Area of NP Testing Research	Trials	Comments
Diagnostic and triage in the acute setting	BNP Study – Maisel 2002 [12]	Landmark trial for BNP testing in acutely dyspneic patients.
	Lainchbury 2003 [17]	First study demonstrating value of NT-proBNP testing for evaluation of acute dyspnea. Results comparing BNP and NT-proBNP were equivalent.
	Bayes-Genis 2005 [16]	NT-proBNP also useful for short-term prognostication.
	Mueller 2004 [18]	BNP and NT-proBNP equivalent for diagnostic evaluation of dyspnea.
	Mueller 2006 [24]	Utility of BNP-guided evaluation and triage for improving diagnosis and reducing costs.
	REDHOT – Maisel 2004 [14]	Showed BNP superior to clinical assessment of heart failure severity.
	PRIDE – Januzzi 2005 [19]	Landmark NT-proBNP assessment. NT-proBNP superior to clinical judgment for diagnosis of heart failure.
	ICON – Januzzi 2006 [20]	NT-pro-BNP powerfully diagnostic and prognostic; age stratified cut-points for diagnosis proposed.
Evaluation in the primary care setting	Cowie 1997 [4]	First study to evaluate BNP as a strategy to diagnose heart failure in the outpatient setting.
	Wright 2003 [28]	First study to evaluate the utility of NT-proBNP for a similar strategy.
	Gustafsson 2005 [30]	Initial evaluation of the value of NT-proBNP in the primary care setting as a step prior to referral for echocardiographic evaluation.

(continued)

Table 6.1 (*continued*).

Population screening for LV dysfunction	**Vasan 2002 [33]**	Initial study to suggest BNP is a sub-optimal tool for detecting LV systolic dysfunction in asymptomatic patients.
	Redfield 2004 [34]	Confirmation of the lack of utility of BNP for population screening.
	Costello 2006 [35]	First evidence to suggest NT-proBNP may be superior to BNP for screening purposes.
Cost-effectiveness studies evaluating screening of "at risk" populations	**Mueller 2006 [24], Siebert 2006 [25]**	Analyses showing that BNP and NT-proBNP are a cost-effective approach to guide diagnosis and management of HF in the acute setting.
	Galasko 2006 [36]	Confirmation of the utility of NT-proBNP for screening high-risk subjects in comparison with other diagnostic modalities.

systolic dysfunction [4,9]. Subsequently, BNP was shown to be a better indicator than ANP or NT-proANP for detection of LV systolic dysfunction [10,11].

The use of BNP as a diagnostic tool in the acute clinical setting was further explored by Maisel and colleagues in the Breathing Not Properly Multinational Study, a prospective diagnostic test evaluation study conducted in 1586 participants in 7 centers. In this landmark trial, authors used one of the first rapid diagnostic assays to demonstrate that at a BNP level of 100 ng/L, BNP had 90% sensitivity, 76% specificity, and an accuracy of 83% for the diagnosis of heart failure in patients presenting with dyspnea, with BNP level being more accurate than either NHANES criteria (67% accuracy) or Framingham criteria (73% accuracy) for diagnosing heart failure [12].

The Breathing Not Properly study investigators later compared BNP testing to the clinical judgment of emergency department (ED) physicians for the diagnosis of heart failure and found that for determination of "correct diagnosis" (i.e., acute heart failure versus no acute heart failure), adding BNP to clinical impression enhanced diagnostic accuracy from 74% to 81%. They also noted that for participants with an intermediate (21% to 79%) probability of acute heart failure, BNP at a cutoff of 100 ng/L correctly classified 74% of the cases. This provided evidence supporting the concept that the evaluation of acute dyspnea would be improved by adding BNP testing to clinical judgment [13]. The relationship between clinical judgment and BNP was further explored in the Rapid Emergency Department Heart Failure Trial (REDHOT) study, which confirmed that clinician perception of the severity of heart failure in the ED setting was inadequate, and clearly inferior to that of BNP [14]. In both the Breathing Not Properly and REDHOT studies, BNP correlated very strongly with the severity of heart failure [12,14] and was prognostic [14] for short-term hazard, all important considerations when using these peptides for triage decision making.

Lending further support to the use of BNP in the evaluation of heart failure among dyspneic patients in the ED was a meta-analysis by Wang and colleagues that included 11 studies published between 1994 and July 2005. In predictable statistical fashion, as sensitivity was improved by lowering the threshold value for a positive test result, specificity decreased proportionally. A low serum BNP proved to be the most useful test to exclude heart failure (<100 ng/L; negative likelihood ratio = 0.11; 95% CI, 0.07–0.16), but other values were useful as well, as a BNP greater than 250 ng/L raised the likelihood of heart failure as the correct diagnosis by 4.5 times [15].

Further data supporting the use of natriuretic peptides for evaluation of the dyspneic patient, this time in the form of NT-proBNP, soon followed [16–18]. In several of these studies NT-proBNP and BNP were compared directly, with similar predictive values observed for the two peptides [17,18]. Subsequently, a comparison trial by Mueller and colleagues demonstrated similar results from BNP and NT-proBNP among dyspneic patients [18]. However, the most definitive and largest clinical trial to date seeking to evaluate testing using NT-proBNP in patients with suspected acutely destabilized heart failure was the ProBNP Investigation of Dyspnea in the Emergency Department (PRIDE) study [19], a prospective study of 600 patients. The prevalence of acute heart failure in this cohort was 35%, and similarly to the BNP Multinational study, the use in PRIDE of the emergency room physician's initial clinical assessment together with NT-proBNP was superior to either factor alone and gave the best combination of sensitivity and specificity. In the PRIDE study, NT-proBNP had similar area under the receiver operating characteristic curve as BNP did in the Breathing Not Properly study, and an NT-proBNP cut point of 900 ng/L provided a nearly identical positive predictive value for that reported for BNP in prior studies. Furthermore, NT-proBNP concentrations in PRIDE paralleled the severity of heart failure as well [19].

Expanding on the concept of stratification of natriuretic peptide results, and as suggested previously in the meta-analysis by Wang [15], the PRIDE investigators found that a stratified cut-point approach was likely superior to a single "one size fits all" cut point. Using this strategy, an NT-proBNP <300 ng/L was recommended as the "rule out" cut-point, corresponding to a negative predictive value of 99%. An appreciation of the importance of age as a confounding factor for both NT-proBNP and BNP led to a stratified approach for "rule in" cut-points of 450/900/1800 ng/L for ages <50/50–75/>75 years. This strategy

Table 6.2 Optimal BNP and NT-proBNP cut-points for diagnosis of heart failure in different clinical settings.

Setting	BNP	NT-proBNP
Acute heart failure	100 ng/L [12]	900 ng/L Alternative approach: 450 ng/L (<50 years) 900 ng/L (50–75 years) 1800 ng/L (>75 years) [19,20]
Renal failure	200 ng/L [39]	1200 ng/L [40]
Outpatient evaluation	Unknown (possibly 20–30 ng/L)	125 ng/L (≤75 years) 450 ng/L (>75 year) Manufacturer recommended

preserved sensitivity and specificity, improved positive predictive value, and decreased the number of "gray zone" measurements [19] (see section on gray zone values).

This multiple cut-point approach was subsequently validated in an international collaborative multicenter trial, the International Collaborative of NT-proBNP (ICON) study, which measured NT-proBNP levels among 1256 patients with and without acute heart failure, and utilized bootstrapping statistical techniques to identify optimal cut-points for diagnosis and prognosis [20].

With both BNP and NT-proBNP testing, certain recurrent themes have emerged. First, the sensitivity of the peptides is often superior to that of clinical assessment at the time of first evaluation. Furthermore, concentrations at presentation are often incrementally useful in the context of results from other diagnostic tests such as chest radiography [21] or echocardiography [22]. Randomized studies further suggest that these markers do, in fact, result in fewer incorrect heart failure admissions, shorter hospital lengths of stay, and lower overall costs [23–25]. Table 6.2 classifies the optimal cut-points derived from the main BNP and NT-proBNP clinical trials in different diagnostic settings.

Validated algorithms are now available for use when applying BNP or NT-proBNP testing [26,27], which integrate sound clinical judgment as well as differential diagnoses together with BNP or NT-proBNP results. When applying natriuretic peptide testing, one must keep in mind the complex physiology that determines their synthesis and secretion; if BNP or NT-proBNP are used in isolation of clinical judgment, it is at the peril of confusion and misdirection. Indeed, there are no one-step algorithms for using BNP or NT-proBNP, and oversimplifying their use does a disservice to the patient and clinician.

Primary care

Another promising application for natriuretic peptide testing is in the field of outpatient evaluation in the primary care setting. It is worth noting that several characteristics of heart failure pathophysiology and NP biology make this field particularly challenging. First and foremost is the fact that in the primary care environment, not all patients are clearly symptomatic when they present to the office; second is that the elevation in natriuretic peptide levels seen in these patients is typically an order of magnitude lower than what is seen in the acute setting, and thus factors that may be less important in the emergency department (e.g., gender, body mass index, subtle forms of heart disease) will have a much greater significance in the primary care office. In other words, while in the emergency department setting interpretation of natriuretic peptide concentrations may be done with "broad strokes", in the outpatient clinic the primary care physician should do so with "finer strokes."

The first study to evaluate natriuretic peptide testing for the diagnosis of heart failure in the outpatient setting was done by Cowie and colleagues [4], where researchers measured concentrations of BNP in 122 consecutive patients referred to a rapid-access heart-failure clinic with a potentially new primary-care diagnosis of heart failure. They found that mean concentrations of natriuretic peptides were 5-fold higher in patients with heart failure than in those with other diagnoses. This important finding was later confirmed in a prospective, randomized controlled trial that tested NT-proBNP accuracy in 305 patients presenting to their primary care physician with symptoms of dyspnea and/or peripheral edema [28]. The primary care physician formulated an initial diagnosis based on clinical assessment, and patients then underwent a full evaluation that included echocardiography and NT-proBNP measurements. The diagnostic accuracy improved 21% in the NT-proBNP group versus 8% in the control group ($P = .002$). This study suggested that the main impact of NT-proBNP testing on diagnostic accuracy was on the clinician's ability to correctly rule out heart failure. The number needed to diagnose one episode of heart failure by NT-proBNP measurement was seven patients [28].

From these initial studies it became clear that NT-proBNP and BNP levels were typically higher in those with heart failure than in those without; however, there seemed to be significant overlap between healthy and nonhealthy subjects. It now seems that a clinical distinction should be made by the physician considering natriuretic peptide measurements in the general population. For symptomatic outpatients, natriuretic peptide testing should be used to enhance the correct *elimination* of the diagnosis of heart failure as the cause of symptoms, that is, to rule out heart failure. In doing so, cut-points fashioned for a high negative predictive value should be utilized. These cut-points would therefore have high sensitivity but lower specificity. Studies have, in fact, confirmed the value of the measurement of plasma BNP and NT-proBNP as "rule-out" tests for heart failure in patients referred by their primary care physician to rapid access diagnostic clinics [29], and in those who were referred for echocardiography [30]. This particular study also showed that a low NT-proBNP value was associated with a lower risk of death, independent of age, gender, and left ventricular ejection fraction [30].

Current recommended guidelines now suggest the use of natriuretic peptide testing as a step prior to referral for echocardiographic or specialist evaluation [31,32]. At present, the recommended cut-points for outpatient evaluation are well established for NT-proBNP (see Table 6.2). The optimal outpatient cut-points remain uncertain for BNP, but are certainly well below the recommended cut-point of 100 ng/L, which is best reserved for acutely dyspneic patients in the emergency department setting, and are presumably in the range of 20–30 ng/L.

For asymptomatic patients however, several studies have not found a screening approach to be necessarily useful for application in "apparently well" patients. Evaluation of BNP was done in a community-based prospective cohort of 3177 participants from the Framingham Study who attended a routine examination from 1995 to1998; using an empirically derived cut-point of 36 ng/L, investigators found that a "positive" BNP would lead to 34% of patients being referred for echocardiography, of whom 85% would have negative findings, suggesting that the performance of BNP for detection of left ventricular systolic dysfunction was suboptimal [33]. A higher BNP cutoff of 55 ng/L was later used by Redfield and colleagues in 2042 randomly selected patients out of a population in Olmstead County, Minnesota. Results again showed that using BNP measurements as an initial screen would lead to a referral for echocardiography in 24% of asymptomatic patients, with 96% of these lacking confirmation of systolic dysfunction [34]. An interesting note is that there may be some evidence to suggest that NT-proBNP could be superior to BNP in some subgroups for detecting LV systolic dysfunction [35]. Moreover, several studies suggested that NT-proBNP may be cost effective for this purpose [36]. However, given uncertainty regarding the role of natriuretic peptides for screening asympomatic subjects, further studies are needed before clear recommendations can be made. Future studies should focus in particular on screening those "at risk" for heart failure (such as those patients with advanced diabetes mellitus, long-standing hypertension, or asymptomatic coronary artery disease).

Gray zone values

In general, levels of BNP and NT-proBNP are directly related to the severity of heart failure symptoms and to the severity of the underlying cardiac abnormalities, and they are best viewed as continuous variables. Thus, as with all binary-model quantitative diagnostic tests that require the determination of a cut-off value to label patients as diseased or nondiseased from a range of values, natriuretic peptides, by definition, are subjected to have "gray zone" values— that is, peptide levels that are associated with indeterminate positive predictive values, which in turn lead to difficulty applying the test result in everyday clinical use. Gray zone results are defined as those values that fall in a range between the lower and upper cut-points of certainty for conventional likelihood ratios using conventional pretest probabilities, where anything below that range has a negative predictive value so high that heart failure is very unlikely, while any level above this range will be so elevated that it makes the diagnosis of heart failure nearly certain [37]. In other words, a gray zone NP value will fall in a range that is indeterminate for the diagnosis or exclusion of heart failure. For BNP, the proposed gray zone is from 100 to 500 ng/L, with values that span a range of increasing likelihood for diagnosis of heart failure. However, as a BNP below 100 ng/L does not exclude heart failure (with a negative predictive value of only 89% in the Breathing Not Properly Multinational Study [12]), clinicians should be aware of the potential risk of missing the diagnosis with levels that are under this value. For NT-proBNP, the gray zone has been suggested to span the range between "rule out" (300 ng/L) and the age-adjusted "rule in" values. By adjusting for age, gray zone NT-proBNP values were less frequent, underscoring the importance of age as a frequent cause of intermediate values for natriuretic peptides. It has been argued that the negative predictive value of BNP and NT-proBNP for excluding heart failure is superior to their positive predictive value for identifying the diagnosis.

There are numerous factors that lead to gray zone values among patients without heart failure, including normative physiology, which most notably includes age [38]. Age affects both NT-proBNP and BNP equally with respect to increased values in older patients without clinically overt heart failure; the utility of age stratification for reducing the likelihood for a false attribution of heart failure to an elevated NT-proBNP value in elders has been discussed [20]. In addition, renal failure [39,40], pulmonary diseases such as pulmonary embolism [41] or primary pulmonary hypertension [42], and other cardiac diagnoses such as atrial fibrillation [43] or acute coronary ischemia [44,45] may all lead to elevations of BNP or NT-proBNP in the absence of obvious heart failure.

Conversely, among those with heart failure and BNP or NT-proBNP levels in the gray zone, a higher percentage of nonsystolic heart failure may be observed [14,46], and more mild heart failure symptoms may be present. Also, rising body-mass index (BMI) is associated with a suppressing effect on both BNP and NT-proBNP release [47,48], with up to 20% of patients with acute heart failure and BMI >35 Kg/M2 demonstrating natriuretic peptides below the diagnostic cut-point.

Irrespective of the mechanism, and most importantly, such elevations of natriuretic peptides, while attributed to other diagnoses, are nonetheless relevant from a prognostic perspective (Fig. 6.3) [49,50].

In order to best manage a gray zone measurement, different approaches have been advocated. In one study, clinical variables were examined for their value to assist in correct interpretation of gray zone natriuretic peptide results. In this

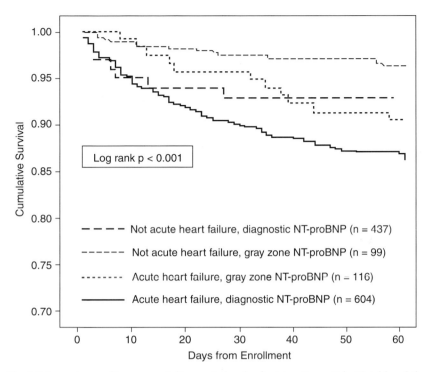

Fig. 6.3 Importance of "gray zone" diagnostic levels of natriuretic peptide. Notably, while "gray zone" NT-proBNP levels were less useful for diagnosis, they were nonetheless useful for prognostic evaluation. Reproduced with permission from [49].

study [49], symptoms and signs consistent with heart failure were more commonly segregated in those gray zone patients who ultimately were diagnosed with heart failure, while those without heart failure were more likely to have histories consistent with pulmonary diseases.

Another strategy for the clinical use of gray zone comes from a prospective cohort study in France of 699 consecutive patients with acute dyspnea who were treated at the emergency department of 3 participating hospitals. Authors formulated a three-zone partition category for a positive, negative, and intermediate zone, with two resulting cutoffs, one to be used for rule out of the diagnostic hypothesis (e.g., that could be used in an emergency department to decide not to admit a patient with mild dyspnea) and another to rule in the diagnosis and undertake a specific treatment. This "middle" zone group would require additional testing to arrive at a final diagnosis. Although it still requires external validation, this approach, initially developed for categorical and ordinal tests, may prove to be useful for other quantitative diagnostic and screening tests as well [37].

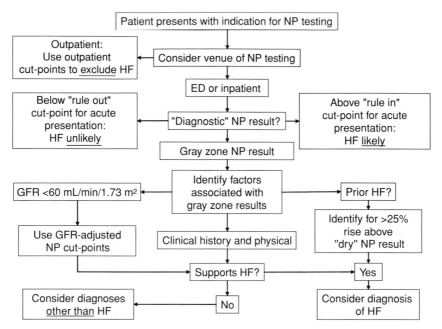

Fig. 6.4 Flow chart algorithm for clinical use of natriuretic peptide results, includes outpatient applications as well as clinical interpretation of "gray zone" values. The recommended cut-points for this various scenarios are found in the corresponding section of the text.

Figure 6.4 depicts a flow chart algorithm for clinical use of natriuretic peptide results, includes outpatient applications as well as clinical interpretation of gray zone values.

Pitfalls

There are three fundamental challenges facing clinicians when it comes to diagnostic testing strategies with natriuretic peptides. The first is related to the various strengths and weaknesses of the commercially available methods for the measurement of the assays. The second has to do with the identification of new heterogenous forms of BNP as well as our lack of knowledge on their role in the pathophysiology of heart failure, and the third is defined by the implications of the common physiologic and comorbid conditions found in patients in whom testing is typically performed.

Analytical pitfalls

Considering the commercially available assays for natriuretic peptide measurement, it is necessary to point out that while the majority of the large-scale clinical trial data for either BNP or NT-proBNP were based on only two assays, there is now a wide range of natriuretic peptide methods commercially available for use. It remains as of yet unclear if each assay delivers the same expected performance that earlier trials have suggested for each peptide. This is of particular relevance for BNP, as most of the immunoassays currently available are based on different antisera, thus leading to a general lack of "harmony" among the various assays; the assays for NT-proBNP are currently all based on the same antibodies, and hence are thought to be interchangeable with respect to their results. Other important analytical considerations worthy of discussion include the importance of rapid turn-around times for the use of natriuretic peptides; for both BNP and NT-proBNP, point-of-care solutions are available. These assays provide rapid turn-around times, but are fraught with higher analytical imprecision, an expected trade-off. Lastly, another pre-analytical issue that is worthy of highlighting is the fact that BNP is temperature sensitive, with the potential for significant degradation of BNP concentrations following phlebotomy if assayed after a prolonged period at all temperatures [51].

Pitfalls in our understanding of natriuretic peptide biology

Even though it is well established that BNP and NT-proBNP levels correlate well with the severity of heart failure, and elevated levels are very sensitive for diagnosis of heart failure, the second major pitfall for natriuretic peptide testing stems from the results of studies that show a discrepancy between plasma concentrations of BNP and a seemingly paradoxic lack of natriuretic peptide activity [52], raising the possibility that there is some disconnection between our measurements of BNP and NT-proBNP and the actual activity of the neurohormonal axis.

There is evidence suggesting two explanations for this discordance. One explanation is the fact that there seems to be several species of low molecular weight BNP molecules (different from the 32 amino acid bioactive BNP) as detected by mass spectroscopy techniques, with an unknown molecular structure. These types of immunoreactive BNP molecules could have a wider array of previously unrecognized biological activity [53]. The other possible explanation is the finding mentioned earlier that there seems to be an unexpected amount of circulating proBNP$_{108}$ (the high molecular weight precursor) that is present in significant amounts in both healthy and diseased individuals [7,8,54]. Prior to these studies, the precursor molecule was not known to be released in significant amounts, and while it does not seem to have significant biological activity, a recent study suggests that these forms seem to constitute much of the circulating immunoreactive BNP in advanced heart failure [8], helping to explain at least in part why there seems to be a state of natriuretic peptide activity deficiency when at the same time our measurements detect high levels of BNP in the plasma. The situation is further complicated by the fact that there seems to be significant cross-detection of some BNP forms by the leading commercial diagnostic assays [8]. Thus, it is reasonable to expect that any result for "BNP" or "NT-proBNP" is likely reflective not just of these analytes but also includes measurement of proBNP$_{108}$ to one degree or another.

Patient-specific factors

The third and possibly most clinically significant pitfall when interpreting BNP and NT-proBNP levels comes from the relatively restricted knowledge regarding the influence of patient-specific physiologic and pathophysiologic factors on the circulating levels of both forms of natriuretic peptides. Table 6.3 summarizes most of the physiologic and comorbid conditions that influence NP levels.

As noted earlier, the effect of age on BNP or NT-proBNP values has been demonstrated in several studies. In a healthy reference sample of subjects with normal LV function who were free of comorbid conditions, Wang and colleagues reported that the strongest predictors of higher natriuretic peptide levels were older age and female gender; while age remains important in acute heart failure, female gender appears to be less important [55]; however, when considering application of BNP or NT-proBNP testing to larger and larger populations, the gender-specific influences on natriuretic peptide levels (thought to potentially be reflective of androgenic effects [56]) are important to consider. Another study with an even more elderly cohort (mean age of 83 years) further confirmed that age (with associated "normative aging processes" such as hypertension and subclinical cardiac diastolic abnormalities) was an independent factor affecting BNP concentrations [57].

As noted previously, several studies have confirmed the impact of obesity on natriuretic peptide levels independently from that of hypertension, diabetes, and other characteristics [58–60]. This relationship appears to be present despite higher left ventricular end-diastolic pressures in obese subjects [61], and affects both BNP and NT-proBNP. An excellent example of the clinical ramifications of this finding are seen in a study that found decreased levels of BNP and NT-proBNP with increasing BMI across clinical strata of normal (<25 kg/m2), overweight (25–29.9 kg/m2), and obese ($>$ or $= 30$ kg/m2) patients [55]. Despite this finding, recent data confirm that NT-proBNP retains strong positive predictive value across BMI strata without the need to adjust cut-points for different weight results [62].

Another common comorbid condition that seems to influence the levels of both BNP and NT-proBNP is renal insufficiency. The underlying reason(s) for linear elevations of both BNP and NT-proBNP (the latter being slightly more affected by renal insufficiency at the most severe ranges of chronic kidney disease) relates both to potentially reduced clearance of the peptides, but also to the marked increase in structural heart disease among patients with chronic kidney disease—such as left ventricular hypertrophy, valve disease, arrhythmia, pulmonary hypertension, and ischemic heart disease [63,64]—as well as to the fluid overload with hypertension and consequent neurohormonal activation seen in these patients.

Table 6.3 Summary of important modifiers of natriuretic peptide concentrations.

Modifier	BNP	NT-proBNP	Comments on mechanism or utility
Age	↑	↑	Correlation with HF persists an age-stratified analyses.
Female gender	↑	↑	Strong correlation with gender is lost in those with acute heart failure.
Obesity	↓↓	↓	BNP more affected given higher levels of clearance receptors in fatty tissue.
Renal failure	↑↑	↑↑↑	NT-proBNP shows slightly stronger correlation to renal function in the range of most severe kidney dysfunction; clinical implication appears minimal compared to BNP, however.
Aortic valve disease	↑	↑	Possible utility for identifying value replacement candidates and in post-op follow-up.
Mitral valve disease	↑	↑	Same as above, levels may be good estimates of hemodynamics. May predict atrial fibrillation onset.
Atrial fibrillation	↑	↑	Suspected direct release by fibrillating myocytes.
Myocardial ischemia	↑	↑	Probably from impaired wall relaxation and contractility and myocardial hypoxia.
Pregnancy	↑	↑	Minor physiologic elevation. Pronounced increase seen in pre-eclampsia and cardiomyopathy.
Neonatal state	↑	↑	Physiologic increase from early volume shifts.
Diabetes mellitus	↑	↑	Strongly associated with micro-albuminuria.
Pulmonary hypertension, including pulmonary embolism	↑	↑	Released due to RV strain and closely related to degree of ventricular dysfunction.
Critical illness	↑↑↑↑	↑↑↑↑	Increase in hemodynamic counterregulatory mechanisms. Useful to guide management and as predictors of mortality.
Intracranial hemorrhage and embolic stroke	↑	↑	May be related to cerebral-mediated cardiac dysfunction.

The degree of renal dependence on clearance of both BNP and NT-proBNP remains a hotly contested topic. Although observational studies show trends toward more effect of chronic kidney disease on NT-proBNP among patients with glomerular filtration rate (GFR) measurements in the lowest ranges, this observation is by no means universal, with some studies showing very similar proportional effects of renal disease on both peptides [65]. Further, mechanistic studies actually argue for a generally similar dependence on renal clearance for both BNP and NT-proBNP [66]. Irrespective of the mechanism, elevation of BNP or NT-proBNP among patients with end-stage renal disease is profoundly prognostic, arguing for more "signal" than "noise".

Using natriuretic peptides for the evaluation of the dyspneic patient with suspected heart failure who also suffers from chronic kidney disease is a challenging prospect. The BNP Multinational Study was pivotal in establishing the correlations between GFR and BNP in those with and without heart failure, indeed establishing that chronic kidney disease does appear to influence the optimum cut-points for BNP in the diagnosis of acute heart failure in dyspneic subjects. The investigators argued that as CKD stage advances, a higher cut-point of BNP (in the range of 200 ng/L) is needed [39]. Similar findings were later reported for the use of NT-proBNP in dyspneic subjects; in this analysis, the clinical results of NT-proBNP testing were similar to those reported for BNP in patients with renal failure, although univariable correlations between GFR and NT-proBNP were higher than those previously reported for BNP [40]. Importantly, NT-proBNP remains highly prognostic for death in those with chronic kidney disease—if not more so than in those with preserved renal function—arguing that elevations of NT-proBNP in patients with chronic kidney disease are important, and should not be discarded [40]. In summary, renal dysfunction has important effects on levels of both BNP and NT-proBNP but these tests remain useful for risk stratification and for diagnosis across the range of renal function. However, clinicians must interpret elevated natriuretic peptide values with caution when detected in the context of chronic kidney disease, particularly among patients with very advanced renal failure, where levels of natriuretic peptides approaching or exceeding the range consistent with "heart failure" may be observed in the absence of the diagnosis.

Lastly, the effects of *prior* heart failure on circulating concentrations of BNP and NT-proBNP may interfere with interpretation of these peptides when such a patient may present with acute symptoms suggestive of heart failure. This is an area where clinical judgment is necessary to adequately assess such patients. However, it is established that BNP and NT-proBNP concentrations among those with acutely destabilized heart failure are typically considerably higher than those patients with chronic stable diagnoses of heart failure; accordingly, it is worthwhile to compare present values for either peptide with prior values. Given the assumed biological variability of BNP and NT-proBNP to be around 25% [66] and no higher than 40%, a change larger than this amount should be interpreted as being consistent with a significant change from the so-called "dry" BNP or NT-proBNP value.

References

1 De Bold AJ, Borenstein HB, Veress AT et al. A rapid and potent natriuretic response to intravenous injection of atrial myocardial extract in rats. *Life Sci* 1981; **28**: 89–94.

2 Yasue H, Yoshimura M, Sunida H et al. Localization and mechanism of secretion of B type natriuretic peptide in comparison with those of A type natriuretic peptide in normal subjects and those with heart failure. *Circulation* 1994; **90**: 195–203.

3 Komatsu Y, Nakao K, Suga S et al. Ctype natriuretic peptide (CNP) in rats and humans. *Endocrinology* 1991; **129**: 1104–1106.

4 Cowie MR, Struthers AD, Wood DA et al. Value of natriuretic peptides in assessment of patients with possible new heart failure in primary care. *Lancet* 1997; **350**: 1347–1351.

5 Yamamoto K, Burnett JC, Jougasaki M et al. Superiority of brain natriuretic peptide as a hormonal marker of ventricular systolic and diastolic dysfunction and ventricular hypertrophy. *Hypertension* 1996; **28**: 988–994.

6 Vanderheyden M, Bartunek I, Goethals M. Brain and other natriuretic peptides: molecular aspects, *Eur J Heart Fail* 2004; **6**: 261–268.

7 Yandle TG, Richards AM, Gilbert A et al. Assay of brain natriuretic peptide (BNP) in human plasma: evidence for high molecular weight BNP as a major plasma component in heart failure. *J Clin Endocrinol Metab* 1993; **76**: 832–838.

8 Liang F, O'Rear J, Schellenberger U et al. Evidence for functional heterogeneity of circulating B-type natriuretic peptide. *J Am Coll Cardiol* 2007; **49**: 1071–1078.

9 Davis M, Espiner E, Richards G et al. Plasma brain natriuretic peptide in assessment of acute dyspnea. *Lancet* 1994; **343**: 440–444.

10 Clerico A, Lervasi G, Del Chicca MG et al. Circulating levels of cardiac natriuretic peptides (ANP and BNP) measured by highly sensitive and specific immunoradiometric assays in normal subjects and in patients with different degrees of heart failure. *J Endocrinol Invest* 1998; **21**: 170–179.

11 McDonagh TA, Robb SD, Murdoch DR et al. Biochemical detection of left-ventricular systolic dysfunction. *Lancet* 1998; **351**: 9–13.

12 Maisel AS, Krishnaswamy P, Nowak RM et al. Rapid measurement of B-type natriuretic peptide in the emergency diagnosis of heart failure. *N Engl J Med* 2002; **347**: 161–167.

13 McCullough PA, Nowak RM, McCord J et al. B-type natriuretic peptide and clinical judgment in emergency diagnosis of heart failure: analysis from Breathing Not Properly (BNP) Multinational Study. *Circulation* 2002; **106**: 416–422.

14 Maisel A, Hollander JE, Guss D et al. Primary results of the Rapid Emergency Department Heart Failure Outpatient Trial (REDHOT). A multicenter study of B-type natriuretic peptide levels, emergency department decision making, and outcomes in patients presenting with shortness of breath. *J Am Coll Cardiol* 2004; **44**: 1328–1333.

15 Wang CS, FitzGerald JM, Schulzer M et al. Does this dyspneic patient in the emergency department have congestive heart failure? *JAMA* 2005; **294**: 1944–1956.

16 Bayes-Genis A, Lopez L, Zapico E et al. NT-ProBNP reduction percentage during admission for acutely decompensated heart failure predicts long-term cardiovascular mortality. *J Card Fail* 2005; **11**: S3–S8.

17 Lainchbury JG, Campbell E, Frampton CM et al. Brain natriuretic peptide and n-terminal brain natriuretic peptide in the diagnosis of heart failure in patients with acute shortness of breath. *J Am Coll Cardiol* 2003; **42**: 728–735.

18 Mueller T, Gegenhuber A, Poelz W et al. Biochemical diagnosis of impaired left ventricular ejection fraction—comparison of the diagnostic accuracy of brain natriuretic peptide (BNP) and amino terminal proBNP (NT-proBNP). *Clin Chem Lab Med* 2004; **42**: 159–163.

19 Januzzi JL Jr, Camargo CA, Anwaruddin S et al. The N-terminal pro-BNP investigation of dyspnea in the emergency department (PRIDE) study. *Am J Cardiol* 2005; **95**: 948–954.

20 Januzzi JL, van Kimmenade R, Lainchbury J et al. NT-proBNP testing for diagnosis and short-term prognosis in acute destabilized heart failure: an international pooled analysis of 1256 patients: the International Collaborative of NT-proBNP Study. *Eur Heart J* 2006; **27**: 330–337.

21 Knudsen CW, Omland T, Clopton P et al. Diagnostic value of B-type natriuretic peptide and chest radiographic findings in patients with acute dyspnea. *Am J Med* 2004; **116**: 363–368.

22 Chen AA, Wood MJ, Krauser DG et al. NT-proBNP levels, echocardiographic findings, and outcomes in breathless patients: results from the ProBNP Investigation of Dyspnoea in the Emergency Department (PRIDE) echocardiographic substudy. *Eur Heart J* 2006; **27**: 839–845.

23 Mueller C, Scholer A, Laule-Kilian K et al. Use of B-type natriuretic peptide in the evaluation and management of acute dyspnea. *N Engl J Med* 2004; **350**: 647–654.

24 Mueller C, Laule-Kilian K, Schindler C et al. Cost-effectiveness of B-type natriuretic peptide testing in patients with acute dyspnea. *Arch Intern Med* 2006; **166**: 1081–1087.

25 Siebert U, Januzzi JL Jr, Beinfeld MT et al. Cost-effectiveness of using N-terminal pro-brain natriuretic peptide to guide the diagnostic assessment and management of dyspneic patients in the emergency department. *Am J Cardiol* 2006; **98**: 800–805.

26 Maisel A. Algorithms for using B-type natriuretic peptide levels in the diagnosis and management of congestive heart failure. *Crit Path Cardiol* 2002; **1**: 67–73.

27 Baggish A, Cameron R, Anwaruddin S et al. A clinical and biochemical critical pathway for the evaluation of patients with suspected acute congestive heart failure: the ProBNP Investigation of Dyspnea in the Emergency Department (PRIDE) Algorithm. *Crit Path Cardiol* 2004; **3**: 171–176.

28 Wright SP, Doughty RN, Pearl A et al. Plasma amino-terminal pro-brain natriuretic peptide and accuracy of heart-failure diagnosis in primary care: a randomized, controlled trial. *J Am Coll Cardiol* 2003; **42**: 1793–1800.

29 Zaphiriou A, Robb S, Murray-Thomas T et al. The diagnostic accuracy of plasma BNP and NT-proBNP in patients referred from primary care with suspected heart failure: results of the UK natriuretic peptide study. *Eur J Heart Fail* 2005; **7**: 537–541.

30 Gustafsson F, Steensgaard-Hansen F, Badskjaer J et al. Diagnostic and prognostic performance of N-terminal ProBNP in primary care patients with suspected heart failure. *J Card Fail* 2005; **11**: S15–S20.

31 Brady AJ, Poole-Wilson PA. ESC-CHF guidelines for the aspirational and the practical. *Heart* 2006; **92**: 437–440.

32 Fuat A, Murphy JJ, Hungin AP et al. The diagnostic accuracy and utility of a B-type natriuretic peptide test in a community population of patients with suspected heart failure. *Br J Gen Pract* 2006; **56**: 327–333.

33 Vasan RS, Benjamin EJ, Larson MG et al. Plasma natriuretic peptides for community screening for left ventricular hypertrophy and systolic dysfunction: the Framingham heart study. *JAMA* 2002; **288**: 1252–1259.

34 Redfield MM, Rodeheffer RJ, Jacobsen SJ et al. Plasma brain natriuretic peptide to detect preclinical ventricular systolic or diastolic dysfunction: a community-based study. *Circulation* 2004; **109**: 3176–3181.

35 Costello-Boerrigter LC, Boerrigter G, Redfield MM et al. Amino-terminal pro-B-type natriuretic peptide and B-type natriuretic peptide in the general community: determinants and detection of left ventricular dysfunction. *J Am Coll Cardiol* 2006; **47**: 345–353.

36 Galasko GI, Barnes SC, Collinson P et al. What is the most cost-effective strategy to screen for left ventricular systolic dysfunction: natriuretic peptides, the electrocardiogram, hand-held echocardiography, traditional echocardiography, or their combination? *Eur Heart J* 2006; **27**: 193–200.

37 Coste J, Jourdain P, Pouchot J. A gray zone assigned to inconclusive results of quantitative diagnostic tests: Application to the use of brain natriuretic peptide for diagnosis of heart failure in acute dyspneic patients. *Clin Chem* 2006; **52**: 2229–2235.

38 Knudsen CW, Clopton P, Westheim A et al. Predictors of elevated B-type natriuretic peptide concentrations in dyspneic patients without heart failure: an analysis from the breathing not properly multinational study. *Ann Emerg Med* 2005; **45**: 573–580.

39 McCullough PA, Duc P, Omland T et al. B-type natriuretic peptide and renal function in the diagnosis of heart failure: an analysis from the Breathing Not Properly Multinational Study. *Am J Kidney Dis* 2003; **41**: 571–579.

40 Anwaruddin S, Lloyd-Jones DM, Baggish A et al. Renal function, congestive heart failure, and amino-terminal pro-brain natriuretic peptide measurement: results from the ProBNP Investigation of Dyspnea in the Emergency Department (PRIDE) Study. *J Am Coll Cardiol* 2006; **47**: 91–97.

41 Melanson SE, Laposata M, Camargo CA Jr et al. Combination of D-dimer and amino-terminal pro-B-type natriuretic peptide testing for the evaluation of dyspneic patients with and without acute pulmonary embolism. *Arch Pathol Lab Med* 2006; **130**: 1326–1329.

42 Nagaya N, Nishikimi T, Uematsu M et al. Plasma brain natriuretic peptide as a prognostic indicator in patients with primary pulmonary hypertension. *Circulation* 2000; **102**: 865–870.

43 Morello A, Lloyd-Jones DM, Chae CU et al. Association of atrial fibrillation and amino-terminal pro-brain natriuretic peptide concentrations in dyspneic subjects with and without acute heart failure: results from the ProBNP Investigation of Dyspnea in the Emergency Department (PRIDE) study. *Am Heart J* 2007; **153**: 90–97.

44 de Lemos JA, Morrow DA, Bentley JH et al. The prognostic value of B-type natriuretic peptide in patients with acute coronary syndromes. *N Engl J Med* 2001; **345**: 1014–1021.

45 James SK, Lindback J, Tilly J et al. Troponin-T and N-terminal pro-B-type natriuretic peptide predict mortality benefit from coronary revascularization in acute coronary syndromes: a GUSTO-IV substudy. *J Am Coll Cardiol* 2006; **48**: 1146–1154.

46 O'Donoghue M, Chen A, Baggish AL et al. The effects of ejection fraction on N-terminal ProBNP and BNP levels in patients with acute CHF: analysis from the ProBNP Investigation of Dyspnea in the Emergency Department (PRIDE) study. *J Card Fail* 2005; **11**: S9–S14.

47 Krauser DG, Lloyd-Jones DM, Chae CU et al. Effect of body mass index on natriuretic peptide levels in patients with acute congestive heart failure: a ProBNP Investigation of Dyspnea in the Emergency Department (PRIDE) substudy. *Am Heart J* 2005; **149**: 744–750.

48 Mehra MR, Uber PA, Park MH et al. Obesity and suppressed B-type natriuretic peptide levels in heart failure. *J Am Coll Cardiol* 2004; **43**: 1590–1595.

49 van Kimmenade RR, Pinto YM, Bayes-Genis A et al. Usefulness of intermediate amino-terminal pro-brain natriuretic peptide concentrations for diagnosis and prognosis of acute heart failure. *Am J Cardiol* 2006; **98**: 386–390.

50 Brenden CK, Hollander JE, Guss D et al. Gray zone BNP levels in heart failure patients in the emergency department: results from the Rapid Emergency Department Heart Failure Outpatient Trial (REDHOT) multicenter study. *Am Heart J* 2006; **151**: 1006–1011.

51 Yeo KT, Wu AH, Apple FS et al. Multicenter evaluation of the Roche NT-proBNP assay and comparison to the Biosite Triage BNP assay. *Clin Chim Acta* 2003; **338**: 107–115.

52 Goetze JP, Kastrup J, Rehfeld JF. The paradox of increased natriuretic hormones in congestive heart failure patients: does the endocrine heart also fail in heart failure? *Eur Heart J* 2003; **24**: 1471–1472.

53 Hawkridge AM, Heublein DM, Bergen HR et al. Quantitative mass spectral evidence for the absence of circulating brain natriuretic peptide (BNP-32) in severe human heart failure. *Proc Natl Acad Sci USA* 2005; **102**: 17442–17447.

54 Giuliani I, Rieunier F, Larue C. Assay for measurement of intact B-type natriuretic peptide prohormone in blood. *Clin Chem* 2006; **52**: 1054–1061.

55 Krauser DG, Chen AA, Tung R et al. Neither race nor gender influences the usefulness of amino-terminal pro-brain natriuretic peptide testing in dyspneic subjects: a ProBNP Investigation of Dyspnea in the Emergency Department (PRIDE) substudy. *J Card Fail* 2006; **12**: 452–457.

56 Chang AY, Abdullah SM, Jain T et al. Associations among androgens, estrogens, and natriuretic peptides in young women: observations from the Dallas Heart Study. *J Am Coll Cardiol* 2007; **49**: 109–116.

57 Sayama H, Nakamura Y, Saito N et al. Why is the concentration of plasma brain natriuretic peptide in elderly inpatients greater than normal? *Coron Artery Dis* 1999; **10**: 537–540.

58 Redfield MM, Rodeheffer RJ, Jacobsen SJ et al. Plasma brain natriuretic peptide concentration: impact of age and gender. *J Am Coll Cardiol* 2002; **40**: 976–982.

59 Wang TJ, Larson MG, Levy D et al. Impact of obesity on plasma natriuretic peptide levels. *Circulation* 2004; **109**: 594–600.

60 Das SR, Drazner MH, Dries DL et al. Impact of body mass and body composition on circulating levels of natriuretic peptides: results from the Dallas Heart Study. *Circulation* 2005; **112**: 2163–2168.

61 Taylor JA, Christenson RH, Rao K et al. B-type natriuretic peptide and N-terminal pro B-type natriuretic peptide are depressed in obesity despite higher left ventricular end diastolic pressures. *Am Heart J* 2006; **152**: 1071–1076.

62 Bayes-Genis A, Lloyd-Jones DM, van Kimmenade RR et al. Effect of body mass index on diagnostic and prognostic usefulness of amino-terminal pro-brain natriuretic peptide in patients with acute dyspnea. *Arch Intern Med* 2007; **167**: 400–407.

63 Takami Y, Horio T, Iwashima Y et al. Diagnostic and prognostic value of plasma brain natriuretic peptide in nondialysis-dependent CRF. *Am J Kidney Dis* 2004; **44**: 420–428.

64 DeFilippi CR, Fink JC, Nass CM. N-terminal pro-B-type natriuretic peptide for predicting coronary disease and left ventricular hypertrophy in asymptomatic CKD not requiring dialysis. *Am J Kidney Dis* 2005; **46**: 35–44.

65 Austin WJ, Bhalla V, Hernandez-Arce I et al. Correlation and prognostic utility of B-type natriuretic peptide and its amino-terminal fragment in patients with chronic kidney disease. *Am J Clin Pathol* 2006; **126**: 506–512.

66 Schou M, Dalsgaard MK, Clemmesen O et al. Kidneys extract BNP and NT-proBNP in healthy young men. *J Appl Physiol* 2005; **99**: 1676–1680.

Chapter 7

Biomarkers for risk stratification in patients with heart failure

W. H. Wilson Tang

Introduction

Biomarker evaluation has become increasingly useful in establishing the "phenotype" of patients with heart failure with respect to the prediction of their clinical courses (i.e., determination of risks of subsequent deterioration or the need for further intervention). In the clinical setting, biomarker evaluation provides a window into the disease mechanism(s) that drives clinical outcomes. However, few interventions have been rigorously tested using biomarkers as part of their indication or exclusion criteria.

This chapter discusses several cardiac-specific biomarkers as well as commonly used tests that may provide important prognostic information for patients with heart failure. A large body of literature on biomarkers is available demonstrating valuable prognostic information for patients with heart failure, but many such biomarkers are only available on a research basis (see Table 7.1 for a partial listing). Hence, this discussion will be restricted to biomarkers that can be assessed through commercial assays and laboratory tests readily available to practicing clinicians.

Cardiac-specific biomarkers for risk stratification
Natriuretic peptides
Natriuretic peptide testing has been extensively studied as an aid to the diagnosis of heart failure in the acute setting (see chapter 6). There is also a growing body of literature supporting the utility of natriuretic peptide testing for risk stratification across the spectrum of heart failure. (see Table 7.2)

Biomarkers in Heart Disease, 1st edition. Edited by James A. de Lemos.
© 2008 American Heart Association, ISBN: 978-1-4051-7571-5

Table 7.1 Selected research-based biochemical markers for risk stratification of heart failure reported in the literature.

Neurohormones
Catecholamines (norepinephrine, epinephrine)
Renin, angiotensin converting enzyme (ACE) activity, angiotensin II, aldosterone
A-type, C-type, N-terminal pro A-type, mid-regional pro A-type natriuretic peptides
Endothelin-1
Vasopressin/copeptin
Cardiotrophin-1
Adrenomedullin and mid-regional pro-adrenomedullin
Urotensin-II
Urocortin

Inflammatory biomarkers
Galectin-3
Soluble ST2 receptor
Tumor necrosis factor alpha (TNFα) and receptors
Interleukin-6 (IL-6)
Growth differentiation factor 15 (GDF-15)
Osteopontin

Metabolic biomarkers
Leptin
Adiponectin
Ghrelin
Insulin-like growth factor-1 (IGF-1)

Other Miscellaneous Biomarkers
G-Protein Coupled Receptor Kinase-2 (GRK-2)
Myotrophin
Apelin
Fatty acid binding protein

Natriuretic peptide testing in acute heart failure
The majority of studies have focused on admission levels of natriuretic peptides, largely because many observational series have test results available during the admission time frame. The largest study to date included a subset of 48,629 subjects enrolled in the Acute Decompensated Heart Failure National Registry (ADHERE) with B-type natriuretic peptide (BNP) levels evaluated within 24 hours of admission. There was a near-linear relationship between increasing quartiles of BNP and in-hospital mortality: 1.9% for BNP <430 pg/mL, 2.8% for BNP 430–839 pg/mL, 3.8% for BNP 840–1729 pg/mL, and 6.0% for BNP >1729 pg/mL (p < 0.0001, Fig. 7.1) [1]. Furthermore, increasing quartiles of BNP

Table 7.2 National Academy of Clinical Biochemistry Laboratory Medicine Practice Guidelines: Recommendations for Use of Biochemical Markers for Risk Stratification of Heart Failure [2].

Class IIa
- Blood BNP or NT-proBNP testing can provide a useful addition to clinical assessment in selected situations when additional risk stratification is required. (Level of Evidence: A)

- Serial blood BNP or NT-proBNP concentrations may be used to track changes in risk profiles and clinical status among patients with heart failure in selected situations where additional risk stratification is required. (Level of Evidence: B)

Class IIb
- Cardiac troponin testing can identify patients with heart failure at increased risk beyond the setting of acute coronary syndromes. (Level of Evidence: B)

Class III
- Routine blood biomarker testing for the sole purpose of risk stratification in patients with heart failure is not warranted. (Level of Evidence: B)

independently predicted mortality in patients with reduced and preserved systolic function.

Although a direct relationship between changes in natriuretic peptide levels and changes in hemodynamic [3] or volume status [4] cannot be precisely defined, changes in plasma levels of natriuretic peptides during treatment have been observed to track with risk of subsequent mortality after discharge and readmission. Plasma natriuretic peptide levels often fall rapidly following diuretic and vasoactive therapy in patients with decompensated heart failure, although these changes may vary widely [5]. Those who died or had to be readmitted within 30 days were more likely to have an increase in serial plasma BNP values, whereas those who did not experience adverse clinical events were more likely to have a downward trend in their serial plasma BNP values [6]. In a separate investigation in elderly patients, the poorest prognosis was observed in patients who did not achieve a reduction of at least 40% of their baseline BNP values (Hazard Ratio [HR] 4.03, 95% confidence interval [CI] 1.50–10.84) [7]. However, the frequency and range of changes in natriuretic peptide levels that would constitute clinical significance remains unclear, as extrapolations from optimal intervals and ranges have only been suggested for stable heart failure patients [8].

If plasma natriuretic peptide levels can predict long-term clinical outcomes, the ability to modulate plasma levels during hospital admission for decompensated heart failure may lead to better clinical outcomes. Logically, plasma natriuretic peptide levels drawn at the time of discharge provide important

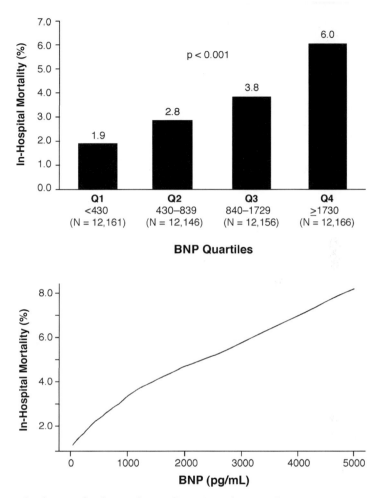

Fig. 7.1 Prediction of in-hospital mortality using admission B-type natriuretic peptide (BNP) levels in patients with acute decompensated heart failure across quartiles (*Upper panel*) and as continuous variable (*Lower panel*) in the Acute Decompensated Heart Failure National Registry (ADHERE). Adapted from [1].

information regarding the probability of rehospitalization in patients admitted for decompensated heart failure. This hypothesis has been tested in a study by Logeart and colleagues, who have demonstrated lower rates of rehospitalization in patients with lower predischarge plasma BNP levels compared to higher predischarge levels. In their study cohort, after adjustment for baseline covariables, the HRs were 5.1 [95% CI 2.8–9.1] for BNP levels 350–700 ng/L and 15.2 [95% CI 8.5–27] for BNP levels >700 ng/L, compared with BNP levels <350 ng/L (Fig. 7.2) [9]. These conclusions have been validated in subsequent

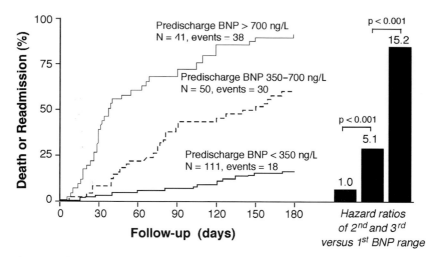

Fig. 7.2 Risk stratification of predischarge plasma B-type natriuretic peptide (BNP) levels and risk of readmissions following discharge for heart failure hospitalization. Adapted from [9].

studies in the general medical ward [10] and in the elderly population [11], where comorbidities and confounding factors may be more prevalent. Whether predischarge values can provide a stronger prognostic value than admission values remains highly debated.

Elevated natriuretic peptide levels may also signify adverse long-term consequences. In the 1-year follow-up of the PRIDE (ProBNP Investigation of Dyspnea in the Emergency Department) study, an aminoterminal proBNP (NT-proBNP) concentration >986 pg/mL at presentation was the single strongest predictor of 1-year mortality (HR 2.88, 95% CI 1.64–5.06, p < 0.001; Fig. 7.3), even independent of a diagnosis of heart failure [12].

Natriuretic peptide testing in chronic heart failure

The prognostic value of BNP, both baseline and serial measurements, consistently extends to the chronic heart failure population [13]. Studies have advocated the use of natriuretic peptide testing in patient selection for cardiac transplantation [14], implantation of cardiac defibrillators [15], and cardiac resynchronization therapy (as well as for tracking changes in clinical status) [16,17]. In direct comparative studies, some evidence suggests a slightly stronger prognostic value for NT-proBNP over BNP testing in predicting long-term outcomes [18]. However, generally speaking, for prognostic purposes all the natriuretic peptide assays have shown concordant results, and they are often used interchangeably.

Serial BNP or NT-proBNP concentrations may also be used to track changes in risk profiles and clinical status among patients with heart failure in selected

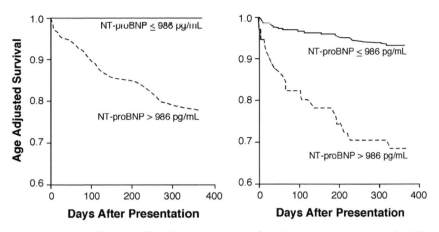

Fig. 7.3 Risk stratification of baseline aminoterminal pro-B-type natriuretic peptide (NT-proBNP) levels in patients with acute decompensated heart failure with (*Left panel*) and without (*Right panel*) a history of heart failure in the Pro-BNP Investigation of Dyspnea in the Emergency Department (PRIDE) study. Adapted from [12].

situations where additional risk stratification is required [13] (Fig. 7.4). However, the absolute values of the ranges in different risk strata reported in the literature vary considerably, depending on the patient population. Indeed, even when natriuretic peptide levels were intermediate in the diagnosis of heart failure, their long-term prognostic values remained robust [19]. Although natriuretic peptides may correlate with symptom status in the outpatient setting, in some cases they may not have a direct relationship with changes in health status [20].

Cardiac troponins

Detectable circulating cardiac troponin represents evidence of myocyte necrosis or injury. Apart from its primary role in defining acute coronary syndromes, there have been extensive investigations into the prognostic role of cardiac troponin levels in patients with heart failure.

Cardiac troponin testing in acute heart failure

In patients presenting with acute heart failure, cardiac troponin testing has been used as part of the clinical work-up to rule out myocardial ischemia as the primary etiology (refer to chapters 1 and 3). In decompensated states, some patients may present with transient or persistent elevation of serum cardiac troponin I (cTnI) or troponin T (cTnT) levels in the absence of any obvious myocardial ischemia, even in the absence of overt impairment of cardiac systolic function

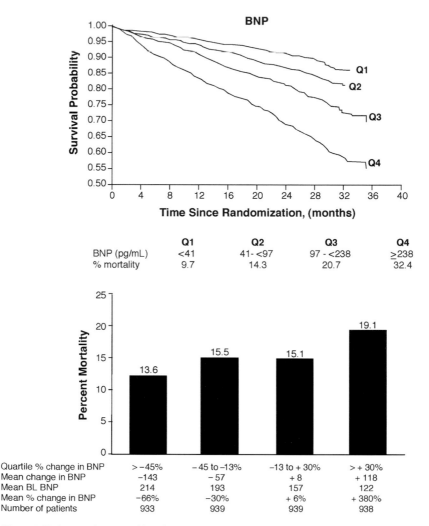

Fig. 7.4 Risk stratification of baseline B-type natriuretic peptide (BNP, *Upper panel*) and relative changes in serial (*Lower panel*) BNP levels in patients with chronic heart failure from the Valsartan in Heart Failure Trial (Val-HeFT). Adapted from [13].

[21]. Detectable cTnT or cTnI levels in this setting have been associated with poor long-term outcomes [22–24] (Fig. 7.5). Furthermore, persistently increased cTnT levels (>0.020 ng/mL) are predictive of higher rates of death and hospital readmission for decompensated heart failure, which may indicate ongoing myocardial damage [25,26].

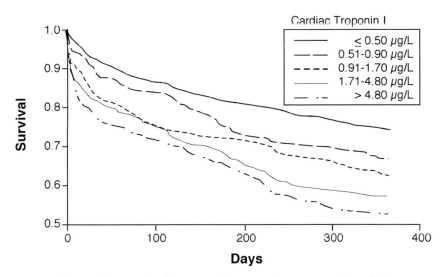

Fig. 7.5 Risk stratification of cardiac troponin I in acute decompensated heart failure across different cut-off values. Adapted from [24].

Cardiac troponin testing in chronic heart failure

In the setting of advanced heart failure, elevated serum troponin levels have been associated with poor long-term prognosis even following adjustment for BNP levels [27]. It is interesting to note that almost one-quarter of patients in the outpatient setting were found to have detectable cTnT levels, and about 17% had persistent elevation over 1 year—both had noticeably worse outcomes [26,28] (Fig. 7.6). However, the utility of routine assessment of serum troponin levels in patients with chronic heart failure remains to be determined.

Noncardiac biomarkers for risk stratification
Standard laboratory testing
Sodium

Serum sodium has long been recognized as an important prognostic marker in patients with heart failure due to its relation with volume homeostasis. Hyponatremia is often a manifestation of volume-overloaded state, whereas hypernatremia can be due to dehydration (such as overzealous diuresis or salt-wasting phenomenon). Both extremes are detrimental to long-term prognosis. Hyponatremia (<134 mEq/L), in particular, has shown to predict adverse outcomes [29]. In the OPTIME-CHF (Outcomes of a Prospective Trial of Intravenous Milrinone for Exacerbations of Chronic Heart Failure) study, every 3 mEq/L reduction in serum sodium on admission predicted a worse 60-day mortality (HR 1.18, 95% CI: 1.03–1.36, p = 0.018) [30]. This was evident in the highest quartile

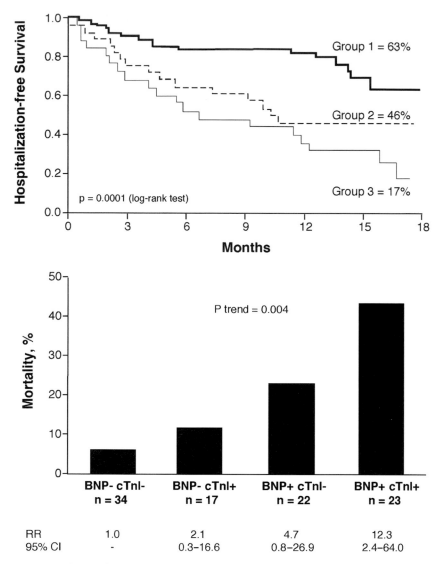

Fig. 7.6 Risk stratification using serial cardiac troponin T (cTnT) levels in chronic heart failure. *Upper panel:* Prognostic value according to persistent cTnT <0.02 ng/mL (Group 1), single cTnT ≥0.02 ng/mL (Group 2), or persistent cTnT ≥0.02 ng/mL (Group 3). Adapted from Perna et al. (25). *Lower panel:* Prognostic value in combination with plasma B-type natriuretic peptide (BNP) assessment. Cut-off values are above (+) or below (−) median levels (cTnI 0.04 ng/mL, Dade-Behring; BNP 485 pg/mL, Biosite). Adapted from [27].

($\leq$135 mEq/L), which had in-hospital mortality of 6%, 60-day mortality of 16%, and 60-day rehospitalization rate of 41% [30].

Blood urea nitrogen, creatinine, and cystatin C

Renal insufficiency has been shown repeatedly to be associated with heightened mortality risk in patients with chronic heart failure [31]. In the acute heart failure setting, worsening renal function often portends poorer survival. In the ADHERE registry, two of the three most important predictors for in-hospital mortality were blood urea nitrogen (BUN) and serum creatinine [32]. In particular, worsening renal function can predict both in-hospital mortality and length of stay, as even an increased creatinine of 0.1 mg/dL was associated with worse outcome [33]. The sensitivity for predicting death using changes in serum creatinine decreased from 92% to 65% as the threshold was raised from 0.1 to 0.5 mg/dL. At a threshold of a 0.3 mg/dL increase, sensitivity was 81% and specificity was 62% for death, and adding the requirement of final creatinine of $\geq$1.5 mg/dL provided improved specificity [32]. Most studies have identified a rise of 0.3–0.5 mg/dL in serum creatinine (occurring in about 30% of patients admitted for decompensated heart failure) as associated with poorer long-term prognosis [34].

Cystatin C is a low molecular weight cysteine protease inhibitor that is produced and released at a constant rate from all nucleated cells. Because cystatin C is freely filtered at the glomeruli and metabolized within the proximal tubules, cystatin C can provide sensitive estimation of renal function independent of body mass. Although cystatin C is available commercially in some laboratory platforms, availability is still limited. Nevertheless, the prognostic role of cystatin C in heart failure has been evaluated in the elderly population and in patients undergoing cardiac catheterization. In both cases, elevated cystatin C was found to be more closely associated with mortality than serum creatinine. Plasma cystatin C levels have also been found to predict long-term mortality in patients with heart failure in the setting of normal serum creatinine levels. Recent data from the Cardiovascular Health Study have suggested that cystatin C may predict increased risk of developing heart failure [35]. Cystatin C above-median (1.30 mg/L) was associated with a 3-fold increase in 1-year mortality risk (adjusted HR 3.2, 95% CI 2.0–5.3, p < 0.0001). In this study cohort, cystatin C levels during admission for decompensated heart failure may also provide important prognostic information even in patients with "normal" serum creatinine [36]. These effects were consistent across gender and age groups, and irrespective of heart failure etiology.

Total cholesterol

Patients with heart failure may have lower total cholesterol levels as their disease states advance (especially in cachectic states). Hence, it is still unclear whether low cholesterol levels signify poor metabolic states or whether other confounding factors may be influencing this relationship. Low total cholesterol levels as well as various lipoprotein levels have been associated with poorer long-term outcomes [37], while paradoxically statin therapy did not cause worse outcomes [38]. In the heart failure cohort derived from the Intermountain Heart Collaborative Study Registry (LVEF ≤40% or clinical diagnoses of heart failure, n = 1646), mortality was reduced for quartile 3 versus quartile 1 of total cholesterol (HR 0.66, p = 0.027). However, subanalysis found this association predominantly in patients who were using statin therapy (n = 848, death = 16.3%) [39]. Clearly, the relationship between cholesterol and heart failure outcomes is complex, and likely a risk marker rather than a risk factor.

Hemoglobin
Relatively mild degrees of anemia can be directly associated with worsening symptoms, lower functional status, and poorer survival as seen in the PRAISE (Prospective Randomized Amlodipine Survival Evaluation) trial database. It can be extrapolated that for each 1 g/dL decrease below 15 g/dL hemoglobin, there is about a 3–11% increase in mortality [40]. Lower hemoglobin was often associated with more impaired hemodynamic profile, higher blood urea nitrogen and creatinine, as well as lower albumin, total cholesterol, and body mass index. After adjusting for known heart failure prognostic factors, low hemoglobin remained an independent predictor of mortality (Fig. 7.7, relative risk 1.13, 95% CI 1.05–1.22, p < 0.01 for each decrease of 1 g/dL) [41]. In contrast, in 552 patients with new-onset heart failure, 18% of patients had hemoglobin levels <11.5 g/dL, but after adjustments for clinical variables, there was no independent association between baseline hemoglobin and survival [42].

Even in stable ambulatory patients with chronic heart failure, development of new onset anemia can be prevalent and associated with poor outcomes. In the COMET (Carvedilol or Metoprolol Evaluation Trial), incident (new-onset) anemia occurred at a rate of 14.2% at year 1 and 27.5% at year 5 of follow-up, particularly in those with advanced age and lower body mass index, higher diuretic dosage, higher creatinine and potassium levels, and lower serum sodium levels [43]. There is also evidence that the subjective experience of fatigue is associated with anemia even after adjusting for potential confounding factors, including NYHA class. Higher rates of hospitalization for heart failure and greater left ventricular mass index have also been associated with lower hemoglobin levels. Furthermore, lower hemoglobin levels have been associated with higher natriuretic peptide levels and renal impairment, whereas resolution of anemia has been associated with improvement in these abnormalities. Both systolic and diastolic heart failure have similar adverse long-term clinical outcomes, and the presence of anemia may even be associated with higher mortality rates in patients with diastolic heart failure.

Few studies have evaluated the prognostic impact of changes in hemoglobin levels on the natural history of heart failure, let alone the influence of heart

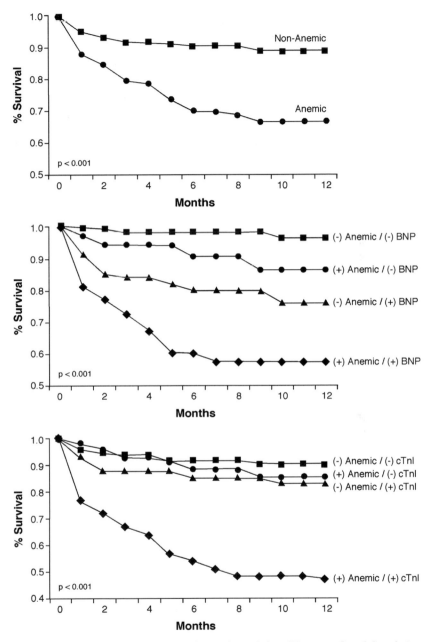

Fig. 7.7 Prognostic value of anemia in chronic heart failure (*Upper panel*) and the relationship between anemia, B-type natriuretic peptide (BNP), and cardiac troponin I (cTnI) in chronic heart failure (*Lower panel*). Cut-off values are median levels (cTnI: 0.04 ng/mL, Dade-Behring; BNP: 485 pg/mL, Biosite). Anemia was defined as hemoglobin <13 mg/dL (male) and <12 mg/dL (female). Adapted from Ralli et al. [44].

failure treatments on changes in hemoglobin levels and outcomes. In Val-HeFT (Valsartan in Heart Failure Trial), those in the quartile with the biggest decline in hemoglobin over 12 months had the greatest risk of subsequent hospitalization (HR 1.41, 95% CI 1.07–1.85, p = 0.014), morbid events (HR 1.47, 95% CI 1.18–1.84, p = 0.001), and death (HR 1.6, 95% CI 1.16–2.2, p = 0.004) compared with the quartile that exhibited the least change in hemoglobin over 12 months [45]. Furthermore, improvement in hemoglobin levels, regardless of the presence or absence of underlying anemia, was associated with lower mortality rates.

In addition, other hematologic parameters in the complete blood count may also provide prognostic information in patients with heart failure. For example, red cell distribution width (RDW, a measurement of the variability of red cell size) is a measure of nutritional deficiency affecting red blood cell production. Data derived from two separate chronic heart failure population (CHARM database and the Duke Databank) found RDW to be a relatively robust marker of long-term mortality in the heart failure population [46].

Inflammatory and oxidative stress biomarkers
Increasing data support a role for inflammation and oxidative stress in the pathophysiology of heart failure. However, ongoing attempts to characterize this "inflammatory phenotype" have been challenged by the lack of commercially available and specific immunoassays, as well as effective therapeutic strategies proven to be beneficial in their anti-inflammatory actions.

Leukocyte and lymphocyte counts
In a post hoc analysis of the Studies of Left Ventricular Dysfunction (SOLVD) study, subclinical inflammation has been associated with worsening heart failure outcomes [47]. In particular, after controlling for important covariates, each increase in leukocyte count of $1000/mm^3$ was significantly associated with an increased risk of all-cause mortality (HR 1.05, p < 0.001). However, this association was primarily found in patients with ischemic cardiomyopathy. Relative lymphocyte count has also emerged as an important prognostic factor influencing long-term outcomes [48–50].

Uric acid
Uric acid is a metabolic by-product of purine metabolism from xanthine oxidase activity, and may increase in the failing circulation because of increased generation, decreased excretion, or both. Xanthine oxidase generates reactive oxygen species, which likely contribute to tissue damage and disease progression. There has been a long-standing recognition that elevated serum uric acid is a marker of chronic inflammation [51], and may be associated with impaired diastolic performance [52], hemodynamic alterations [53], and poorer outcomes in both acute [54] and chronic heart failure settings [55]. Serum uric acid levels ≥565 μmol/L predicted mortality (HR 7.14; p < 0.0001), and appeared

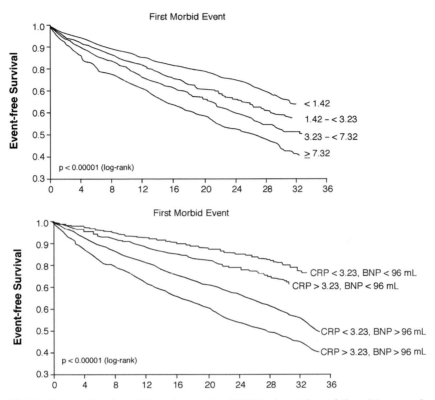

Fig. 7.8 Prognostic value of C-reactive protein (CRP) in chronic heart failure (*Upper panel*) and in combination with B-type natriuretic peptide (BNP, *Lower panel*) in the Valsartan in Heart Failure Trial (Val-HeFT). Adapted from [57].

synergistic with reduced left ventricular ejection fraction and peak ventilatory oxygen uptake in predicting 12-month mortality [55].

C-reactive protein
C-reactive protein, (CRP) a hepatocyte-derived inflammatory cytokine, is elevated in some patients with heart failure. Elevated CRP can portend poor outcomes in the setting of acute decompensated heart failure [56] as well as in chronic heart failure [57–59] (Fig. 7.8). Elevated CRP has also been associated with increased risk of developing incident heart failure [60]. In the Framingham Heart Study for elderly subjects without a history of myocardial infarction, a serum CRP level ≥ 5 mg/dL was associated with a 2.8-fold increased risk of heart failure (p = 0.02) [61]. Furthermore, in the dialysis population, persistently elevated CRP levels have been associated with cardiac hypertrophy and dysfunction [62]. Shah and colleagues reported the characteristics of CRP in a mixed

patient population referred for nonemergent cardiac catheterization (only 36% having a history of heart failure, with mean left ventricular ejection fraction 57 ±19%). In this series, patients with CRP > 3mg/L demonstrated a trend toward larger left atrial volume indices and a greater likelihood of diastolic dysfunction, although neither reached statistical significance [62]. However, Shah and colleagues reported a significant correlation between increased CRP levels and elevated left ventricular end-diastolic pressures (p = 0.0005) [63], and CRP levels have been reported to correlate with disease severity in patients with diastolic heart failure [64].

Myeloperoxidase
Myeloperoxidase (MPO) is a leukocyte-derived enzyme that can produce a cascade of reactive oxidative species, including hypochlorous acid and other reactive oxidant species, which may ultimately lead to lipid peroxidation, direct scavenging of nitric oxide, and nitric oxide synthase (NOS) inhibition. Plasma MPO testing has been approved for risk stratification for acute coronary syndromes (see chapter 5), and its prognostic value appeared synergistic with left ventricular ejection fraction in patients with a history of myocardial infarction [65]. Studies also suggest plasma MPO levels are elevated in patients with chronic systolic heart failure [66], and elevated MPO levels provide good diagnostic value in community-based screening for cardiac dysfunction [67]. In animal studies, preservation of left ventricular function has been observed in MPO-deficient mice following myocardial infarction [68], suggesting that MPO may provide a mechanistic link between inflammation, oxidant stress, and impaired cardiac remodeling. Plasma MPO levels were found to be higher in patients with more advanced HF as determined by detailed echocardiographic evaluation, and may provide prognostic value in predicting long-term clinical outcomes, even after adjustment for commonly used prognostic variables [69] (Fig. 7.9).

Current controversies

End-point selection: What justifies the "risk" to be stratified?
Although prediction of adverse clinical outcomes has been the primary strategy for investigators to demonstrate the clinical utility of a biomarker, few have been utilized in everyday clinical practice for this purpose. The main reason is that while distinguishing a patient's risk provides a snapshot, the assumption is that the natural history of disease progression will not be altered. Also, the "negative predictive value" of biomarkers in risk stratification has been less emphasized but may be clinically useful—the determination of a low-risk state is perhaps as important for patient reassurance and monitoring of clinical stability.

The possibility that changes in a specific biomarker can predict an event or a clinical condition is merely a direct association, and may not imply causality or

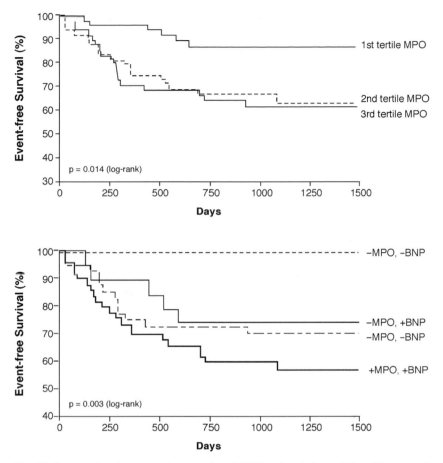

Fig. 7.9 Prognostic value of myeloperoxidase (MPO) in chronic heart failure (*Upper panel*) and in combination with B-type natriuretic peptide (BNP, *Lower panel*). Cut-offs are above (+) or below (−) levels (MPO: 271 pM, PrognostiX; BNP: 65 pg/mL, Christchurch research assay). Adapted from [69].

the possibility of reversal following an intervention. "Risk markers" are common, and can only be distinguished from a "risk factor" when specific treatments targeting the biomarker are available and can lead to alteration in the natural history of the condition. Even when such conditions are met, there is still no guarantee that the biomarker reflects the intended mechanistic insight. Therefore, even though "hard end-points" may provide an attractive splay of Kaplan-Meier curves, the true utility of a biomarker remains its ability to provide information for therapeutic decisions or interventions. Uric acid assessment is a good example—specifically, raising uric acid by direct infusion [70] or lowering uric acid by probenecid without altering the oxidative stress processes (or xanthine oxidase activity) [71] will not influence the underlying pathophysiology (and likely the long-term outcomes). The clinical utility of risk stratification therefore needs to be proven in contrast to simply establishing statistical significance.

Analysis selection: Is there adequate accounting for confounders?

As presented in this chapter, the large majority of clinical studies have provided their data in one of three ways—by illustrating a graded increase in risk of adverse outcomes via Kaplan-Meier curve analyses or by quantifying the event rates based on above or below cut-off values of one or several biomarkers with post hoc analyses. These techniques are often plagued with inherited biases, and may not illustrate potential confounding factors that contribute to the underlying differences between different cohorts. Multivariable analysis can only adjust variables that are known to be potential confounders. The true test of the clinical utility of the prognostic value still relies on the process of validation either in a different patient database or prospectively in illustrating the reliability of the prediction. Therefore, like any other areas of research, only consistency and concordance of results (such as in the case of natriuretic peptides and cardiac troponin) can build confidence in the findings and the conclusions.

Patient selection: Are the data generalizable in different populations?

Biomarker studies are often retrospective observational series or post hoc analyses of stored samples from large-scale clinical trials. Although efforts have been made to provide a mechanistic understanding of the pathophysiology of acute heart failure, the majority of biomarker-based studies have been performed in the chronic heart failure population. Only in rare cases was prospective collection with assessment of outcomes conducted, and even less often in randomized controlled trials. Many of these data are aggregated, and the subjects included are largely restricted to those who fulfilled the clinical trial inclusion/exclusion criteria. This means that in a large majority of cases, a biomarker's ability to stratify short- and long-term risks may differ in the broader range of patients seen in clinical practices. The applicability of a specific biomarker to different patient populations can only become a reality when the assay is commercially available so that their diagnostic and prognostic abilities can be tested. So far, the prognostic value of natriuretic peptide testing has been consistent, but the diagnostic ranges and test intervals are still debated for specific purposes. Even in situations where confounding factors may influence the absolute values of the assay (such as in the setting of obesity), the prognostic value of natriuretic peptide testing remained robust [72].

Assay selection: Are all assays created equal?

The greater technical challenge is reproducibility of results, which requires harmonization of assays developed in different diagnostic assay platforms.

Research-based assays often have very different diagnostic accuracies and inter-/intra-assay variabilities compared with commercially available assays, and different sample collection and processing procedures may influence some assays. Moreover, assay development may yield changes over time. For example, different generations of cardiac troponin assays have yielded different value ranges and perhaps different insights. In fact, with the highest sensitivity of the latest generation, the majority of patients with chronic heart failure have detectable cardiac troponin I levels.

In the case of natriuretic peptide assessment, the three different assays commercially available may have a 10–25% difference in their reported absolute values. Many of the earlier works in natriuretic peptides utilized the Shionogi assay or the Christchurch assay, which have different absolute values based on different antibodies and techniques used. Furthermore, there is no direct conversion between BNP and NT-proBNP levels when tested in different situations. In the overall scheme of risk stratification and global assessment of biomarker levels, resolving difficulties in establishing agreement among laboratory specialists and clinicians regarding who has high, intermediate, or low risk is paramount.

Another challenge in interpreting the prognostic value of a specific biomarker is assessing its contribution relative to other existing or cardiac-specific biomarkers. Although many clinical biomarkers carry prognostic value when analyzed alone, the relative contributions of biomarkers may differ, sometimes being synergistic and sometimes not [44]. One interesting example comes from a direct comparison between the prognostic value of admission NT-proBNP and BUN in a cohort of patients admitted for decompensated heart failure [73]. In multivariate regression analysis, the predictive values of BUN and NT-pro-BNP were very similar: the hazard ratio for NT-pro-BNP greater than the median was 1.81 (95% CI, 1.02–3.23, $p = 0.044$), and the hazard ratio for BUN greater than the median was 1.83 (95% CI, 1.03–3.24, $p = 0.039$), but analysis of the associations between NT-pro-BNP, BUN, and 30-day death or readmission revealed that BUN was a better predictor of outcomes (HR 3.15, 95% CI 1.29–7.66, $p = 0.012$) than NT-pro-BNP (HR 1.44, 95% CI 0.62–3.39, $p = 0.399$), consistent with findings from the ADHERE registry [32]. This came in direct contrast to other studies illustrating that the combination of NT-proBNP with measures of renal function better predicts short-term outcome in acute heart failure than either parameter alone [74]. Therefore, despite the abundance of literature on this topic, routine assessment of specific cardiac biomarkers in combination with standard measures for risk stratification still needs further refinement.

Conclusions

Until the past decade, clinical monitoring and management of patients with heart failure have relied heavily on physical evaluation and physiologic measurements, coupled with clinical acumen, in order to determine the likelihood that patients may do well or do poorly. Some drugs are used to relieve symptoms, yet many life-saving therapies are given in a "one-size-fits-all" approach. The emergence of biomarkers provides a new dimension in assessing the severity and progression of the underlying disease state. The ultimate "holy grail" for heart failure biomarkers is to identify one that can define the disease. Most likely, the same biomarker would also provide important prognostic information of the disease state, as it would likely be involved in the pathophysiologic process as a mediator or an end product. However, the most important aspect for risk stratification is the ability of biomarkers to determine who would benefit from an intervention. In the case of cardiac troponin, an elevated cTnT or cTnI defines the presence of acute coronary syndrome and myocardial infarction, and further defines which patients may need specific interventions (e.g., prompt invasive coronary evaluation or the use of glycoprotein IIb/IIIa antagonists during coronary stenting).

At present, there is still no biomarker in acute and chronic heart failure that fulfills all of these roles, although natriuretic peptide and cardiac troponin testing hold promise. However, many of the controversies surrounding the use of biomarkers for risk stratification in heart failure are not unique to the heart failure population. The latest guidelines have suggested their user in selected cases where risk stratification can be helpful [74]. Nevertheless, it is still necessary to define the prognostic value of a specific biomarker test in terms of its ability not only to predict the probability of a future clinical event, but to add to clinical decision making in managing heart failure.

Acknowledgments

I would like to thank Kevin Shrestha for his editorial assistance with the manuscript.

Dr Tang has previously served as consultant for Biosite Diagnostics, Inc., and has received research support from Abbott Diagnostics, Inc.

References

1 Fonarow GC, Peacock WF, Phillips CO, Givertz MM, Lopatin M. Admission B-type natriuretic peptide levels and in-hospital mortality in acute decompensated heart failure. *J Am Coll Cardiol* 2007; **49**: 1943–1950.

2 Tang WH, Francis GS, Morrow DA, Newby LK, Canon CP, Jesse RL et al. National Academy of Clinical Biochemistry Laboratory Medicine Practice Guidelines: Clinical Utilization of Cardiac Biomarker Testing in Heart Failure. *Circulation* 2007; **116**: e99–109.

3 O'Neill JO, Bott-Silverman CE, McRae AT, 3rd, Troughton RW, Ng K, Starling RC et al. B-type natriuretic peptide levels are not a surrogate marker for invasive hemodynamics during management of patients with severe heart failure. *Am Heart J* 2005; **149**: 363–369.

4 James KB, Troughton RW, Feldschuh J, Soltis D, Thomas D, Fouad-Tarazi F. Blood volume and brain natriuretic peptide in congestive heart failure: a pilot study. *Am Heart J* 2005; **150**: 984.

5 Kazanegra R, Cheng V, Garcia A, Krishnaswamy P, Gardetto N, Clopton P et al. A rapid test for B-type natriuretic peptide correlates with falling wedge pressures in patients treated for decompensated heart failure: a pilot study. *J Card Fail* 2001; **7**: 21–29.

6 Cheng V, Kazanagra R, Garcia A, Lenert L, Krishnaswamy P, Gardetto N et al. A rapid bedside test for B-type peptide predicts treatment outcomes in patients admitted for decompensated heart failure: a pilot study. *J Am Coll Cardiol* 2001; **37**: 386–391.

7 Cournot M, Leprince P, Destrac S, Ferrieres J. Usefulness of in-hospital change in B-type natriuretic peptide levels in predicting long-term outcome in elderly patients admitted for decompensated heart failure. *Am J Geriatr Cardiol* 2007; **16**: 8–14.

8 Wu AH, Smith A, Apple FS. Optimum blood collection intervals for B-type natriuretic peptide testing in patients with heart failure. *Am J Cardiol* 2004; **93**: 1562–1563.

9 Logeart D, Thabut G, Jourdain P, Chavelas C, Beyne P, Beauvais F et al. Predischarge B-type natriuretic peptide assay for identifying patients at high risk of re-admission after decompensated heart failure. *J Am Coll Cardiol* 2004; **43**: 635–641.

10 Verdiani V, Nozzoli C, Bacci F, Cecchin A, Rutili MS, Paladini S et al. Pre-discharge B-type natriuretic peptide predicts early recurrence of decompensated heart failure in patients admitted to a general medical unit. *Eur J Heart Fail* 2005; **7**: 566–571.

11 Valle R, Prevaldi C, D'Eri A, Fontebasso A, Giovinazzo P, Noventa F et al. B-type natriuretic peptide predicts postdischarge prognosis in elderly patients admitted due to cardiogenic pulmonary edema. *Am J Geriatr Cardiol* 2006; **15**: 202–207.

12 Januzzi JL, Jr., Sakhuja R, O'Donoghue M, Baggish AL, Anwaruddin S, Chae CU et al. Utility of amino-terminal pro-brain natriuretic peptide testing for prediction of 1-year mortality in patients with dyspnea treated in the emergency department. *Arch Intern Med* 2006; **166**: 315–320.

13 Anand IS, Fisher LD, Chiang YT, Latini R, Masson S, Maggioni AP et al. Changes in brain natriuretic peptide and norepinephrine over time and mortality and morbidity in the Valsartan Heart Failure Trial (Val-HeFT). *Circulation* 2003; **107**: 1278–1283.

14 Gardner RS, Ozalp F, Murday AJ, Robb SD, McDonagh TA. N-terminal pro-brain natriuretic peptide. A new gold standard in predicting mortality in patients with advanced heart failure. *Eur Heart J* 2003; **24**: 1735–1743.

15 Verma A, Kilicaslan F, Martin DO, Minor S, Starling R, Marrouche NF et al. Preimplantation B-type natriuretic peptide concentration is an independent predictor of future appropriate implantable defibrillator therapies. *Heart* 2006; **92**: 190–195.

16 Pitzalis MV, Iacoviello M, Di Serio F, Romito R, Guida P, De Tommasi E et al. Prognostic value of brain natriuretic peptide in the management of patients receiving cardiac resynchronization therapy. *Eur J Heart Fail* 2006; **8**: 509–514.

17 Yu CM, Fung JW, Zhang Q, Chan CK, Chan I, Chan YS et al. Improvement of serum NT-ProBNP predicts improvement in cardiac function and favorable prognosis after cardiac resynchronization therapy for heart failure. *J Card Fail* 2005; **11**: S42–46.

18 Masson S, Latini R, Anand IS, Vago T, Angelici L, Barlera S et al. Direct comparison of B-type natriuretic peptide (BNP) and amino-terminal proBNP in a large population of patients with chronic and symptomatic heart failure: the Valsartan Heart Failure (Val-HeFT) data. *Clin Chem* 2006; **52**: 1528–1538.

19 van Kimmenade RR, Pinto YM, Bayes-Genis A, Lainchbury JG, Richards AM, Januzzi JL, Jr. Usefulness of intermediate amino-terminal pro-brain natriuretic peptide concentrations for diagnosis and prognosis of acute heart failure. *Am J Cardiol* 2006; **98**: 386–390.

20 Luther SA, McCullough PA, Havranek EP, Rumsfeld JS, Jones PG, Heidenreich PA et al. The relationship between B-type natriuretic peptide and health status in patients with heart failure. *J Card Fail* 2005; **11**: 414–421.

21 Macin SM, Perna ER, Cimbaro Canella JP, Augier N, Riera Stival JL, Cialzeta J et al. Increased levels of cardiac troponin-T in outpatients with heart failure and preserved systolic function are related to adverse clinical findings and outcome. *Coron Artery Dis* 2006; **17**: 685–691.

22 Gattis WA, O'Connor CM, Hasselblad V, Adams KF, Jr., Kobrin I, Gheorghiade M. Usefulness of an elevated troponin-I in predicting clinical events in patients admitted with acute heart failure and acute coronary syndrome (from the RITZ-4 trial). *Am J Cardiol* 2004; **93**: 1436–1437, A10.

23 Missov E, Mair J. A novel biochemical approach to congestive heart failure: cardiac troponin T. *Am Heart J* 1999; **138**: 95–99.

24 You JJ, Austin PC, Alter DA, Ko DT, Tu JV. Relation between cardiac troponin I and mortality in acute decompensated heart failure. *Am Heart J* 2007; **153**: 462–470.

25 Del Carlo CH, Pereira-Barretto AC, Cassaro-Strunz C, Latorre Mdo R, Ramires JA. Serial measure of cardiac troponin T levels for prediction of clinical events in decompensated heart failure. *J Card Fail* 2004; **10**: 43–48.

26 Perna ER, Macin SM, Canella JP, Augier N, Stival JL, Cialzeta JR et al. Ongoing myocardial injury in stable severe heart failure: value of cardiac troponin T monitoring for high-risk patient identification. *Circulation* 2004; **110**: 2376–2382.

27 Horwich TB, Patel J, MacLellan WR, Fonarow GC. Cardiac troponin I is associated with impaired hemodynamics, progressive left ventricular dysfunction, and increased mortality rates in advanced heart failure. *Circulation* 2003; **108**: 833–838.

28 Hudson MP, O'Connor CM, Gattis WA, Tasissa G, Hasselblad V, Holleman CM et al. Implications of elevated cardiac troponin T in ambulatory patients with heart failure: a prospective analysis. *Am Heart J* 2004; **147**: 546–552.

29 Packer M, Lee WH, Kessler PD, Medina N, Yushak M, Gottlieb SS. Identification of hyponatremia as a risk factor for the development of functional renal insufficiency during converting enzyme inhibition in severe chronic heart failure. *J Am Coll Cardiol* 1987; **10**: 837–844.

30 Klein L, O'Connor CM, Leimberger JD, Gattis-Stough W, Pina IL, Felker GM et al. Lower serum sodium is associated with increased short-term mortality in hospitalized patients with worsening heart failure: results from the Outcomes of a Prospective Trial of Intravenous Milrinone for Exacerbations of Chronic Heart Failure (OPTIME-CHF) study. *Circulation* 2005; **111**: 2454–2460.

31 Hindnavis V, Tang WH. Current and novel pharmacological approaches to renal insufficiency in heart failure. Minerva *Cardioangiol* 2006; **54**: 753–762.

32 Fonarow GC, Adams KF, Jr., Abraham WT, Yancy CW, Boscardin WJ. Risk stratification for in-hospital mortality in acutely decompensated heart failure: classification and regression tree analysis. *JAMA* 2005; **293**: 572–580.

33 Gottlieb SS, Abraham W, Butler J, Forman DE, Loh E, Massie BM et al. The prognostic importance of different definitions of worsening renal function in congestive heart failure. *J Card Fail* 2002; **8**: 136–141.

34 Forman DE, Butler J, Wang Y, Abraham WT, O'Connor CM, Gottlieb SS et al. Incidence, predictors at admission, and impact of worsening renal function among patients hospitalized with heart failure. *J Am Coll Cardiol* 2004; **43**: 61–67.

35 Sarnak MJ, Katz R, Stehman-Breen CO, Fried LF, Jenny NS, Psaty BM et al. Cystatin C concentration as a risk factor for heart failure in older adults. *Ann Intern Med* 2005; **142**: 497–505.

36 Lassus J, Harjola VP, Sund R, Siirila-Waris K, Melin J, Peuhkurinen K et al. Prognostic value of cystatin C in acute heart failure in relation to other markers of renal function and NT-proBNP. *Eur Heart J* 2007; **15**: 1841–1847.

37 Horwich TB, Hamilton MA, Maclellan WR, Fonarow GC. Low serum total cholesterol is associated with marked increase in mortality in advanced heart failure. *J Card Fail* 2002; **8**: 216–224.

38 Horwich TB, MacLellan WR, Fonarow GC. Statin therapy is associated with improved survival in ischemic and non-ischemic heart failure. *J Am Coll Cardiol* 2004; **43**: 642–648.

39 May HT, Muhlestein JB, Carlquist JF, Horne BD, Bair TL, Campbell BA et al. Relation of serum total cholesterol, C-reactive protein levels, and statin therapy to survival in heart failure. *Am J Cardiol* 2006; **98**: 653–658.

40 Mozaffarian D, Nye R, Levy WC. Anemia predicts mortality in severe heart failure: the prospective randomized amlodipine survival evaluation (PRAISE). *J Am Coll Cardiol* 2003; **41**: 1933–1939.

41 Horwich TB, Fonarow GC, Hamilton MA, MacLellan WR, Borenstein J. Anemia is associated with worse symptoms, greater impairment in functional capacity and a significant increase in mortality in patients with advanced heart failure. *J Am Coll Cardiol* 2002; **39**: 1780–1786.

42 Kalra PR, Collier T, Cowie MR, Fox KF, Wood DA, Poole-Wilson PA et al. Haemoglobin concentration and prognosis in new cases of heart failure. *Lancet* 2003; **362**: 211–212.

43 Komajda M, Anker SD, Charlesworth A, Okonko D, Metra M, Di Lenarda A et al. The impact of new onset anaemia on morbidity and mortality in chronic heart failure: results from COMET. *Eur Heart J* 2006; **27**: 1440–1446.

44 Ralli S, Horwich TB, Fonarow GC. Relationship between anemia, cardiac troponin I, and B-type natriuretic peptide levels and mortality in patients with advanced heart failure. *Am Heart J* 2005; **150**: 1220–1227.

45 Anand IS, Kuskowski MA, Rector TS, Florea VG, Glazer RD, Hester A et al. Anemia and change in hemoglobin over time related to mortality and morbidity in patients with chronic heart failure: results from Val-HeFT. *Circulation* 2005; **112**: 1121–1127.

46 Allen LA, Felker GM, Pocock SJ, Shaw LK, McMurray JJV, Pfeffer MA et al. Red Cell Distribution Width as a Novel Prognostic Marker in Heart Failure: Data From the CHARM Program and the Duke Databank [Abstract 835-6]. *J Am Coll Cardiol* 2007; **49**: 88A.

47 Cooper HA, Exner DV, Waclawiw MA, Domanski MJ. White blood cell count and mortality in patients with ischemic and nonischemic left ventricular systolic dysfunction (an analysis of the Studies Of Left Ventricular Dysfunction [SOLVD]). *Am J Cardiol* 1999; **84**: 252–257.

48 Acanfora D, Gheorghiade M, Trojano L, Furgi G, Pasini E, Picone C et al. Relative lymphocyte count: a prognostic indicator of mortality in elderly patients with congestive heart failure. *Am Heart J* 2001; **142**: 167–173.

49 Ommen SR, Hodge DO, Rodeheffer RJ, McGregor CG, Thomson SP, Gibbons RJ. Predictive power of the relative lymphocyte concentration in patients with advanced heart failure. *Circulation* 1998; **97**: 19–22.

50 Huehnergarth KV, Mozaffarian D, Sullivan MD, Crane BA, Wilkinson CW, Lawler RL et al. Usefulness of relative lymphocyte count as an independent predictor of death/urgent transplant in heart failure. *Am J Cardiol* 2005; **95**: 1492–1495.

51 Leyva F, Anker SD, Godsland IF, Teixeira M, Hellewell PG, Kox WJ et al. Uric acid in chronic heart failure: a marker of chronic inflammation. *Eur Heart J* 1998; **19**: 1814–1822.

52 Cicoira M, Zanolla L, Rossi A, Golia G, Franceschini L, Brighetti G et al. Elevated serum uric acid levels are associated with diastolic dysfunction in patients with dilated cardiomyopathy. *Am Heart J* 2002; **143**: 1107–1111.

53 Kittleson MM, St John ME, Bead V, Champion HC, Kasper EK, Russell SD et al. Increased levels of uric acid predict haemodynamic compromise in patients with heart failure independently of B-type natriuretic peptide levels. *Heart* 2007; **93**: 365–367.

54 Cengel A, Turkoglu S, Turfan M, Boyaci B. Serum uric acid levels as a predictor of in-hospital death in patients hospitalized for decompensated heart failure. *Acta Cardiol* 2005; **60**: 489–492.

55 Anker SD, Doehner W, Rauchhaus M, Sharma R, Francis D, Knosalla C et al. Uric acid and survival in chronic heart failure: validation and application in metabolic, functional, and hemodynamic staging. *Circulation* 2003; **107**: 1991–1997.

56 Mueller C, Laule-Kilian K, Christ A, Brunner-La Rocca HP, Perruchoud AP. Inflammation and long-term mortality in acute congestive heart failure. *Am Heart J* 2006; **151**: 845–850.

57 Anand IS, Latini R, Florea VG, Kuskowski MA, Rector T, Masson S et al. C-reactive protein in heart failure: prognostic value and the effect of valsartan. *Circulation* 2005; **112**: 1428–1434.

58 Windram JD, Loh PH, Rigby AS, Hanning I, Clark AL, Cleland JG. Relationship of high-sensitivity C-reactive protein to prognosis and other prognostic markers in outpatients with heart failure. *Am Heart J* 2007; **153**: 1048–1055.

59 Ronnow BS, Reyna SP, Muhlestein JB, Horne BD, Allen Maycock CA, Bair TL et al. C-reactive protein predicts death in patients with non-ischemic cardiomyopathy. *Cardiology* 2005; **104**: 196–201.

60 Kardys I, Knetsch AM, Bleumink GS, Deckers JW, Hofman A, Stricker BH et al. C-reactive protein and risk of heart failure. The Rotterdam Study. *Am Heart J* 2006; **152**: 514–520.

61 Vasan RS, Sullivan LM, Roubenoff R, Dinarello CA, Harris T, Benjamin EJ et al. Inflammatory markers and risk of heart failure in elderly subjects without prior myocardial infarction: the Framingham Heart Study. *Circulation* 2003; **107**: 1486–1491.

62 Kim BS, Jeon DS, Shin MJ, Kim YO, Song HC, Lee SH et al. Persistent elevation of C-reactive protein may predict cardiac hypertrophy and dysfunction in patients maintained on hemodialysis. *Am J Nephrol* 2005; **25**: 189–195.

63 Shah SJ, Marcus GM, Gerber II, McKeown BH, Vessey JC, Jordan MV et al. High sensitivity C-reactive protein and parameters of left ventricular dysfunction. *J Card Fail* 2006; **12**: 61–65.

64 Michowitz Y, Arbel Y, Wexler D, Sheps D, Rogowski O, Shapira I et al. Predictive value of high sensitivity CRP in patients with diastolic heart failure. *Int J Cardiol* 2007; Apr 27; doi: 10.1016/j.ijcard.2007.02.037.

65 Mocatta TJ, Pilbrow AP, Cameron VA, Senthilmohan R, Frampton CM, Richards AM et al. Plasma concentrations of myeloperoxidase predict mortality after myocardial infarction. *J Am Coll Cardiol* 2007; **49**: 1993–2000.

66 Tang WH, Brennan ML, Philip K, Tong W, Mann S, Van Lente F et al. Plasma myeloperoxidase levels in patients with chronic heart failure. *Am J Cardiol* 2006; **98**: 796–799.

67 Ng LL, Pathik B, Loke IW, Squire IB, Davies JE. Myeloperoxidase and C-reactive protein augment the specificity of B-type natriuretic peptide in community screening for systolic heart failure. *Am Heart J* 2006; **152**: 94–101.

68 Askari AT, Brennan ML, Zhou X, Drinko J, Morehead A, Thomas JD et al. Myeloperoxidase and plasminogen activator inhibitor 1 play a central role in ventricular remodeling after myocardial infarction. *J Exp Med* 2003; **197**: 615–624.

69 Tang WH, Tong W, Troughton RW, Martin MG, Shrestha K, Borowski A et al. Prognostic value and echocardiographic determinants of plasma myeloperoxidase levels in chronic heart failure. *J Am Coll Cardiol* 2007; **49**: 2364–2370.

70 Waring WS, Adwani SH, Breukels O, Webb DJ, Maxwell SR. Hyperuricaemia does not impair cardiovascular function in healthy adults. *Heart* 2004; **90**: 155–159.

71 George J, Carr E, Davies J, Belch JJ, Struthers A. High-dose allopurinol improves endothelial function by profoundly reducing vascular oxidative stress and not by lowering uric acid. *Circulation* 2006; **114**: 2508–2516.

72 Horwich TB, Hamilton MA, Fonarow GC. B-type natriuretic peptide levels in obese patients with advanced heart failure. *J Am Coll Cardiol* 2006; **47**: 85–90.

73 Shenkman HJ, Zareba W, Bisognano JD. Comparison of prognostic significance of amino-terminal pro-brain natriuretic Peptide versus blood urea nitrogen for predicting events in patients hospitalized for heart failure. *Am J Cardiol* 2007; **99**: 1143–1145.

74 van Kimmenade RR, Januzzi JL, Jr., Baggish AL, Lainchbury JG, Bayes-Genis A, Richards AM et al. Amino-terminal pro-brain natriuretic Peptide, renal function, and outcomes in acute heart failure: redefining the cardiorenal interaction? *J Am Coll Cardiol* 2006; **48**: 1621–1627.

Chapter 8

Natriuretic peptides for disease monitoring in patients with chronic heart failure

Richard W. Troughton and A. Mark Richards

Rationale for monitoring clinical status and guiding therapy with BNP/NT-ProBNP

Optimizing medical therapy for individual patients remains one of the major challenges of heart failure (HF) management [1]. Guidelines recommend titrating proven therapies, including angiotensin converting enzyme (ACE)-inhibitors and beta blockers, to doses achieved in landmark studies [2]. Adherence to these targets is associated with improved outcomes in clinical trials and in observational studies [3,4], but for a variety of reasons adherence to guidelines and use of effective medications at optimal doses is frequently not achieved in real-world populations [2,5–8]. One contributing reason is the lack of a validated objective marker to guide optimal drug dosing for individual patients [9]. In particular, there is no guide to optimal diuretic therapy. As a result, some high-risk patients may receive suboptimal treatment, while others may be overtreated particularly with loop diuretics [10]. There is an acknowledged need for effective heart failure monitoring strategies but, as yet, no agreement about the best method [1,11,12]. In most settings clinical status is monitored primarily by gross indicators, like weight and physical examination. Although some physical examination findings have prognostic value, they do not accurately reflect central hemodynamic disturbance or cardiac dysfunction [13,14]. Symptom self-reporting, 6-minute walk, or echocardiography with assessment of left ventricular (LV) filling pressures could all be used in combination with regular clinical assessment, but each has limitations, particularly with regard to resource constraints, and none is validated for routine monitoring [1,2]. Implantable hemodynamic monitoring systems may soon be available, but none are currently

Biomarkers in Heart Disease, 1st edition. Edited by James A. de Lemos.
© 2008 American Heart Association, ISBN: 978-1-4051-7571-5

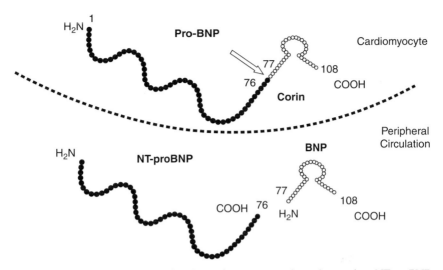

Fig. 8.1 Pro-BNP synthesized within the cardiomyocyte is cleaved to produce NT-proBNP and BNP, which are the major molecular forms secreted into the circulation. Adapted from [26] with permission.

approved and only a small proportion of patients are likely to be eligible for these devices [15,16].

In contrast, biomarkers now play a pivotal role in the management of cardiovascular diseases and guide treatment of many conditions [17]. Obvious examples are LDL cholesterol as a target in hyperlipidemia, or plasma glucose in diabetes mellitus. Troponin elevation may also guide early intervention in the acute coronary syndrome context. For chronic heart failure, the B-type natriuretic peptides stand out as potential biomarkers for monitoring and optimizing heart failure therapy. They are established diagnostic markers for HF—now endorsed in all heart failure guidelines—and powerful markers of cardiac dysfunction and prognosis [18–21].

The **B-type natriuretic peptides** are secreted predominantly from cardiac myocytes and the major source is the LV, although significant atrial and right ventricular secretion may occur in advanced heart failure [22]. Synthesis of the BNP prohormone (proBNP, 1-108aa) is stimulated primarily by cardiomyocyte stretch (Fig. 8.1) [23–25] but also is modulated by many factors including ischemia and neurohumoral activation. Proteolytic cleavage of proBNP, largely within the myocytes, produces 2 major circulating molecular forms, the bioactive BNP (77-108) and its corresponding amino-terminal component, NT-proBNP (1-76) that are secreted in a 1:1 ratio and can be detected in the peripheral circulation [24,26]. BNP has a shorter half-life due to active clearance by neutral endopeptidase and natriuretic peptide C-type receptors. Levels of the more stable NT-proBNP are therefore higher than BNP by a factor of 5–10-fold [27]. Plasma levels increase with higher LV pressure or with volume loading and reflect the severity of LV dysfunction, correlating inversely with LV ejection fraction and positively with indices of LV mass and filling pressure [24,28]. Higher levels are seen with increasing severity of symptomatic impairment and cardiac dysfunction [29].

Wide variation in BNP and NT-proBNP levels occurs among patients with stable symptomatic HF despite similar severity of cardiac dysfunction [22,30,31]. Levels of both peptides are higher in women, lower in obese subjects, and increase with age, renal dysfunction, and atrial fibrillation [31–34]. In renal dysfunction reduced renal clearance is a factor as the transcardiac gradient is similar in patients with impaired versus those with normal renal function [31]. LV diastolic function, RV systolic function, and mitral regurgitation are also important determinants of BNP levels, presumably reflecting left atrial and RV production in more advanced HF [22]. The majority of interindividual variation in peptide levels is explained by differences in LV systolic and diastolic function, RV function, renal function, and age [22]. Hereditary factors may contribute to a proportion of residual variation in BNP levels [35]. The relationship of BNP/NT-proBNP levels to many indices of cardiac and end organ dysfunction mean that they act as a marker of global status, rather than as indicators of a single cardiac parameter, such as left atrial pressure. Appropriate evaluation of BNP/NT-proBNP levels therefore depends on careful interpretation in the context of all the factors that influence levels [36]. Greater understanding of the factors influencing BNP and NT-proBNP levels has led to use of more appropriate cut-point levels for accurate HF diagnosis, depending on age and other factors [37]. These factors should also inform the choice of appropriate cut-points or targets for monitoring and guiding treatment.

Potential roles for BNP/NT-ProBNP in monitoring and guiding treatment of heart failure

BNP/NT-ProBNP as a marker of hemodynamic indices

In stable patients with cardiovascular disease, BNP and NT-ProBNP levels correlate positively with indices of LV filling pressure at the time of routine cardiac catheterization [38]. In acute decompensated HF, improvements in clinical status, LV filling pressure, cardiac output, and systemic vascular resistance are usually accompanied by concordant falls in BNP or NT-proBNP levels [39–41]. However, in acute HF, *absolute* levels of BNP or NT-proBNP do not appear to correlate strongly with hemodynamic indices either at baseline or after treatment [39–41]. This finding suggests that threshold BNP or NT-proBNP values may provide limited hemodynamic information. In contrast, in one study where repeated BNP measurements were taken during 48–72 hours of hemodynamically guided treatment, the fall in BNP levels during treatment correlated significantly with the fall in pulmonary capillary wedge pressure (PCWP) in the subgroup of patients who improved during treatment [39]. Plasma BNP fell further in the subsequent 24–48 hours despite no further changes in PCWP during that time, indicating a lag between hemodynamic compensation and trough BNP levels. This delayed response has been reported elsewhere and is consistent with constitutive secretion of BNP.

Although routine use of a pulmonary artery catheter to guide treatment of acute HF is no longer indicated [42], serial monitoring of BNP and NT-proBNP combined with clinical assessment could identify patients not responding to therapy for whom invasive hemodynamic assessment may be helpful to plan further interventions [11,42].

Data from studies with implantable hemodynamic devices that measure or estimate left atrial pressure provide some insight into the relationship of BNP and NT-proBNP to hemodynamic indices in ambulant HF subjects [15,16]. One such study involved the permanently implanted Chronicle™ device that estimates pulmonary artery diastolic (ePAD) from right ventricular pressure at the time of pulmonary valve opening [16]. Serial measurements of ePAD and simultaneous NT-proBNP levels were taken during 10-month follow-up. Baseline levels of NT-proBNP differed among the 19 patients studied and there was significant variation in serial NT-proBNP levels and ePAD and other hemodynamic indices during follow-up. For the whole group data no significant relationship existed between NT-proBNP levels and either ePAD or RV systolic pressure at any time point. However, within patient analyses demonstrated significant positive correlations between NT-proBNP and estimated ePAD, suggesting that within individual patients, variation in NT-proBNP levels relates strongly to changes in hemodynamic status [16]. These findings suggest that although absolute levels of BNP and NT-proBNP cannot be used as surrogates for LV filling pressures, *changes* in levels provide more accurate information regarding changes in hemodynamic indices.

Serial monitoring of BNP/NT-proBNP: Incremental value for risk stratification

In cross-sectional observational studies, BNP and NT-proBNP are among the most powerful independent predictors of mortality and HF events. This finding has been consistently demonstrated in large studies across the spectrum of HF from stage A patients at risk for developing HF to stage D patients with advanced symptomatic disease. A single measurement of a BNP predicts mortality and hospitalization for HF independent of left ventricular ejection fraction (LVEF), symptomatic class, age, and other key determinants of survival [18,43,44].

Studies demonstrate that serial measurements of BNP or NT-proBNP provide independent prognostic information that is incremental to single baseline values [19,40,45]. In the Val-HEFT neurohumoral substudy, changes in BNP and NT proBNP levels during follow-up independently predicted survival in 4300 patients [44]. Patients with levels above the median at baseline but below the

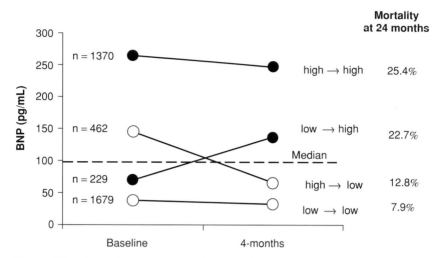

Fig. 8.2 Mortality at 2 years among subjects in the Val-HEFT study was predicted by serial BNP measurement. Highest mortality occurred in patients with above median BNP at 4 months regardless of the baseline BNP level. Lower mortality was seen in subjects with below median BNP at 4 months. Adapted from [44] with permission.

median at 4 months had 2-year mortality risks similar to those with low peptide levels at both time points, whereas those with below-median baseline levels that rose above the median at 4 months had mortality rates that approximated those with persistently elevated levels (Fig. 8.2) [44].

In the outpatient setting, Maeda et al. measured BNP levels at baseline and 3 months after optimization of therapy in 102 patients recently hospitalized with severe HF. Although BNP levels fell after therapy was optimized, 3-month BNP levels remained the strongest independent predictor of subsequent mortality [20]. Serial BNP or NT-proBNP levels measured during follow-up appear to reflect the distance from most recent HF decompensation, but act as powerful predictors of subsequent prognosis [45,46].

Among patients admitted with acute HF the highest mortality and rehospitalization rates occur in patients for whom BNP or NT-proBNP levels increase despite active treatment. A fall in BNP or NT-proBNP of 30% or more from admission to discharge is associated with best outcomes [19,45]. Whereas BNP or NT-ProBNP levels at admission are useful for the accurate diagnosis and early management of HF, predischarge peptide levels provide the strongest prediction of subsequent risk following discharge [21,37,45,47]. Whether routine predischarge testing alters management or outcomes is currently being tested.

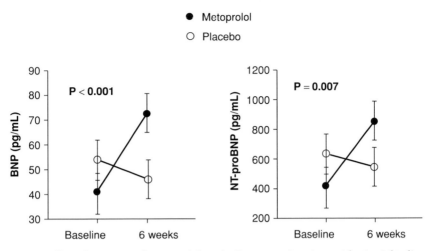

Fig. 8.3 Effect of initiation of metoprolol on the B-type natriuretic peptides in eight clinically stable patients with systolic heart failure and receiving stable ACE inhibitor and diuretic doses. Introduction of metoprolol was associated with a doubling in BNP and NT-proBNP levels reflecting changes in secretion and clearance despite clinical stability. Adapted from [53] with permission.

Changes in BNP/NT-proBNP in response to treatment

Plasma levels of BNP and NT-proBNP can be used to monitor the response to therapy in HF [18,48–50]. BNP or NT proBNP levels fall following institution of diuretic and vasodilator therapy [49,51], whereas withdrawal of diuretics is associated with a rise in peptide levels [52]. ACE inhibitors and angiotensin receptor blockers cause a fall in natriuretic peptide levels [18,49].

The response to beta-blockers is more complex. Commencement of metoprolol in stable mild HF is associated with an initial rise in BNP and NT-proBNP levels that reflects changes in secretion and clearance and is not associated with clinical decompensation (Fig. 8.3) [53]. Peptide levels then fall during longer-term beta-blocker therapy, paralleling reverse LV remodeling seen with these agents [54]. Similar data has been demonstrated for carvedilol (Fig. 8.4) [48,55], although there is some evidence that newer vasodilator beta-blockers may cause an initial fall in BNP [56].

Plasma BNP and NT-proBNP levels also reflect the response to biventricular pacing. In the CARE-HF study, patients who received cardiac resynchronization therapy had significantly lower NT-proBNP levels at 3- and 18-month follow-up than did patients in the placebo arm (Fig. 8.5) [57]. Greater reductions in NT-proBNP were seen in clinical responders than nonresponders. Changes in

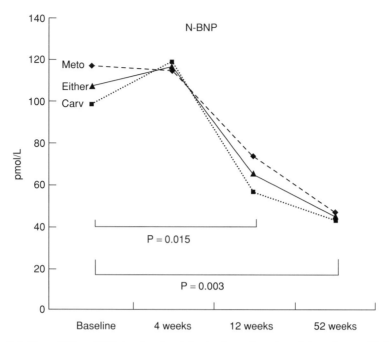

Fig. 8.4 Mean NT-proBNP levels after introduction of metoprolol and carvedilol in patients with stable systolic heart failure, demonstrating an early rise in peptide levels followed by a later fall. Adapted from [55] with permission.

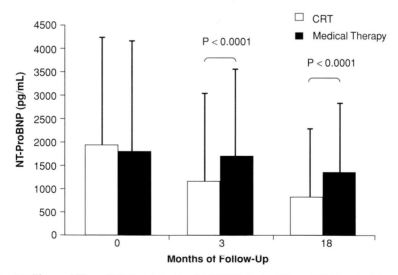

Fig. 8.5 Plasma NT-proBNP levels in the CARE-HF study. NT-proBNP levels at 3- and 18-month follow-up were significantly lower in the cardiac resynchronization therapy (CRT) group compared to the medical therapy. Adapted from [57] with permission.

NT-proBNP levels during follow-up correlated with changes in LV volumes and ejection fraction [57].

Prediction of response to therapy

Many studies have shown that BNP or NT-proBNP levels identify HF subjects with greatest risk for adverse outcomes during treatment and follow-up [18,43,44,50].

Further evidence suggests that these peptides may also identify patients that benefit most from proven therapies. The neurohumoral substudy of the ANZ Heart Failure Trial involved 415 patients with ischemic cardiomyopathy and LVEF below 45% who were randomized to treatment with placebo or carvedilol in addition to background ACE inhibitors and loop diuretic therapy. The study found a reduction in the combined end-point of death and hospital admission for patients treated with carvedilol. Prerandomization BNP and NT-proBNP predicted outcome irrespective of treatment group [50]. In addition, the greatest benefit from treatment with carvedilol was seen in patients with above-median peptide levels, whereas outcomes for patients with below-median levels of BNP treated with carvedilol were similar to those treated with placebo [50]. In the larger COPERNICUS study a similar pattern was seen, with a trend toward greater absolute benefit from carvedilol in the subgroup of patients with the highest NT-proBNP concentrations [48].

Treatment of heart failure guided by BNP/NT-proBNP levels

Because BNP/NT-proBNP levels are such powerful markers of the severity of cardiac dysfunction, prognosis, and of response to therapy, treatment targeted to lower levels of these peptides could potentially lead to improved clinical outcomes.

In the first study to assess the concept of titrating treatment to lower BNP levels, Murdoch et al. randomized patients to treatment guided by BNP levels or by clinical status. They demonstrated that BNP-guided treatment could lower BNP below levels seen with clinically guided therapy (Fig. 8.6). Lower BNP levels were achieved by titration of ACE inhibitor to nearly twice usual target doses and by increased diuretic doses [49].

In a second randomized pilot study, the effect of NT-proBNP guided treatment of HF on clinical outcomes was assessed in 69 patients with a history of decompensated HF, current NYHA class II–IV symptoms, and LVEF <40% [51]. Subjects were randomized to have therapy adjusted according to a preset algorithm either based solely on clinical status or according to serial levels of NT-proBNP. In the NT–proBNP-guided group, treatment was titrated to achieve an NT-proBNP level below 200 p mol/L (approximately 1700 ng/L). Levels above this target triggered increases in therapy even when there was no clinical evidence of decompensation or volume overload. When clinical or NT-proBNP targets were not met, doses of loop diuretic, ACE inhibitor, spironolactone,

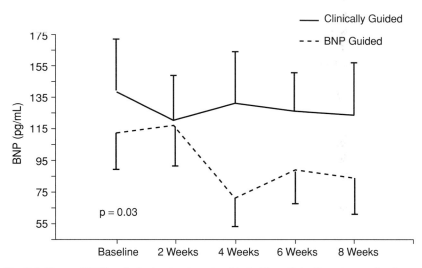

Fig. 8.6 Plasma BNP levels during treatment guided either clinically or targeted to lower BNP levels. Adapted from [49] with permission.

long-acting nitrate, and other vasodilators were increased according to a pre-determined sequence. At follow-up, NT-proBNP levels fell significantly in the hormone-guided group but not in the clinical group. At a median of 9.5 months follow-up, the primary end-point of death, cardiovascular admission, or HF decompensation was significantly lower in the hormone-guided group (Fig. 8.7). There were 19 events in the NT–proBNP-guided group compared to 54 events in the control group (p = 0.02).

Subsequently a larger French multicenter study ("STARS-BNP") studied 220 patients with symptomatic systolic HF (NYHA II–IV, LVEF <45%) recruited in 21 hospitals and randomized to clinically guided treatment or to treatment guided to lower BNP levels below 100 pg/mL [58]. During a median of 15 months follow-up, there were significantly fewer events (death or HF hospi-talization) in the BNP group compared to the clinical group (25 versus 57; p < 0.001). Beyond 3 months, medications were increased more often in the BNP group, for whom doses of ACE inhibitor and beta-blocker medications were significantly higher. Patients in the BNP group were seen on average twice as often for planned clinical review to titrate medication, but they were less likely to require review for clinical decompensation. At the end of the study, one-third of patients in the BNP group had BNP levels below 100 pg/mL.

The "STARBRITE" study, enrolled 130 patients from three centers in the United States [59]. Subjects with systolic HF (LVEF < 35%) were recruited during admission for HF decompensation and were randomized to outpatient treatment guided by predischarge BNP level or by clinical congestion score.

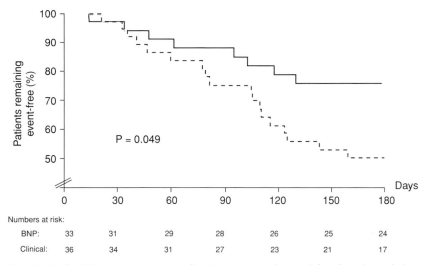

Fig. 8.7 Kaplan-Meier event curves indicating patients alive and free from heart failure event. There was a significantly lower probability of events in the group whose treatment was adjusted according to serial measurements of plasma NT-proBNP [51]. Reproduced from [51] with permission from Elsevier.

At 90 days the BNP group exhibited no difference in days alive and out of hospital, but had lower BNP values (p = 0.02) with no significant difference in creatinine or systolic blood pressure. The study may have been limited by relatively short follow-up period that may not have allowed time for the BNP-guided strategy to affect the clinical end-point. Additionally, predischarge BNP level—although providing an individualized target—may not be the best target for BNP-guided treatment as levels may continue to fall for days and even weeks following an acute decompensation, or after further titration of ACE inhibitor or diuretic therapy. However, one important finding noted by the STARBRITE investigators was that subjects with BNP-guided treatment were more likely to receive target doses of ACE inhibitor (P < 0.05) and beta-blocker medications (p = 0.07) and were less likely to receive increases in diuretic drugs. Hence, treatment guided by BNP was associated with greater use of evidence-based drugs, possibly because persistently elevated BNP levels served as a reminder to investigators to optimize therapy.

The concept of NT–proBNP- or BNP-guided treatment of HF is being tested in at least five larger studies, of which three have published methods papers [59–61]. The BNP-Assisted Treatment To LEssen Serial CARdiac REadmissions and Death ("BATTLE-SCARRED") study has randomized 350 patients with pre-served or impaired ejection fraction to "usual care," intensive clinically guided therapy, or NT-proBNP-guided therapy, with stratification based on age above and below 75 years [61].

Whether therapy should be guided by a uniform BNP or NT-proBNP target for all patients or by individualized targets is a matter for debate. Knowledge of a patient's BNP or NT-proBNP level when clinically stable is very useful for monitoring, as an increase of >20% for NT-proBNP is indicative of an important clinical change and likely decompensation [62,63]. Use of individualized "dry-weight" levels as a target for treatment titration, however, is less likely to trigger intensification of treatment even if levels are high and indicative of greater risk for adverse events. Use of a uniform target based on levels associated with increased risk or clinical decompensation may be preferable, as this is likely to trigger treatment intensification in more patients. Although this approach could potentially lead to more adverse effects, including greater rates of azotemia or symptomatic hypotension, this has not been reported as a significant problem in the pilot studies performed to date [51,58,59]. However, this remains a concern if this strategy is employed more broadly, especially where patient monitoring is not as intense as in the clinical trials. Thus, treatment titration should be performed in the context of careful assessment of clinical status and biochemical indices of renal function and electrolyte balance [51,58,59].

In regard to frequency of measurement in the outpatient setting, testing every 3 months as modeled in the titration studies should be considered, with more frequent measurements up to biweekly being appropriate in unstable patients or following treatment titration [51,58,59]. In the acute setting, current data would support measurement at admission, to facilitate accurate early diagnosis, and at time of discharge to improve risk stratification and potentially guide follow-up decision making [19,37,64].

Intra-individual variability in BNP and NT-ProBNP levels and implications for disease monitoring

Although it is clear from many studies that repeated measurements of BNP and NT-proBNP have significant clinical value as markers of risk [19,20,40,41,43,44,51], recent studies demonstrate significant variation between serial measurements of BNP or NT-proBNP, even in clinically stable subjects [65,66]. Variations in serial peptide levels reflect measurement precision (analytical variability) as well as changes in secretion and clearance (biological variability). Analytical variability is a function of specific assay and peptide characteristics [2,67], whereas biological variability reflects the complex network of hemodynamic and neurohumoral stimuli and counterregulatory mechanisms that control peptide secretion and clearance [68].

For serial levels of either peptide to allow monitoring or guidance of therapy, variability in patients with clinically stable HF needs to be low enough that changes reflect genuine alterations in cardiac status. Significant random or "unexplained" biological variation could potentially confound the use of serial peptide measurements to adjust treatment [69]. Initial concerns in this regard have been largely set to rest by recent studies [62,63,65,66,70].

Earliest studies of variability in serial BNP and NT-proBNP levels were performed in small cohorts of normal and clinically stable HF subjects [65,66]. Wu et al. measured peptide levels in 8 normal subjects on 4 occasions at 2-week intervals. Absolute levels of BNP and NT-proBNP were low and intra-individual coefficients of variation (CV) measured 33% for NT-proBNP and of 48–56% for BNP depending on the assay used [66]. Based on these data, the minimum percent change that would indicate an alteration greater than background biological variation (with 95% confidence) was calculated at 92% for NT-proBNP and 129–168% for BNP. These findings are unlikely to be relevant to the HF setting, as in healthy subjects peptide levels are low and very small absolute changes in peptide levels can result in high proportional changes that are not biologically significant [69].

Bruins et al. assessed 43 stable HF subjects with serial measurements taken under standardized conditions within 1 day, on consecutive days and weekly over 6 consecutive weeks [65]. Total CV for within day, day-to-day, and week-to-week samples were 12%, 27%, and 41% for BNP and 9%, 20%, and 35% for NT-proBNP. Corresponding minimum percent change values for within day, day-to-day, and week-to-week samples were 32%, 74%, and 113% for BNP and 25%, 55%, and 98% for NT-proBNP [65].

Larger cohorts have been studied and clinical stability has been more rigorously defined [62,63,70]. Schou et al. selected 20 patients who had been clinically stable according to 22 strict inclusion and exclusion criteria [63]. The intra-individual CV over a 1-week interval was 15% for BNP and 8% for NT-proBNP, with an analytical CV of 3% for BNP and 1% for NT-proBNP. Based on these measurements, minimum percent change values of 43% for BNP and 23% for NT-proBNP could be calculated. Cortes et al. demonstrated similar results in 74 clinically stable patients with measurements of NT-proBNP at 12 and 24 months from baseline [70]. More than a 22% change in levels exceeded background biological variation.

It is clear from several studies that the degree of variability in BNP or NT-proBNP levels is related to the degree of peptide elevation at baseline [62,63,71]. The percentage variability on serial testing is lower at higher starting peptide levels. Above NT-proBNP levels of 1000 pg/mL, which is just below the target level in NT–proBNP-guided treatment studies, the percentage variability in serial tests is <30% and below 10% in truly stable patients (Fig. 8.8) [63,71].

These findings suggest that the degree of variability in serial BNP or NT-proBNP levels in stable HF subjects is low enough to allow these peptides to be used as a clinically valuable monitoring tool [69].

Analytical factors contribute only a small part of the total background variation in peptide levels. Biological variation that is more than three times the analytical imprecision of the assay in use should be regarded as clinically

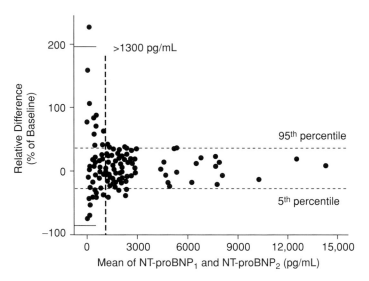

Fig. 8.8 Variability in NT-proBNP levels taken 2 weeks apart in clinically stable subjects with heart failure demonstrating that the degree of variability is lower when peptide levels are higher and above levels used to titrate therapy in treatment studies. Adapted from [71] with permission.

significant [68]. In this context immunoassays with the lowest analytical imprecision will allow detection of smaller changes in BNP concentrations that may be clinically relevant [66–68]. There has been recent interest in the presence of alternative molecular forms of BNP and NT-proBNP [26]. Whether this contributes to overall variability is uncertain, but it is unlikely to be a major factor given the low total biological variability reported earlier. Data from newer assays that look at more stable midregional portions of the NT-proBNP or NT-proANP molecule may be helpful in this regard [72].

Biological variation is the major determinant of total variability and this does not appear to be random but reflects clinically relevant alterations in peptide secretion due to active physiological processes including altered hemodynamic loading conditions, activation of multiple neurohormonal and immunological factors including angiotensin II, endothelin, and norepinephrine as well as myocardial ischemia [65–68]. These factors are dynamic and contribute actively to cardiac remodeling and end-organ dysfunction in heart failure.

With regard to hemodynamic loading, implantable hemodynamic devices demonstrate significant daily variation in indices of LV filling pressure, particularly in the setting of ischemia [15,16]. Changes in NT-proBNP levels correlate strongly with changes in filling pressure measured by implantable devices implying that clinically undetected hemodynamic decompensation may be an important determinant of peptide variability [16].

Conclusion

Evidence indicates that BNP and NT-proBNP can facilitate monitoring of clinical status and may be useful to guide optimization of HF therapy. Plasma levels reflect the severity of symptoms and overall cardiac dysfunction and predict the likelihood of HF events or death. Serial BNP/NT-proBNP testing in hospital or the community identifies the response to therapy and provides incremental risk stratification over a single baseline level. Peptide levels fall the further a patient is from his or her most recent decompensation but continue to provide a powerful estimate of subsequent risk of HF events or death. Intra-individual variation in serial samples taken from stable patients appears modest and does not seem to mitigate the clinical utility of serial testing. A change of >20% for NT-proBNP generally indicates a significant change beyond background variability and reflects a change in clinical status. BNP and NT-proBNP levels fall with effective diuretic, vasodilator, and longer-term beta-blocker therapy, but levels after treatment optimization still predict adverse outcomes. Peptide levels may also identify patients most likely to benefit from intensified medical therapy. Studies indicate that titrating medical therapy to achieve BNP or NT-proBNP levels below a target range is associated with more optimal use of proven medications and may improve clinical outcomes compared to empiric strategies. These data suggest that serial BNP/NT-proBNP testing may be useful for monitoring response to therapy, determining risk of future adverse events, and potentially for guiding optimal medical therapy.

References

1 Tang WH, Francis GS. The difficult task of evaluating how to monitor patients with heart failure. *J Card Fail* 2005; **11**: 422–424.
2 Hunt SA. ACC/AHA 2005 guideline update for the diagnosis and management of chronic heart failure in the adult: a report of the American College of Cardiology/American Heart Association Task Force on Practice Guidelines (Writing Committee to Update the 2001 Guidelines for the Evaluation and Management of Heart Failure). *J Am Coll Cardiol* 2005; **46**: e1–82.
3 Granger BB, Swedberg K, Ekman I et al. Adherence to candesartan and placebo and outcomes in chronic heart failure in the CHARM programme: double-blind, randomised, controlled clinical trial. *Lancet* 2005; **366**: 2005–2011.
4 Komajda M, Lapuerta P, Hermans N et al. Adherence to guidelines is a predictor of outcome in chronic heart failure: the MAHLER survey. *Eur Heart J* 2005; **26**: 1653–1659.
5 Lenzen MJ, Boersma E, Reimer WJ et al. Under-utilization of evidence-based drug treatment in patients with heart failure is only partially explained by dissimilarity to patients enrolled in landmark trials: a report from the Euro Heart Survey on Heart Failure. *Eur Heart J* 2005; **26**: 2706–2713.
6 Swedberg K, Cleland J, Dargie H et al. Guidelines for the diagnosis and treatment of chronic heart failure: executive summary (update 2005): The Task Force for the

Diagnosis and Treatment of Chronic Heart Failure of the European Society of Cardiology. *Eur Heart J* 2005; **26**: 1115–1140.

7 Hlatky MA. Underuse of evidence-based therapies. *Circulation* 2004; **110**: 644–645.

8 Stafford RS, Radley DC. The underutilization of cardiac medications of proven benefit, 1990 to 2002. *J Am Coll Cardiol* 2003; **41**: 56–61.

9 Nicholls MG, Lainchbury JG, Richards AM et al. Brain natriuretic peptide-guided therapy for heart failure. *Ann Med* 2001; **33**: 422–427.

10 van Kraaij DJ, Jansen RW, Bouwels LH et al. Furosemide withdrawal improves postprandial hypotension in elderly patients with heart failure and preserved left ventricular systolic function. *Arch Intern Med* 1999; **159**: 1599–1605.

11 Nohria A, Tsang SW, Fang JC et al. Clinical assessment identifies hemodynamic profiles that predict outcomes in patients admitted with heart failure. *J Am Coll Cardiol* 2003; **41**: 1797–1804.

12 Nicholls MG, Richards AM. Disease monitoring of patients with chronic heart failure. *Heart* 2007; **93**: 519–523.

13 Drazner MH, Rame JE, Stevenson LW et al. Prognostic importance of elevated jugular venous pressure and a third heart sound in patients with heart failure. *N Engl J Med* 2001; **345**: 574–581.

14 Stevenson LW, Perloff JK. The limited reliability of physical signs for estimating hemodynamics in chronic heart failure. *JAMA* 1989; **261**: 884–888.

15 McClean D, Aragon J, Jamali A et al. Noninvasive calibration of cardiac pressure transducers in patients with heart failure: an aid to implantable hemodynamic monitoring and therapeutic guidance. *J Card Fail* 2006; **12**: 568–576.

16 Braunschweig F, Fahrleitner-Pammer A, Mangiavacchi M et al. Correlation between serial measurements of N-terminal pro brain natriuretic peptide and ambulatory cardiac filling pressures in outpatients with chronic heart failure. *Eur J Heart Fail* 2006; **8**: 797–803.

17 Mo VY, De Lemos JA. Individualizing therapy in acute coronary syndromes: using a multiple biomarker approach for diagnosis, risk stratification, and guidance of therapy. *Curr Cardiol Rep* 2004; **6**: 273–278.

18 Anand IS, Fisher LD, Chiang YT et al. Changes in brain natriuretic peptide and norepinephrine over time and mortality and morbidity in the Valsartan Heart Failure Trial (Val-HeFT). *Circulation* 2003; **107**: 1278–1283.

19 Bettencourt P, Azevedo A, Pimenta J et al. N-terminal-pro-brain natriuretic peptide predicts outcome after hospital discharge in heart failure patients. *Circulation* 2004; **110**: 2168–2174.

20 Maeda K, Tsutamoto T, Wada A et al. High levels of plasma brain natriuretic peptide and interleukin-6 after optimized treatment for heart failure are independent risk factors for morbidity and mortality in patients with congestive heart failure. *J Am Coll Cardiol* 2000; **36**: 1587–1593.

21 Maisel AS, Krishnaswamy P, Nowak RM et al. Rapid measurement of B-type natriuretic peptide in the emergency diagnosis of heart failure. *N Engl J Med* 2002; **347**: 161–167.

22 Troughton RW, Prior DL, Pereira JJ et al. Plasma B-type natriuretic peptide levels in systolic heart failure: importance of left ventricular diastolic function and right ventricular systolic function. *J Am Coll Cardiol* 2004; **43**: 416–422.

23 Yasue H, Yoshimura M, Sumida H et al. Localization and mechanism of secretion of B-type natriuretic peptide in comparison with those of A-type natriuretic peptide in normal subjects and patients with heart failure. *Circulation* 1994; **90**: 195–203.

24 Mukoyama M, Nakao K, Hosoda K et al. Brain natriuretic peptide as a novel cardiac hormone in humans. Evidence for an exquisite dual natriuretic peptide system, atrial natriuretic peptide and brain natriuretic peptide. *J Clin Invest* 1991; **87**: 1402–1412.

25 Iwanaga Y, Nishi I, Furuichi S et al. B-type natriuretic peptide strongly reflects diastolic wall stress in patients with chronic heart failure: comparison between systolic and diastolic heart failure. *J Am Coll Cardiol* 2006; **47**: 742–748.

26 Lam CS, Burnett JC Jr., Costello-Boerrigter L et al. Alternate circulating pro-B-type natriuretic peptide and B-type natriuretic peptide forms in the general population. *J Am Coll Cardiol* 2007; **49**: 1193–1202.

27 Lainchbury JG, Campbell E, Frampton CM et al. Brain natriuretic peptide and n-terminal brain natriuretic peptide in the diagnosis of heart failure in patients with acute shortness of breath. *J Am Coll Cardiol* 2003; **42**: 728–735.

28 Nishikimi T, Yoshihara F, Morimoto A et al. Relationship between left ventricular geometry and natriuretic peptide levels in essential hypertension. *Hypertension* 1996; **28**: 22–30.

29 Lee SC, Stevens TL, Sandberg SM et al. The potential of brain natriuretic peptide as a biomarker for New York Heart Association class during the outpatient treatment of heart failure. *J Card Fail* 2002; **8**: 149–154.

30 Tang WH, Girod JP, Lee MJ et al. Plasma B-type natriuretic peptide levels in ambulatory patients with established chronic symptomatic systolic heart failure. *Circulation* 2003; **108**: 2964–2966.

31 Tsutamoto T, Wada A, Sakai H et al. Relationship between renal function and plasma brain natriuretic peptide in patients with heart failure. *J Am Coll Cardiol* 2006; **47**: 582–586.

32 Redfield MM, Rodeheffer RJ, Jacobsen SJ et al. Plasma brain natriuretic peptide concentration: impact of age and gender. *J Am Coll Cardiol* 2002; **40**: 976–982.

33 Wang TJ, Larson MG, Levy D et al. Impact of obesity on plasma natriuretic peptide levels. *Circulation* 2004; **109**: 594–600.

34 Knudsen CW, Omland T, Clopton P et al. Impact of atrial fibrillation on the diagnostic performance of B-type natriuretic peptide concentration in dyspneic patients: an analysis from the breathing not properly multinational study. *J Am Coll Cardiol* 2005; **46**: 838–844.

35 Wang TJ, Larson MG, Levy D et al. Heritability and genetic linkage of plasma natriuretic peptide levels. *Circulation* 2003. **108**: 13–16.

36 Nishikimi T, Matsuoka H. Routine measurement of natriuretic peptide to guide the diagnosis and management of chronic heart failure. *Circulation* 2004; **109**: e325–326.

37 Januzzi JL, van Kimmenade R, Lainchbury J et al. NT-proBNP testing for diagnosis and short-term prognosis in acute destabilized heart failure: an international pooled analysis of 1256 patients: the International Collaborative of NT-proBNP Study. *Eur Heart J* 2006; **27**: 330–337.

38 Richards AM, Crozier IG, Yandle TG et al. Brain natriuretic factor: regional plasma concentrations and correlations with haemodynamic state in cardiac disease. *Br Heart J* 1993; **69**: 414–417.

39 Kazanegra R, Cheng V, Garcia A et al. A rapid test for B-type natriuretic peptide correlates with falling wedge pressures in patients treated for decompensated heart failure: a pilot study. *J Card Fail* 2001; **7**: 21–29.

40 Johnson W, Omland T, Hall C et al. Neurohormonal activation rapidly decreases after intravenous therapy with diuretics and vasodilators for class IV heart failure. *J Am Coll Cardiol* 2002; **39**: 1623–1629.

41 Knebel F, Schimke I, Pliet K et al. NT-ProBNP in acute heart failure: correlation with invasively measured hemodynamic parameters during recompensation. *J Card Fail* 2005; **11**: S38–41.

42 Stevenson LW. Are hemodynamic goals viable in tailoring heart failure therapy? Hemodynamic goals are relevant. *Circulation* 2006; **113**: 1020–1027, 1033.

43 Latini R, Masson S, Anand I et al. The comparative prognostic value of plasma neurohormones at baseline in patients with heart failure enrolled in Val-HeFT. *Eur Heart J* 2004; **25**: 292–299.

44 Latini R, Masson S, Wong M et al. Incremental prognostic value of changes in B-type natriuretic peptide in heart failure. *Am J Med* 2006; **119**: 70 e23–30.

45 Cheng V, Kazanagra R, Garcia A et al. A rapid bedside test for B-type peptide predicts treatment outcomes in patients admitted for decompensated heart failure: a pilot study. *J Am Coll Cardiol* 2001; **37**: 386–391.

46 Nishikimi T, Matsuoka H. Plasma brain natriuretic peptide levels indicate the distance from decompensated heart failure. *Circulation* 2004; **109**: e329–330.

47 Bettencourt P, Frioes F, Azevedo A et al. Prognostic information provided by serial measurements of brain natriuretic peptide in heart failure. *Int J Cardiol* 2004; **93**: 45–48.

48 Hartmann F, Packer M, Coats AJ et al. Prognostic impact of plasma N-terminal probrain natriuretic peptide in severe chronic congestive heart failure: a substudy of the Carvedilol Prospective Randomized Cumulative Survival (COPERNICUS) trial. *Circulation* 2004; **110**: 1780–1786.

49 Murdoch DR, McDonagh TA, Byrne J et al. Titration of vasodilator therapy in chronic heart failure according to plasma brain natriuretic peptide concentration: randomized comparison of the hemodynamic and neuroendocrine effects of tailored versus empirical therapy. *Am Heart J* 1999; **138**: 1126–1132.

50 Richards AM, Doughty R, Nicholls MG et al. Neurohumoral prediction of benefit from carvedilol in ischemic left ventricular dysfunction. Australia-New Zealand Heart Failure Group. *Circulation* 1999; **99**: 786–792.

51 Troughton RW, Frampton CM, Yandle TG et al. Treatment of heart failure guided by plasma aminoterminal brain natriuretic peptide (N-BNP) concentrations. *Lancet* 2000; **355**: 1126–1130.

52 Braunschweig F, Linde C, Eriksson MJ et al. Continuous haemodynamic monitoring during withdrawal of diuretics in patients with congestive heart failure. *Eur Heart J* 2002; **23**: 59–69.

53 Davis ME, Richards AM, Nicholls MG et al. Introduction of metoprolol increases plasma B-type cardiac natriuretic peptides in mild, stable heart failure. *Circulation* 2006; **113**: 977–985.

54 Doughty RN, Whalley GA, Walsh HA et al. Effects of carvedilol on left ventricular remodeling after acute myocardial infarction: the CAPRICORN Echo Substudy. *Circulation* 2004; **109**: 201–206.

55 Fung JW, Yu CM, Yip G et al. Effect of beta blockade (carvedilol or metoprolol) on activation of the renin-angiotensin-aldosterone system and natriuretic peptides in chronic heart failure. *Am J Cardiol* 2003; **92**: 406–410.

56 Sanderson JE, Chan WW, Hung YT et al. Effect of low dose beta blockers on atrial and ventricular (B type) natriuretic factor in heart failure: a double blind, randomised comparison of metoprolol and a third generation vasodilating beta blocker. *Br Heart J* 1995; **74**: 502–507.

57 Fruhwald FM, Fahrleitner-Pammer A, Berger R et al. Early and sustained effects of cardiac resynchronization therapy on N-terminal pro-B-type natriuretic peptide in patients with moderate to severe heart failure and cardiac dyssynchrony. *Eur Heart J* 2007; **28**: 1592–1597.

58 Jourdain P, Jondeau G, Funck F et al. Plasma brain natriuretic peptide-guided therapy to improve outcome in heart failure: the STARS-BNP Multicenter Study. *J Am Coll Cardiol* 2007; **49**: 1733–1739.

59 Shah MR, Claise KA, Bowers MT et al. Testing new targets of therapy in advanced heart failure: the design and rationale of the Strategies for Tailoring Advanced Heart Failure Regimens in the Outpatient Setting: BRain NatrIuretic Peptide Versus the Clinical CongesTion ScorE (STARBRITE) trial. *Am Heart J* 2005; **150**: 893–898.

60 Brunner-La Rocca HP, Buser PT, Schindler R et al. Management of elderly patients with congestive heart failure–design of the Trial of Intensified versus standard Medical therapy in Elderly patients with Congestive Heart Failure (TIME-CHF). *Am Heart J* 2006; **151**: 949–955.

61 Lainchbury JG, Troughton RW, Frampton CM et al. NTproBNP-guided drug treatment for chronic heart failure: design and methods in the "BATTLESCARRED" trial. *Eur J Heart Fail* 2006; **8**: 532–538.

62 Schou M, Gustafsson F, Kjaer A et al. Long-term clinical variation of NT-proBNP in stable chronic heart failure patients. *Eur Heart J* 2007; **28**: p. 177–182.

63 Schou M, Gustafsson F, Nielsen PH et al. Unexplained week-to-week variation in BNP and NT-proBNP is low in chronic heart failure patients during steady state. *Eur J Heart Fail* 2007; **9**: 68–74.

64 Logeart D, Thabut G, Jourdain P et al. Predischarge B-type natriuretic peptide assay for identifying patients at high risk of re-admission after decompensated heart failure. *J Am Coll Cardiol* 2004; **43**: 635–641.

65 Bruins S, Fokkema MR, Romer JW et al. High intraindividual variation of B-type natriuretic peptide (BNP) and amino-terminal proBNP in patients with stable chronic heart failure. *Clin Chem* 2004; **50**: 2052–2058.

66 Wu AH, Smith A, Wieczorek S et al. Biological variation for N-terminal pro- and B-type natriuretic peptides and implications for therapeutic monitoring of patients with congestive heart failure. *Am J Cardiol* 2003; **92**: 628–631.

67 Apple FS, Panteghini M, Ravkilde J et al. Quality specifications for B-type natriuretic peptide assays. *Clin Chem* 2005; **51**: 486–493.

68 Clerico A, Zucchelli GC, Pilo A et al. Clinical relevance of biological variation of B-type natriuretic peptide. *Clin Chem* 2005; **51**: 925–926.

69 Richards AM. Variability of NT-proBNP levels in heart failure: implications for clinical application. *Heart* 2007; **93**: 899–900.

70 Cortes R, Rivera M, Salvador A et al. Variability of NT-proBNP plasma and urine levels in patients with stable heart failure: a 2-year follow-up study. *Heart* 2007; **93**: 957–962.

71 Araujo JP, Azevedo A, Lourenco P et al. Intra-individual variation of amino-terminal pro-B-type natriuretic peptide levels in patients with stable heart failure. *Am J Cardiol* 2006; **98**: 1248–1250.

72 Gegenhuber A, Struck J, Dieplinger B et al. Comparative evaluation of B-type natriuretic peptide, mid-regional pro-A-type natriuretic peptide, mid-regional pro-adrenomedullin, and Copeptin to predict 1-year mortality in patients with acute destabilized heart failure. *J Card Fail* 2007; **13**: 42–49.

PART III

Biomarkers for Screening in Ambulatory Populations

Chapter 9

C-Reactive Protein

Amit Khera

Introduction

Cardiovascular disease (CVD) has been the leading cause of death in the United States every year since 1900, except for during the influenza pandemic of 1918. Despite the great impact of preventive efforts, currently approximately 900,000 people succumb to CVD each year, and this illness accounts for more deaths than the next 4 leading causes combined, including all cancers [1]. Ultimately, the best treatment for this illness is to prevent its occurrence. Advances in the understanding of risk factors for CVD over the past half century have led to substantial reductions in CVD mortality rates. However, the rate of decline in CVD has slowed, raising valid questions regarding the effectiveness of current preventive strategies: as a result, there is growing interest in novel strategies for heart disease prevention and screening. Various candidates for improvement in CVD screening have been proposed, of which C-reactive protein (CRP) testing appears the most promising.

Limitations of current methods for population screening of heart disease

Two different but complementary approaches have been utilized for the prevention of CVD [2]. The *population-based* strategy attempts to shift the distribution of risk factors in the entire population to a lower average level (i.e., shifting the mean blood pressure), often utilizing public health measures. An alternative preventive strategy for CVD is termed the *high-risk* strategy [2], which involves setting a threshold of risk and focusing treatment strategies on individuals who

Biomarkers in Heart Disease, 1st edition. Edited by James A. de Lemos.
© 2008 American Heart Association, ISBN: 978-1-4051-7571-5

exceed this risk; such as treating blood pressure in a patient once he or she is considered hypertensive. Traditional medical practice centers on this approach, which has several advantages, including providing interventions that are targeted to the individual, thereby creating a more favorable risk-benefit ratio. Importantly, this strategy also improves cost-effectiveness of various therapies.

Individual risk factors perform poorly as screening tests for CVD, as the distribution of individual risk factors overlaps substantially between those with and without CVD. It has been demonstrated repeatedly that almost half of all myocardial infarctions (MI) occur in patients with normal cholesterol levels [3,4], and approximately 20% of those suffering from coronary events have none of the conventional risk factors for this illness [5]. The limitations of individual risk factors have led to the concept of global risk assessment in the form of predictive equations, with the Framingham Risk Score being the currently recommended standard for assessing CVD risk in the U.S. adult population [6,7]. Despite the many advantages of the Framingham Risk Score, it has become increasingly evident that this algorithm has limited accuracy in predicting CVD risk, particularly among women [8,9], young people [10], and various ethnic groups [11]. Several lines of evidence suggest that CRP testing may enhance CVD risk assessment in ambulatory populations, and overcome some of the limitations of current CV risk assessment strategies.

Biology and chemical properties of C-reactive protein

Discovered in 1930 by Tillett and Francis [12], CRP is a pentameric 23 kDa member of the pentraxin family of plasma proteins that was originally named for its ability to precipitate the C-polysaccharide of *Streptococcus pneumonia* [13]. It is a nonspecific systemic acute phase reactant protein involved in innate immunity, activating the classical complement pathway, stimulating phagocytes, and binding to immunoglobulin receptors [14]. Recently, CRP has stimulated interest as a barometer of inflammatory processes related to CVD. Importantly, CRP elevation is not specific for atherosclerotic disease and can occur with a broad range of inflammatory stimuli such as infection, autoimmune diseases, malignancy, and trauma. In response to these stimuli, plasma levels of CRP can potentially increase greater than 10,000-fold [13]. CRP is produced predominantly in the liver, although other sources such as adipose tissue and vascular smooth muscle cells have been described [15–17].

Several biologic and chemical properties of CRP contribute to its appeal as a clinically useful biomarker (Table 9.1). CRP levels are quite stable in plasma, with a half-life of approximately 19 hours, and they have no diurnal variation [13]. The correlation of CRP levels over time in individuals is approximately 0.6, which is similar to that for low-density lipoprotein (LDL) levels, and frozen samples are stable for extended periods [18]. In addition, CRP measurement does not require the fasting state.

Table 9.1 Clinical and biochemical properties of C-reactive protein applicable to clinical use.

Half-life	19 hours
Diurnal variation	No
Correlation of levels over time	r = 0.6
Fasting sample required	No
Commercially available assay	Yes
Assay standardized	Partially
Clinical reference range reported	Yes (<1-low, 1–3-intermediate, >3 mg/L high relative risk)

The initial utility of CRP for CVD risk assessment was hampered because the threshold of detection of older assays (>5 mg/L) was above the typical range of CRP levels in the general population. This deficiency was remedied by introducing newer, high-sensitivity assays that could detect values within the "normal" range of <3 mg/L [19]. Currently, there are several commercially available assays that can reliably measure CRP levels in this range, including point of care assays. Although there is some variability in CRP values between these testing methods [20], ongoing efforts by the Centers for Disease Control should result in further standardization of these assays [21].

C-reactive protein and cardiovascular events

Inflammation is intimately linked to atherosclerotic disease [22]. It plays a critical role in all stages of the atherosclerotic process including initiation, progression, and complications (including plaque rupture and the development of acute coronary syndromes). Given this relationship, markers of inflammation should increase in relation to activity of atherosclerotic disease. Indeed, an early case report from the 1940s described elevations of CRP following acute MI [23]. Several studies reported decades later similarly described higher CRP levels in subjects with acute coronary syndromes, and an association with worse outcomes in those with the highest levels [24–27]. These intriguing findings left unclear whether CRP elevations were in response to the coronary events and to myocardial damage, or whether they reflected the underlying pathophysiologic process. Also, the prognostic value of CRP in primary prevention populations was not known.

The Multiple Risk Factor Intervention Trial (MRFIT) provided the first prospective evidence for a link between CRP and the risk of vascular events [28]. In this nested case-control study, those in the highest quartile of CRP compared with those in the lowest had a more than 4-fold increased risk of coronary heart disease death, an effect limited to smokers. Confirmation of these findings were reported the following year in a larger nested case-control sample of over 1000 subjects from the Physicians' Health Study [29]. In this cohort of initially healthy U.S. male physicians, plasma CRP levels in the 4th quartile were associated with an almost 3-fold increase in the risk of MI (odds ratio 2.9, 95% confidence interval 1.8–4.6), and 2-fold increase in the risk of stroke (OR 1.9, 95% CI 1.1–3.3). Importantly, these findings were independent of other CV risk factors and were observed among both smokers and nonsmokers.

Since these initial reports, more than 25 prospective studies (Fig. 9.1) have confirmed the association between higher CRP levels and increased risk of incident CV events in populations initially free of clinically evident disease. In addition to MI [29–36] and stroke [35,37], higher CRP levels have been linked to the risk of a diverse range of CV end-points including coronary death [28,38], peripheral arterial disease [39], and sudden death [40]. These relationships have been observed in cohorts of men and women [28,29,34,41], in various populations in Europe and the United States [4,30,32,33,38,42], and in epidemiologic cohort studies as well as clinical trials [43,44]. Importantly, in a few large prospective studies such as the Framingham Heart Study and the Rotterdam Study of older individuals, higher CRP levels were not associated with an increased risk of CV events after accounting for other risk factors [45,46]. A meta-analysis of 11 studies performed prior to 2000 revealed an adjusted odds ratio of 2.0 for CV events with CRP levels in the top third compared with the bottom third [31], while a recent updated meta-analysis of 22 trials revealed a more modest odds ratio of 1.5 [47].

CRP also provides predictive information for CV disease beyond that conveyed by lipid measures and other more established risk factors. Analyses from the Women's Health Study demonstrated that while both CRP and LDL cholesterol levels were predictive of incident CV events, the increment in risk with higher quartiles of CRP was greater than that with higher LDL levels [4,48]. In addition, CRP was able to further stratify risk among those with high or low LDL levels (Fig. 9.2). Subsequent analyses in the same cohort revealed that CRP measures provided additional predictive value among tertiles of apolipoprotein B_{100} and non-HDL cholesterol [48]. CRP has also been shown to stratify CV risk among subjects with the metabolic syndrome in various cohorts [49,50].

As the Framingham Risk Score is the standard of CV risk assessment in the United States, a relevant question is whether CRP provides additional prognostic information to this algorithm. Several studies have explored this question with conflicting results and interpretations. When gauged by a statistical parameter termed the c-statistic, CRP appears to provide little to no incremental value to CV risk assessment based upon traditional risk factors [45–47,51]. In the largest nested case-control study of CRP to date, investigators from the

Study   Outcome

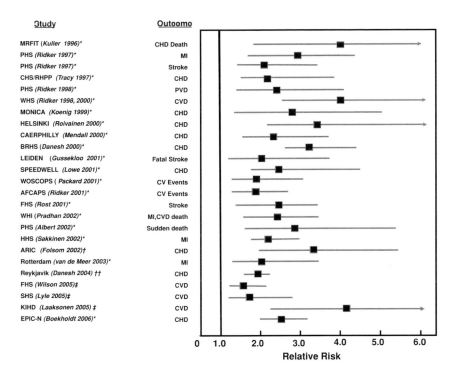

Fig. 9.1 Prospective studies of C-reactive protein and cardiovascular events.
CHD = coronary heart disease; MI = myocardial infarction; PAD = peripheral artery
disease; CV = cardiovascular; MRFIT = Multiple Risk Factor Intervention Trial; PHS =
Physicians' Health Study; CHS = Cardiovascular Health Study; RHPP = Rural Health
Promotion Project; WHS = Women's Health Study; MONICA = MONItoring trends
and determinants In CArdiovascular disease; HELSINKI = Helsinki Heart Study; CAER-
PHILLY = Caerphilly Heart Study; BRHS = British Regional Heart Study; LEIDEN = Lei-
den Heart Study; SPEEDWELL = Speedwell Heart Study; WOSCOPS = West of Scotland
Coronary Prevention Study; AFCAPS = Air Force Coronary Atherosclerosis Prevention
Study; FHS = Framingham Heart Study; WHI = Women's Health Initiative; and HHS
= Honolulu Heart Study; ARIC = Atherosclerosis Risk in Communities Study; SHS =
Strong Heart Study; KIHD = Kuopio Ischemic Heart Disease Risk Factor Study; EPIC-
N = European Prospective Investigation in Cancer and Nutrition * relative risk upper v.
lower quartile; † relative risk upper v. lower quintile; †† relative risk upper v. lower tertile;
‡ relative risk CRP >3mg/L v. <1mg/L
(Adapted from [49] with permission).

Reykjavik Study demonstrated that those in the top third of CRP values had
a modest increased odds of CV events compared with those in the bottom
third (OR 1.45, 95% CI 1.25–1.68) after accounting for other CV risk factors.
This magnitude of increased CV risk was less than that conveyed by cholesterol

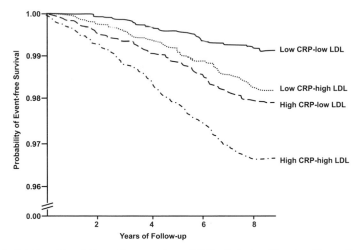

Fig. 9.2 Relationship of C-reactive protein and LDL cholesterol levels with cardiovascular events. High and low values for C-reactive protein (CRP) and low-density lipoprotein cholesterol (LDL) represent above and below the median values. Data are from the Women's Health Study (27,939 women) [4].

levels, smoking, or systolic blood pressure, and there was minimal change in the c-statistic when CRP was added to these other variables (increase from 0.64 to 0.65) [47]. However, more than 10 large epidemiologic studies have shown that CRP levels predict CV risk after adjustment for these risk factors [52], and others have demonstrated that CRP levels can stratify risk within categories of the Framingham Risk Score [30,53,54]. In summary, while in aggregate population studies support a modest increased hazard for CV events (~50% increase in relative risk after adjustment for risk factors) comparing the highest versus lowest CRP levels, this increment in risk does not appear to materially influence typical measures of discrimination. This unresolved issue contributes to the controversy regarding the clinical use of CRP, as will be discussed in a later section of this chapter.

C-reactive protein and atherosclerosis

Various biologic mechanisms explain how CRP may reflect CV risk. Activated leukocytes in the evolving atheroma release a host of cytokines, including interleukin-6 (IL-6), tumor necrosis factor α, and interleukin-1 [22]. These cytokines then act on the liver to stimulate release of acute phase response proteins including CRP, serum amyloid A, and fibrinogen, with IL-6 being the principal cytokine stimulating CRP release from the liver [13]. Vascular smooth muscle cells, endothelial cells, and adipocytes may also directly produce CRP,

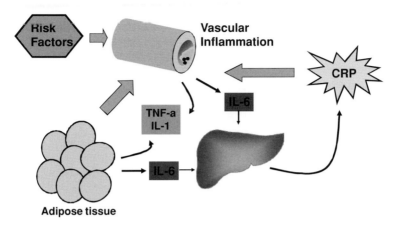

Fig. 9.3 Potential mechanisms for the association between C-reactive protein and cardiovascular events. 1) Atherosclerosis risk factors promote atherogenesis and vascular inflammation with the release of cytokines such as interleukin 6 (IL-6), tumor necrosis factor alpha (TNF-α), and interleukin 1 (IL-1) from activated leukocytes. IL-6 stimulates C-reactive protein (CRP) release from the liver. 2) Adipose tissue directly promotes atherosclerosis and also is a major source of IL-6, which increases CRP levels. These are parallel events without a direct relationship between CRP and vascular disease. 3) CRP derived from various sources directly promotes vascular disease. (Adapted from [55] with permission).

although the contribution of these sources to circulating levels is unknown [15–17]. One prevailing hypothesis of how CRP reflects vascular risk is that vascular inflammation, stimulated by various risk factors and other insults, results in CRP production in the liver that is measurable in the blood (Fig. 9.3) [55]. As such, CRP may be more closely associated with rupture-prone, inflammatory plaques than with the overall burden of atherosclerotic disease [56]. However, this paradigm is too simplistic, and CRP elevations and atherothrombosis may reflect parallel events with a common stimulus. Indeed, obesity and other metabolic risk factors may both promote atherosclerotic disease [57] and stimulate CRP release, as up to one-third of circulating IL-6 derives from adipose tissue and measures of obesity are highly correlated with CRP levels [58,59]. In addition, CRP derived from various sources may itself be a culprit in vascular risk.

An area of contention is whether or not CRP itself is directly involved in the atherosclerotic process. Several lines of evidence suggest that CRP may be a *risk factor* for CVD rather than just a *risk marker*. In vitro cell culture experiments and animal studies have provided insights as to how CRP may promote atherothrombosis including inducing the expression of cellular adhesion molecules, suppressing endothelial nitric oxide synthase, and increasing levels of endothelin 1, chemokines, and PAI-1 [60,61]. In addition to these effects

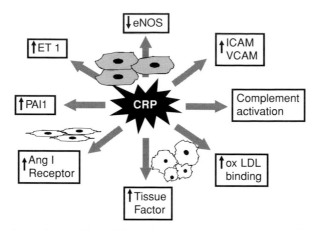

Fig. 9.4 Proatherosclerotic effects of C-reactive protein. C-reactive protein (CRP) adversely affects endothelial cell function by decreasing endothelial nitric oxide synthase (eNOS) expression, upregulating cellular adhesion molecules such as ICAM and VCAM, and increasing the release of endothelin-1(ET-1) and plasminogen activator inhibitor 1 (PAI-1). CRP also increases the number of angiotensin type 1 (Ang 1) receptors on vascular smooth muscle cells and affects macrophage function by inducing the secretion of tissue factor and enhancing oxidized LDL binding.

on endothelial cells, CRP can adversely affect vascular smooth muscle cell function, and can alter monocyte and macrophage activity by promoting tissue factor secretion and uptake of oxidized LDL (Fig. 9.4) [60,61]. Subsequently, two studies from the same group of investigators demonstrated that exogenous CRP given as a single bolus to healthy volunteers activated coagulation and thrombosis pathways as measured by prothrombin and PAI-1 levels, and was proinflammatory, resulting in increases in monocyte chemoattractant protein (MCP)-1 and IL-8 levels [62,63]. However, the validity of many of these earlier studies have been recently questioned as possible effects of lipopolysaccharide and azide contaminants that are commonly found in commercially prepared CRP preparations [64,65].

Transgenic mice studies offer additional insights into these issues by providing models of endogenous CRP production. An initial experiment by Paul et al. utilized mice genetically engineered to overexpress human CRP on the background of apo E deficiency; they reported that aortic atherosclerotic lesions were larger in the CRP transgenic mice compared with those without the transgene [66]. Despite this intriguing finding, two subsequent investigations of CRP transgenic mice have found no increase in atherosclerosis, despite higher CRP levels in these animals [67,68]. Human genetic studies of CRP have also provided conflicting reports as well (Table 9.2). Miller et al. resequenced the CRP gene in 192 subjects in the Women's Health Study and identified 6 sequence polymorphisms

Table 9.2 Association studies of *CRP* gene polymorphisms with coronary heart disease.

Study	Design	Number of CHD events	Association with CRP Levels	Association with CHD Events
Physicians' Health Study [69]	Nested case-control	610 cases	Yes	No
Framingham Heart Study [71]	Cohort	52 incident 210 prevalent	Yes	No
Rotterdam Study [70]	Cohort	584 incident	Yes	No
Cardiovascular Health Study [73]	Cohort	490 incident	Yes	Yes
NHANES [92]	Cohort	235 prevalent	Yes	Possibly
European Cohorts [93]	Nested case-control	985 cases	Yes	No

that were consistently related to CRP levels in additional cohorts [69]. However, none of these variants were associated with CV events in a direction consistent with their effect on CRP in over 1300 cases and controls from the Physicians' Health Study. Similar null genetic studies of CRP have been reported by other investigators [70–72]. Investigators from the Cardiovascular Health Study evaluated the relationships of five single-nucleotide polymorphisms in the CRP gene to CRP levels, subclinical atherosclerosis, and CV events. The investigators found three polymorphisms to be associated with CV events in whites, and one in blacks, suggesting a causal role for CRP in these events [73]. Novel CRP inhibitors currently under development will provide additional opportunities to explore the role of CRP in atherothrombosis [74]. Regardless of any etiologic role in atherogenesis, CRP may still be an important risk marker for CVD.

C-reactive protein for population screening

Given the increasingly evident shortcomings of the Framingham Risk Score, novel strategies for CV risk assessment are being sought. CRP testing has emerged as a leading candidate to enhance risk assessment given its biologic characteristics and the wealth of clinical data that has amassed supporting its potential use for this purpose. In 2003, the American Heart Association and Centers for Disease Control (AHA/CDC) issued clinical practice recommendations supporting the use of CRP testing as an adjunct to CV risk assessment in

Table 9.3 Potential strategies for incorporating C-reactive protein into cardiovascular risk assessment.

Strategy	Reference	Result
Measure in subjects at intermediate risk (10–20% 10-year CHD risk) by FRS	AHA/CDC [75]	CRP demonstrated to stratify risk in this group [30,53,54]
Create a CRP-modified FRS	Cook et al. [78]	Reclassification of ~20% of intermediate risk (5–20% 10-year CHD risk) women [78]
Create a novel risk score incorporating CRP	Ridker et al. [80]	Reclassification of ~40–50% of intermediate risk (5–20% 10-year CHD risk) women [80]

select cases [75]. In this statement, CRP was advocated over other inflammatory biomarkers due to its more advanced clinical assay and extensive supporting data. Importantly, clinical cut-points for CRP interpretation were outlined (<1mg/L, lower risk; 1–3 mg/L, intermediate risk; >3 mg/L, higher risk), and the optional use of CRP was recommended for those at intermediate risk (10–20% absolute 10-year risk of coronary heart disease events) by the Framingham Risk Score.

Although this AHA/CDC statement provided some clarification regarding the clinical use of CRP, the appropriate strategy for incorporating this biomarker into CV risk assessment for primary prevention has not been settled (Table 9.3). One potential strategy is to work within the Framingham Risk Score construct, as suggested by the AHA/CDC recommendations. Based upon Bayesian principles and therapeutic decision making, CRP testing may be most informative in those considered intermediate risk by Framingham Risk Score [76]. In this group, high CRP levels may warrant escalation to the high-risk category (>20% 10-year risk) with intensification of preventive therapies, including the use of cholesterol-lowering agents in both sexes and aspirin in women (aspirin is already recommended for men at intermediate risk). Indeed, high CRP levels in this group appear to escalate CV risk beyond the high-risk threshold (>20% 10-year risk), at least in men [53]. In contrast, CRP testing is ineffective as an adjunctive tool in those considered low risk by the Framingham Risk Score, in whom refining risk may result in the most meaningful clinical changes, such as eligibility for statin therapy and aspirin, and in whom traditional risk assessment methods are most problematic [9,10]. The modest relative risk increase with high CRP levels in these subjects would not measurably increase their absolute short-term CV risk. Similarly, CRP testing would add little to clinical decision making for those considered high risk by the Framingham Risk

Score, as preventive therapies should already be maximized in this group, and low CRP levels do not sufficiently lower risk estimates to warrant withdrawing these therapies [77].

Another proposed strategy is to incorporate CRP measures into a modified Framingham Risk Score [78,79]. Ridker et al. analyzed data from over 40,000 participants in the Women's Health Study, a cohort of women ages 45 years and older who were followed for an average of 10 years, to determine the additional utility of adding CRP to Framingham risk covariates [78]. In a derivation cohort of 15,048 women, global CV risk prediction models using Framingham variables and CRP were constructed, with measures of global fit and calibration favoring the inclusion of CRP to enhance the accuracy of these risk prediction algorithms. Furthermore, in a validation cohort of 26,927 women, models including CRP were able to reclassify subjects to higher or lower risk groups within risk categories derived by the traditional Framingham algorithms. Reclassification occurred in approximately 20% of those deemed to be 5–20% 10-year risk by the Framingham Risk Score, but only in 2.1% of those in the lowest risk group (<5% risk), which constituted the vast majority of the participants.

Ridker and colleagues have proposed a novel CV risk prediction algorithm for women, distinct from the Framingham Risk Score, which includes CRP as well as other emerging and traditional CV risk factors [80]. In their analyses, 35 putative risk factors were assessed in a model derivation cohort of 16,400 subjects in the Women's Health Study, and the generated models were tested in a validation cohort of 8158 subjects. A more detailed model including nine variables, as well as a clinically simplified model consisting of age, hemoglobin A1C, current smoking, systolic blood pressure, HDL cholesterol, total cholesterol, CRP, and parental history of MI < age 60 were assessed. Both models improved measures of global fit and calibration compared with traditional Framingham algorithms, and demonstrated modest improvements in discrimination of CV events as measured by the c-statistic. In addition, these new models reclassified 40–50% of women categorized into the 5- <10% and 10- <20% risk groups by Framingham Risk Score into higher or lower risk groups. Similar novel algorithms for CV risk prediction incorporating CRP have not been proposed for men, and validation of these models in women from other cohorts have not been performed.

Controversies regarding the clinical use of C-reactive protein

Few putative CV risk factors have been as extensively and rigorously evaluated as CRP. Despite fairly robust data supporting its predictive ability for incident CV events, the incorporation of CRP into clinical risk assessment for CV disease remains controversial [52,77]. Indeed, the story thus far of CRP and CV risk assessment is illustrative of the challenges facing all new potential risk markers for this purpose. Several unresolved questions contribute to the ongoing debate about the clinical use of CRP including applicability to diverse populations, clarification of its biologic role in atherothrombosis, and incremental value over traditional risk assessment measures.

Currently recommended clinical cut-points of CRP outlined in the AHA/CDC guidelines were derived from >40,000 patients from more than 15 different populations [75]. However, those populations were predominantly derived from homogeneous cohorts with very few ethnic minorities, and lower rates of obesity than in the general U.S. population. Subsequent reports have demonstrated that there are significant ethnic differences in CRP levels, raising questions about the applicability of uniform thresholds of CRP across ethnic groups to denote CV risk [59,81–84]. Investigators in Canada measured CRP in a random sample of 1250 subjects from 4 different ethnic groups and demonstrated marked differences in age- and sex-adjusted mean CRP levels, ranging from 3.74 mg/L among Aboriginals, to 2.59 mg/L in South Asians, 2.06 in Europeans, and 1.18 mg/L among Chinese (p < 0.0001) [84]. In addition, multiple studies performed in the United States have shown that CRP levels are higher in blacks than in whites, with median levels approximately 30% higher [59,81–83]. Although these racial differences in CRP may reflect an increased risk for CV disease known to occur in African Americans, it should be recognized that African Americans do not have a greater burden of atherosclerosis than other ethnic groups, and data assessing the prognostic significance of CRP in different ethnic groups are urgently needed.

Perhaps more unexpected is the current appreciation for gender differences in CRP, with women having higher levels than men [56,83,85]. CRP levels diverge between genders as obesity increases [59], which may explain why gender differences in CRP were not appreciated in studies involving cohorts with a low prevalence of obesity [86,87]. Given that women have lower CV event rates than men, the use of the same CRP threshold to denote higher CV risk (>3 mg/L) may result in overutilization of preventive therapies in women. For example, in the Dallas Heart Study more than 50% of white women had elevated CRP levels compared with approximately 30% of white men (Fig. 9.5) [59]. Thus, CRP risk thresholds may need to be adjusted for different race and gender groups.

Another area of controversy is whether CRP provides additional information regarding CV risk to knowledge of routinely measured risk factors and the Framingham Risk Score. Despite CRP levels tracking closely with traditional risk factors, more than 10 studies have found an independent association between CRP and CV events after adjusting for the components of the Framingham Risk Score [52]. Importantly, *independence* between risk markers does not necessarily signify *incremental* utility. Several studies have utilized the c-statistic, which is analogous to measuring the area under the receiver-operator curve, to evaluate the incremental utility of CRP for the discrimination of incident CV events and have demonstrated minimal difference when CRP is added to Framingham covariates [45–47,51]. In general, a multivariable odds ratio of greater than 3

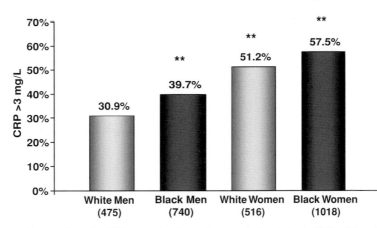

Fig. 9.5 Race and gender differences in C-reactive protein levels in the Dallas Heart Study. ** p-value <0.05 compared with white men [59].

is required for a meaningful change in this c-statistic (from 0.80 to 0.85) [88], while the reported odds ratio for CRP is more modest at around 1.5 [47]. However, the c-statistic may not be the optimal gauge of a risk marker's incremental value, and various other metrics have been suggested including use of alternative indices of global model fit, assessment of calibration, and evaluation of reclassification of risk among risk categories assigned by the Framingham Risk Score [89].

Similar statistical critiques could also be made for traditional risk factors such as low density LDL-c and elevated blood pressure that also provide minimal incremental value for CV risk prediction in multivariable models [47,89]. However, several lines of evidence including in vitro studies, animal models, large-scale observational studies, and clinical trials have confirmed that LDL-c is pathologically implicated in the atherosclerotic process and is a titratable target such that LDL lowering reduces atherosclerotic risk [6]. In contrast, it remains unclear whether CRP is directly involved in atherogenesis and whether lowering CRP modifies CV risk. In the Pravastatin or Atorvastatin Evaluation and Infection Therapy (PROVE IT) study examining intensive versus moderate LDL-c lowering using statin therapy in subjects experiencing acute coronary syndromes, those who achieved CRP levels <2 mg/L at 30 days had a significantly lower risk of CV events than those who achieved higher levels [43]. However, achieved levels do not necessarily reflect the overall reduction in CRP from baseline values, and the extent to which statin-mediated changes CRP can be disentangled from changes in LDL-c remain controversial [90]. Indirectly assessing the merits of targeting elevated CRP levels is the ongoing Justification for the Use of Statins in Primary Prevention: an Intervention Trial Evaluating Rosuvastatin (JUPITER) trial, which is examining whether treatment with statin therapy benefits subjects with elevated CRP levels (>2m/L), but LDL-c levels below current treatment thresholds (<130 mg/dl) [91]. If indeed statins are found to be beneficial in this setting, the study design precludes assessment of whether or not similar benefits exist for those with lower CRP levels.

Conclusions

Existing screening methods for heart disease risk have important limitations, and CRP has been embraced as a leading candidate to improve CV risk assessment. Currently, no other novel biomarker has as robust supporting data for an association with CV events as CRP. Despite several potential approaches, the optimal strategy for incorporating CRP into clinical practice for CV risk assessment remains unclear, and various additional questions must be addressed before this biomarker can be advocated for widespread use as a population screening tool. These challenges are not unique to CRP, but are applicable to all emerging CV risk assessment strategies, including other novel biomarkers, imaging studies, and the use of genetic data. In this way, CRP has served as the catalyst to expand our understanding of CV risk assessment methodology.

References

1 American Heart Assocation. Heart disease and stroke statistics-2006 Update. Dallas, TX: American Heart Association; 2006.

2 Rose G. Sick individuals and sick populations. *Int J Epidemiol* 1985; **14**: 32–8.

3 Castelli WP. Lipids, risk factors and ischaemic heart disease. *Atherosclerosis* 1996; **124**: S1–9.

4 Ridker PM, Rifai N, Rose L, Buring JE, Cook NR. Comparison of C-reactive protein and low-density lipoprotein cholesterol levels in the prediction of first cardiovascular events. *N Engl J Med* 2002; **347**: 1557–1565.

5 Khot UN, Khot MB, Bajzer CT, Sapp SK, Ohman EM, Brener SJ, et al. Prevalence of conventional risk factors in patients with coronary heart disease. *Jama* 2003; **290**: 898–904.

6 Executive Summary of The Third Report of The National Cholesterol Education Program (NCEP) Expert Panel on Detection, Evaluation, and Treatment of High Blood Cholesterol in Adults (Adult Treatment Panel III). *Jama* 2001; **285**: 2486–2497.

7 Wilson PW, D'Agostino RB, Levy D, Belanger AM, Silbershatz H, Kannel WB. Prediction of coronary heart disease using risk factor categories. *Circulation* 1998; **97**: 1837–1847.

8 Michos ED, Nasir K, Braunstein JB, Rumberger JA, Budoff MJ, Post WS, et al. Framingham risk equation underestimates subclinical atherosclerosis risk in asymptomatic women. *Atherosclerosis* 2006; **184**: 201–206.

9 Nasir K, Michos ED, Blumenthal RS, Raggi P. Detection of high-risk young adults and women by coronary calcium and National Cholesterol Education Program Panel III guidelines. *J Am Coll Cardiol* 2005; **46**: 1931–1936.

10 Akosah KO, Schaper A, Cogbill C, Schoenfeld P. Preventing myocardial infarction in the young adult in the first place: how do the National Cholesterol Education Panel III guidelines perform? *J Am Coll Cardiol* 2003; **41**: 1475–1479.

11 Liu J, Hong Y, D'Agostino RB, Sr., Wu Z, Wang W, Sun J, et al. Predictive value for the Chinese population of the Framingham CHD risk assessment tool compared with the Chinese Multi-Provincial Cohort Study. *Jama* 2004; **291**: 2591–2599.

12 Tillett WS, Francis T. Serologic reactions in pneumonia with non-protien somatic fraction of pneumococcus. *J Exp Med* 1930; **52**: 561–585.

13 Pepys MB, Hirschfield GM. C-reactive protein: a critical update. *J Clin Invest* 2003; **111**: 1805–1812.

14 Black S, Kushner I, Samols D. C-reactive Protein. *J Biol Chem* 2004; **279**: 48487–48490.

15 Calabro P, Willerson JT, Yeh ET. Inflammatory cytokines stimulated C-reactive protein production by human coronary artery smooth muscle cells. *Circulation* 2003; **108**: 1930–1932.

16 Ouchi N, Kihara S, Funahashi T, Nakamura T, Nishida M, Kumada M, et al. Reciprocal association of C-reactive protein with adiponectin in blood stream and adipose tissue. *Circulation* 2003; **107**: 671–674.

17 Yasojima K, Schwab C, McGeer EG, McGeer PL. Generation of C-reactive protein and complement components in atherosclerotic plaques. *Am J Pathol* 2001; **158**: 1039–1051.

18 Ridker PM, Rifai N, Pfeffer MA, Sacks F, Braunwald E. Long-term effects of pravastatin on plasma concentration of C-reactive protein. The Cholesterol and Recurrent Events (CARE) Investigators. *Circulation* 1999; **100**: 230–235.

19 Eda S, Kaufmann J, Roos W, Pohl S. Development of a new microparticle-enhanced turbidimetric assay for C-reactive protein with superior features in analytical sensitivity and dynamic range. *J Clin Lab Anal* 1998; **12**: 137–144.

20 Roberts WL, Moulton L, Law TC, Farrow G, Cooper-Anderson M, Savory J, et al. Evaluation of nine automated high-sensitivity C-reactive protein methods: implications for clinical and epidemiological applications. Part 2. *Clin Chem* 2001; **47**: 418–425.

21 Roberts WL. CDC/AHA Workshop on Markers of Inflammation and Cardiovascular Disease: Application to Clinical and Public Health Practice: laboratory tests available to assess inflammation–performance and standardization: a background paper. *Circulation* 2004; **110**: e572–576.

22 Libby P. Inflammation in atherosclerosis. *Nature* 2002; **420**: 868–874.

23 Lofstrom G. Nonspecific capsular swelling in pneumococci. *Acta Med Scand* 1943; **141**: 7–97.

24 Berk BC, Weintraub WS, Alexander RW. Elevation of C-reactive protein in "active" coronary artery disease. *Am J Cardiol* 1990; **65**: 168–172.

25 de Beer FC, Hind CR, Fox KM, Allan RM, Maseri A, Pepys MB. Measurement of serum C-reactive protein concentration in myocardial ischaemia and infarction. *Br Heart J* 1982; **47**: 239–243.

26 Haverkate F, Thompson SG, Pyke SD, Gallimore JR, Pepys MB. Production of C-reactive protein and risk of coronary events in stable and unstable angina. European Concerted Action on Thrombosis and Disabilities Angina Pectoris Study Group. *Lancet* 1997; **349**: 462–466.

27 Liuzzo G, Biasucci LM, Gallimore JR, Grillo RL, Rebuzzi AG, Pepys MB, et al. The prognostic value of C-reactive protein and serum amyloid a protein in severe unstable angina. *N Engl J Med* 1994; **331**: 417–424.

28 Kuller LH, Tracy RP, Shaten J, Meilahn EN. Relation of C-reactive protein and coronary heart disease in the MRFIT nested case-control study. Multiple Risk Factor Intervention Trial. *Am J Epidemiol* 1996; **144**: 537–547.

29 Ridker PM, Cushman M, Stampfer MJ, Tracy RP, Hennekens CH. Inflammation, aspirin, and the risk of cardiovascular disease in apparently healthy men. *N Engl J Med* 1997; **336**: 973–979.

30 Cushman M, Arnold AM, Psaty BM, Manolio TA, Kuller LH, Burke GL, et al. C-reactive protein and the 10-year incidence of coronary heart disease in older men and women: the cardiovascular health study. *Circulation* 2005; **112**: 25–31.

31 Danesh J, Whincup P, Walker M, Lennon L, Thomson A, Appleby P, et al. Low grade inflammation and coronary heart disease: prospective study and updated meta-analyses. *Bmj* 2000; **321**: 199–204.

32 Ford ES, Giles WH. Serum C-reactive protein and fibrinogen concentrations and self-reported angina pectoris and myocardial infarction: findings from National Health and Nutrition Examination Survey III. *J Clin Epidemiol* 2000; **53**: 95–102.

33 Koenig W, Sund M, Frohlich M, Fischer HG, Lowel H, Doring A, et al. C-Reactive protein, a sensitive marker of inflammation, predicts future risk of coronary heart disease in initially healthy middle-aged men: results from the MONICA (Monitoring Trends and Determinants in Cardiovascular Disease) Augsburg Cohort Study, 1984 to 1992. *Circulation* 1999; **99**: 237–242.

34 Ridker PM, Buring JE, Shih J, Matias M, Hennekens CH. Prospective study of C-reactive protein and the risk of future cardiovascular events among apparently healthy women. *Circulation* 1998; **98**: 731–733.

35 Rost NS, Wolf PA, Kase CS, Kelly-Hayes M, Silbershatz H, Massaro JM, et al. Plasma concentration of C-reactive protein and risk of ischemic stroke and transient ischemic attack: the Framingham study. *Stroke* 2001; **32**: 2575–2579.

36 Sakkinen P, Abbott RD, Curb JD, Rodriguez BL, Yano K, Tracy RP. C-reactive protein and myocardial infarction. *J Clin Epidemiol* 2002; **55**: 445–451.

37 Ford ES, Giles WH. Serum C-reactive protein and self-reported stroke: findings from the Third National Health and Nutrition Examination Survey. *Arterioscler Thromb Vasc Biol* 2000; **20**: 1052–1056.

38 Laaksonen DE, Niskanen L, Nyyssonen K, Punnonen K, Tuomainen TP, Salonen JT. C-reactive protein in the prediction of cardiovascular and overall mortality in middle-aged men: a population-based cohort study. *Eur Heart J* 2005; **26**: 1783–1789.

39 Ridker PM, Stampfer MJ, Rifai N. Novel risk factors for systemic atherosclerosis: a comparison of C-reactive protein, fibrinogen, homocysteine, lipoprotein(a), and standard cholesterol screening as predictors of peripheral arterial disease. *Jama* 2001; **285**: 2481–2485.

40 Albert CM, Ma J, Rifai N, Stampfer MJ, Ridker PM. Prospective study of C-reactive protein, homocysteine, and plasma lipid levels as predictors of sudden cardiac death. *Circulation* 2002; **105**: 2595–2599.

41 Ridker PM, Hennekens CH, Buring JE, Rifai N. C-reactive protein and other markers of inflammation in the prediction of cardiovascular disease in women. *N Engl J Med* 2000; **342**: 836–843.

42 Boekholdt SM, Hack CE, Sandhu MS, Luben R, Bingham SA, Wareham NJ, et al. C-reactive protein levels and coronary artery disease incidence and mortality in apparently healthy men and women: the EPIC-Norfolk prospective population study 1993–2003. *Atherosclerosis* 2006; **187**: 415–422.

43 Ridker PM, Cannon CP, Morrow D, Rifai N, Rose LM, McCabe CH, et al. C-reactive protein levels and outcomes after statin therapy. *N Engl J Med* 2005; **352**: 20–28.

44 Ridker PM, Rifai N, Clearfield M, Downs JR, Weis SE, Miles JS, et al. Measurement of C-reactive protein for the targeting of statin therapy in the primary prevention of acute coronary events. *N Engl J Med* 2001; **344**: 1959–1965.

45 van der Meer IM, de Maat MP, Kiliaan AJ, van der Kuip DA, Hofman A, Witteman JC. The value of C-reactive protein in cardiovascular risk prediction: the Rotterdam Study. *Arch Intern Med* 2003; **163**: 1323–1328.

46 Wilson PW, Nam BH, Pencina M, D'Agostino RB, Sr., Benjamin EJ, O'Donnell CJ. C-reactive protein and risk of cardiovascular disease in men and women from the Framingham Heart Study. *Arch Intern Med* 2005; **165**: 2473–2478.

47 Danesh J, Wheeler JG, Hirschfield GM, Eda S, Eiriksdottir G, Rumley A, et al. C-reactive protein and other circulating markers of inflammation in the prediction of coronary heart disease. *N Engl J Med* 2004; **350**: 1387–1397.

48 Ridker PM, Rifai N, Cook NR, Bradwin G, Buring JE. Non-HDL cholesterol, apolipoproteins A-I and B100, standard lipid measures, lipid ratios, and CRP as risk factors for cardiovascular disease in women. *Jama* 2005; **294**: 326–333.

49 Ridker PM, Buring JE, Cook NR, Rifai N. C-reactive protein, the metabolic syndrome, and risk of incident cardiovascular events: an 8-year follow-up of 14 719 initially healthy American women. *Circulation* 2003; **107**: 391–397.

50 Rutter MK, Meigs JB, Sullivan LM, D'Agostino RB, Sr., Wilson PW. C-reactive protein, the metabolic syndrome, and prediction of cardiovascular events in the Framingham Offspring Study. *Circulation* 2004; **110**: 380–385.

51 Folsom AR, Chambless LE, Ballantyne CM, Coresh J, Heiss G, Wu KK, et al. An assessment of incremental coronary risk prediction using C-reactive protein and other novel risk markers: the atherosclerosis risk in communities study. *Arch Intern Med* 2006; **166**: 1368–1373.

52 Ridker PM. C-reactive protein and the prediction of cardiovascular events among those at intermediate risk: moving an inflammatory hypothesis toward consensus. *J Am Coll Cardiol* 2007; **49**: 2129–2138.

53 Koenig W, Lowel H, Baumert J, Meisinger C. C-reactive protein modulates risk prediction based on the Framingham Score: implications for future risk assessment: results from a large cohort study in southern Germany. *Circulation* 2004; **109**: 1349–1353.

54 Ridker PM, Cook N. Clinical usefulness of very high and very low levels of C-reactive protein across the full range of Framingham Risk Scores. *Circulation* 2004; **109**: 1955–1959.

55 Nilsson J. CRP–marker or maker of cardiovascular disease? *Arterioscler Thromb Vasc Biol* 2005; **25**: 1527–1528.

56 Khera A, de Lemos JA, Peshock RM, Lo HS, Stanek HG, Murphy SA, et al. Relationship between C-reactive protein and subclinical atherosclerosis: the Dallas Heart Study. *Circulation* 2006; **113**: 38–43.

57 See R, Abdullah SM, McGuire DK, Khera A, Patel MJ, Lindsey JB, et al. The association of differing measures of overweight and obesity with prevalent atherosclerosis: the Dallas Heart Study. *J Am Coll Cardiol* 2007; **50**: 752–759.

58 Mohamed-Ali V, Goodrick S, Rawesh A, Katz DR, Miles JM, Yudkin JS, et al. Subcutaneous adipose tissue releases interleukin-6, but not tumor necrosis factor-alpha, in vivo. *J Clin Endocrinol Metab* 1997; **82**: 4196–4200.

59 Khera A, McGuire DK, Murphy SA, Stanek HG, Das SR, Vongpatanasin W, et al. Race and gender differences in C-reactive protein levels. *J Am Coll Cardiol* 2005; **46**: 464–469.

60 Verma S, Devaraj S, Jialal I. Is C-reactive protein an innocent bystander or proatherogenic culprit? C-reactive protein promotes atherothrombosis. *Circulation* 2006; **113**: 2135–2150; discussion 50.

61 Jialal I, Devaraj S, Venugopal SK. C-reactive protein: risk marker or mediator in atherothrombosis? *Hypertension* 2004; **44**: 6–11.

62 Bisoendial RJ, Kastelein JJ, Levels JH, Zwaginga JJ, van den Bogaard B, Reitsma PH, et al. Activation of inflammation and coagulation after infusion of C-reactive protein in humans. *Circ Res* 2005; **96**: 714–716.

63 Bisoendial RJ, Kastelein JJ, Peters SL, Levels JH, Birjmohun R, Rotmans JI, et al. Effects of CRP infusion on endothelial function and coagulation in normocholesterolemic and hypercholesterolemic subjects. *J Lipid Res* 2007; **48**: 952–960.

64 Lafuente N, Azcutia V, Matesanz N, Cercas E, Rodriguez-Manas L, Sanchez-Ferrer CF, et al. Evidence for sodium azide as an artifact mediating the modulation of inducible nitric oxide synthase by C-reactive protein. *J Cardiovasc Pharmacol* 2005; **45**: 193–196.

65 Pepys MB, Hawkins PN, Kahan MC, Tennent GA, Gallimore JR, Graham D, et al. Proinflammatory effects of bacterial recombinant human C-reactive protein are caused by contamination with bacterial products, not by C-reactive protein itself. *Circ Res* 2005; **97**: e97–103.

66 Paul A, Ko KW, Li L, Yechoor V, McCrory MA, Szalai AJ, et al. C-reactive protein accelerates the progression of atherosclerosis in apolipoprotein E-deficient mice. *Circulation* 2004; **109**: 647–655.

67 Hirschfield GM, Gallimore JR, Kahan MC, Hutchinson WL, Sabin CA, Benson GM, et al. Transgenic human C-reactive protein is not proatherogenic in apolipoprotein E-deficient mice. *Proc Natl Acad Sci USA* 2005; **102**: 8309–8314.

68 Trion A, de Maat MP, Jukema JW, van der Laarse A, Maas MC, Offerman EH, et al. No effect of C-reactive protein on early atherosclerosis development in apolipoprotein E*3-leiden/human C-reactive protein transgenic mice. *Arterioscler Thromb Vasc Biol* 2005; **25**: 1635–1640.

69 Miller DT, Zee RY, Suk Danik J, Kozlowski P, Chasman DI, Lazarus R, et al. Association of common CRP gene variants with CRP levels and cardiovascular events. *Ann Hum Genet* 2005; **69**: 623–638.

70 Kardys I, de Maat MP, Uitterlinden AG, Hofman A, Witteman JC. C-reactive protein gene haplotypes and risk of coronary heart disease: the Rotterdam Study. *Eur Heart J* 2006; **27**: 1331–1337.

71 Kathiresan S, Larson MG, Vasan RS, Guo CY, Gona P, Keaney JF, Jr., et al. Contribution of clinical correlates and 13 C-reactive protein gene polymorphisms to interindividual variability in serum C-reactive protein level. *Circulation* 2006; **113**: 1415–1423.

72 Zee RY, Ridker PM. Polymorphism in the human C-reactive protein (CRP) gene, plasma concentrations of CRP, and the risk of future arterial thrombosis. *Atherosclerosis* 2002; **162**: 217–219.

73 Lange LA, Carlson CS, Hindorff LA, Lange EM, Walston J, Durda JP, et al. Association of polymorphisms in the CRP gene with circulating C-reactive protein levels and cardiovascular events. *Jama* 2006; **296**: 2703–2711.

74 Pepys MB, Hirschfield GM, Tennent GA, Gallimore JR, Kahan MC, Bellotti V, et al. Targeting C-reactive protein for the treatment of cardiovascular disease. *Nature* 2006; **440**: 1217–1221.

75 Pearson TA, Mensah GA, Alexander RW, Anderson JL, Cannon RO, 3rd, Criqui M, et al. Markers of inflammation and cardiovascular disease: application to clinical and public health practice: A statement for healthcare professionals from the Centers for Disease Control and Prevention and the American Heart Association. *Circulation* 2003; **107**: 499–511.

76 Pasternak RC, Abrams J, Greenland P, Smaha LA, Wilson PW, Houston-Miller N. 34th Bethesda Conference: Task force #1–Identification of coronary heart disease risk: is there a detection gap? *J Am Coll Cardiol* 2003; **41**: 1863–1874.

77 Lloyd-Jones DM, Liu K, Tian L, Greenland P. Narrative review: Assessment of C-reactive protein in risk prediction for cardiovascular disease. *Ann Intern Med* 2006; **145**: 35–42.

78 Cook NR, Buring JE, Ridker PM. The effect of including C-reactive protein in cardiovascular risk prediction models for women. *Ann Intern Med* 2006; **145**: 21–29.

79 Ridker PM, Wilson PW, Grundy SM. Should C-reactive protein be added to metabolic syndrome and to assessment of global cardiovascular risk? *Circulation* 2004; **109**: 2818–2825.

80 Ridker PM, Buring JE, Rifai N, Cook NR. Development and validation of improved algorithms for the assessment of global cardiovascular risk in women: the Reynolds Risk Score. *Jama* 2007; **297**: 611–619.

81 Albert MA, Glynn RJ, Buring J, Ridker PM. C-Reactive protein levels among women of various ethnic groups living in the United States (from the Women's Health Study). *Am J Cardiol* 2004; **93**: 1238–1242.

82 Ford ES, Giles WH, Mokdad AH, Myers GL. Distribution and correlates of C-reactive protein concentrations among adult US women. *Clin Chem* 2004; **50**: 574–581.

83 Lakoski SG, Cushman M, Criqui M, Rundek T, Blumenthal RS, D'Agostino RB, Jr., et al. Gender and C-reactive protein: data from the Multiethnic Study of Atherosclerosis (MESA) cohort. *Am Heart J* 2006; **152**: 593–598.

84 Anand SS, Razak F, Yi Q, Davis B, Jacobs R, Vuksan V, et al. C-reactive protein as a screening test for cardiovascular risk in a multiethnic population. *Arterioscler Thromb Vasc Biol* 2004; **24**: 1509–1515.

85 Woloshin S, Schwartz LM. Distribution of C-reactive protein values in the United States. *N Engl J Med* 2005; **352**: 1611–1613.

86 Rifai N, Ridker PM. Population distributions of C-reactive protein in apparently healthy men and women in the United States: implication for clinical interpretation. *Clin Chem* 2003; **49**: 666–669.

87 Ye X, Yu Z, Li H, Franco OH, Liu Y, Lin X. Distributions of C-reactive protein and its association with metabolic syndrome in middle-aged and older Chinese people. *J Am Coll Cardiol* 2007; **49**: 1798–1805.

88 Pepe MS, Janes H, Longton G, Leisenring W, Newcomb P. Limitations of the odds ratio in gauging the performance of a diagnostic, prognostic, or screening marker. *Am J Epidemiol* 2004; **159**: 882–890.

89 Cook NR. Use and misuse of the receiver operating characteristic curve in risk prediction. *Circulation* 2007; **115**: 928–935.

90 Kinlay S. Low-density lipoprotein-dependent and -independent effects of cholesterol-lowering therapies on C-reactive protein: a meta-analysis. *J Am Coll Cardiol* 2007; **49**: 2003–2009.

91 Ridker PM. Rosuvastatin in the primary prevention of cardiovascular disease among patients with low levels of low-density lipoprotein cholesterol and elevated high-sensitivity C-reactive protein: rationale and design of the JUPITER trial. *Circulation* 2003; **108**: 2292–2297.

92 Crawford DC, Sanders CL, Qin X, Smith JD, Shephard C, Wong M, et al. Genetic variation is associated with C-reactive protein levels in the Third National Health and Nutrition Examination Survey. *Circulation* 2006; **114**: 2458–2465.

93 Casas JP, Shah T, Cooper J, Hawe E, McMahon AD, Gaffney D, et al. Insight into the nature of the CRP-coronary event association using Mendelian randomization. *Int J Epidemiol* 2006; **35**: 922–931.

Chapter 10

Newer markers for population screening: focus on lipoprotein-related markers

Vijay Nambi, Ron C. Hoogeveen, and Christie M. Ballantyne

Introduction

Identification and treatment of major modifiable risk factors for coronary heart disease (CHD) has led to improvements in CHD morbidity and mortality, yet many individuals who have CHD events may not have remarkable risk profiles based on major risk factors alone [1]. Therefore, increasing research interest has been focused on examining whether measurement of other factors may improve CHD risk assessment and perhaps even provide targets of therapy.

For cardiovascular disease prevention, recommended goals, such as those established by the U.S. National Cholesterol Education Program Adult Treatment Panel III (ATP III) guidelines [2], are predicated on the estimated risk of atherosclerotic cardiovascular disease over the next 10 years. In general, treatment decisions in patients classified as low or high risk by traditional risk scores are straightforward. However, patients that are classified as "intermediate" risk may in fact have "indeterminate" risk, and their actual risk may require further assessment to ascertain. Intermediate risk has been variably defined, with some referring to a 10-year calculated risk of 10–20% whereas others consider a 10-year risk of 5–20% as intermediate. It has been noted that ~65% of patients thought to be intermediate risk by traditional risk-stratifying schemes are misclassified and actually belong to the high- or low-risk groups [3]. The estimated percentage of the population considered to be at intermediate risk varies, with some reports suggesting that only 10% of the population have a 10-year risk between 6% and 20% [4], whereas another suggests that 35% of the population may be in this risk range [5].

Biomarkers in Heart Disease, 1st edition. Edited by James A. de Lemos.
© 2008 American Heart Association, ISBN: 978-1-4051-7571-5

Because traditional risk factors are generally effective in identifying risk, newer biomarkers are likely to add only modestly to risk prediction. Individuals who are clearly "low" risk (<5%) are rarely reclassified into a high-risk category. Therefore, we recommend that physicians should first use the risk stratification methods outlined in the current treatment guidelines to classify patients as low, intermediate, or high risk. In individuals determined to be at intermediate risk and for whom the decision for therapy is not clear, biomarkers may be useful to "fine-tune" the management strategy. Among the newer biomarkers that have been evaluated for risk prediction in population-based studies, C-reactive protein (CRP) and lipoprotein-associated phospholipase A_2 (Lp-PLA$_2$) have been approved by the U.S. Food and Drug Administration for assessment of cardiovascular disease risk. In this chapter we review the utility of advanced lipoprotein testing, lipoprotein(a), (Lp(a)) and Lp-PLA$_2$ in screening a population; other markers that have potential utility in screening, including CRP and B-type natriuretic peptide, are reviewed elsewhere in chapters 6 and 9.

Lipoprotein-related biomarkers

Non–high-density lipoprotein cholesterol level

Although ATP III focuses on low-density lipoprotein cholesterol (LDL-C) as the primary target of therapy, the revised guidelines also established non-high density lipoprotein cholesterol (non-HDL-C) as a secondary target of therapy in individuals with high triglycerides (Table 10.1). Non–HDL-C, obtained from the standard lipid panel by subtracting HDL-C from total cholesterol, reflects the combined cholesterol in atherogenic lipoproteins (LDL, very low density lipoprotein [VLDL] remnants, and Lp(a)) and therefore provides a measure of all apo B–containing lipoproteins. A number of studies suggest that non–HDL-C is a stronger risk predictor than LDL-C. In the Lipid Research Clinics Follow-up Study, each 30-mg/dL increment in non–HDL-C was associated with a 19% increase in risk for cardiovascular death, whereas each 30-mg/dL increment in LDL-C was associated with an 8% increase in risk for cardiovascular death [6]. In the Women's Health Study, the relative risk for a cardiovascular event in women with non–HDL-C in the highest quintile (>191.0 mg/dL) was 2.51 (95% confidence interval [CI] 1.69–3.72) relative to the lowest quintile (<39.5 mg/dL) [7]. By comparison, relative risk in women with LDL-C in the highest quintile (>153.9 mg/dL) was 1.62 (95% CI 1.17–2.25).

Apolipoprotein B level

Because the various lipoprotein fractions differ greatly in size and lipid composition, it is critical to understand the distinction between the plasma concentration of lipids and the plasma concentration of lipoprotein particles. For example, VLDL contains mostly triglycerides and is much larger than LDL particles, which contain mostly cholesterol. Furthermore, the half-life and plasma concentrations of LDL particles in the circulation are approximately 9 times greater

Table 10.1 Updated ATP III goals and cut-points for therapy by risk category [2,97].

| Risk category | LDL-C, mg/dL | | | Non-HDL-C, mg/dL |
	Goal	Initiation level for TLC	Consideration level for drug therapy	Goal
CHD or CHD risk equivalents (10-yr risk >20%)	<100 (optional: <70)	≥100	≥100 (<100: drug optional)	<130
2+ risk factors (10-yr risk 10–20%)	<130 (optional: <100)	≥130	≥130 (100–129: drug optional)	<160
2+ risk factors (10-yr risk <10%)	<130	≥130	≥160	<160
0–1 risk factor	<160	≥160	≥190 (160–189: LDL-C–lowering drug optional)	<190

than that of the VLDL particles from which they are metabolically derived [8]. Besides differences in size and lipid composition, different lipoprotein fractions have distinct biological functions and are generally categorized as pro- or anti-atherogenic. The rationale for measurement of apo B is that all lipoprotein fractions considered to be atherogenic, including VLDL, intermediate-density lipoprotein (IDL), LDL, and Lp(a), contain one molecule of apo B per lipoprotein particle. Therefore, in contrast to conventional lipid measures, measurement of apo B levels accurately captures the total number of circulating atherogenic lipoprotein particles. In epidemiological studies apo B has been found to be predictive of future cardiovascular events and in some studies was more predictive than LDL-C [7,9,10]. Furthermore, several clinical trials suggest that apo B is superior to LDL-C in judging the efficacy of statin therapy [11,12].

Measurement of apo B has certain practical advantages over LDL-C, as fasting is not required for accurate measurement of plasma apolipoproteins. Moreover, LDL-C cannot be accurately calculated in patients with triglyceride levels exceeding 400 mg/dL, in whom LDL-C must be determined by nonstandardized direct measurements. In contrast, the measurement of apo B has been automated and standardized.

In the Québec Cardiovascular Study, a 1–standard deviation increment in baseline plasma apo B was associated with a 5-year relative risk for CHD of 1.3 (95% CI 1.04–1.60) after adjustment for triglycerides, HDL-C, and total cholesterol:HDL-C ratio [13]. In the Atherosclerosis Risk in Communities (ARIC) study, apo B level was strongly associated with incident CHD on univariate analysis, with a similar relative risk as LDL-C, but was not associated with CHD in multivariable models that included LDL-C, triglyceride, and HDL-C [14]. In the Women's Health Study, apo B and non–HDL-C were similarly predictive of cardiovascular events, with respective relative risks of 2.50 and 2.51 for the highest compared with the lowest quintile [7].

Optimal assessment of atherogenic lipoprotein levels for risk assessment and targets of therapy

Although the ATP III guidelines continue to focus on LDL-C levels, some investigators have suggested that non–HDL-C or apo B levels might be more useful. Suggested targets for all three parameters have been suggested (Table 10.2). Non–HDL-C is strongly correlated with apo B [15], and unlike apo B, non–HDL-C requires no additional measurement beyond the standard lipid profile. Therefore, in clinical practice, the use of non–HDL-C can be recommended to assess total levels of atherogenic lipoproteins, and in patients with high triglycerides, the ATP III guidelines provide non–HDL-C goals as a secondary target of therapy.

Lipoprotein(a)

Although Lp(a) has been extensively studied in the last four decades, the complexity of the lipoprotein's structure and metabolism has hampered studies to

Table 10.2 Proposed goals for LDL-C, non–HDL-C, and apo B [16].

Risk category	Therapeutic goal, mg/dL		
	LDL-C	Non-HDL-C	Apo B
CHD or CHD risk equivalents	<100	<130	<90
2+ risk factors	<130	<160	<110
0–1 risk factor	<160	<190	<130

define how measurement of Lp(a) should be used in clinical practice. Lp(a) contains a lipoprotein moiety that is similar to LDL in lipid composition and the presence of apo B but contains a unique glycoprotein, apo(a), which is covalently attached to apo B by a single disulfide bond (Fig. 10.1) [17]. The sequence of apo(a) is similar to that of plasminogen [18] (Fig. 10.2). Apo(a) contains a variable number of identically repeated copies of kringle IV type 2 domains, leading to differences in Lp(a) size and molecular weight. The presence of the plasminogen-like moieties in Lp(a) have led investigators to hypothesize that Lp(a) constitutes a unique link between atherosclerosis and thrombosis. Lp(a) is present in atherosclerotic lesions, with plaque accumulation related to levels of Lp(a) in plasma [19].

Levels of Lp(a) have much greater variability in humans than levels of LDL or HDL, and this is believed to be primarily due to production rather than catabolism [20]. In Caucasians, 90% of variability in plasma Lp(a) levels is thought to be determined at the level of the gene, and the number of kringle IV type 2 domain repeats contributes a large amount to the variation in levels [21]. In general, there is an inverse relation between apo(a) isoform size and plasma levels of Lp(a) [22]. However, isoform size does not explain plasma levels for many individuals, as African Americans have higher Lp(a) levels than Caucasians despite similar apo(a) isoform size [23].

The role of Lp(a) in CHD risk has been examined in many studies. A meta-analysis of 27 prospective studies with more than 5000 incident CHD cases and mean follow-up of 10 years showed that Lp(a) levels in the top third were associated with a 70% increase in risk for CHD compared with those in the bottom third [24]. In a case-control analysis from the ARIC study, which included 725 incident CHD cases, Lp(a) was found to be an independent predictor of incident CHD, with a relative risk of 1.17 per standard deviation increase in a model that also included LDL-C, HDL-C, and triglycerides [15]. Lp(a) was also associated with stroke in the ARIC study among women but not men [25]. Several studies have suggested that the risk associated with elevated Lp(a) levels may be augmented in individuals with high levels of LDL-C. In the Prospective Epidemiological Study of Myocardial Infarction (PRIME), Lp(a) levels were

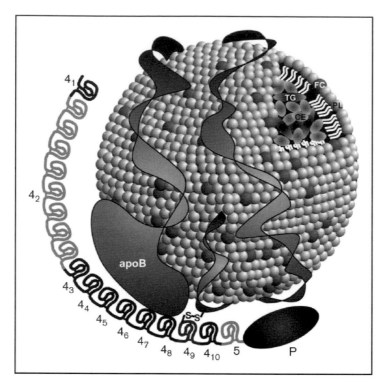

Fig. 10.1 Structure of Lp(a). Lp(a) contains a lipoprotein moiety that is similar to LDL but also contains a unique glycoprotein, apo(a), which is covalently attached to apo B by a single disulfide bond. *Abbreviations:* IV$_2$ = kringle IV type 2 domain; CE = cholesteryl esters; FC = free cholesterol; P = protease; TG = triglycerides. Reprinted with permission from [17].

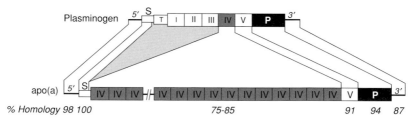

Fig. 10.2 Comparison of plasminogen and apo(a) sequence structure. *Abbreviations:* I, II, III, IV, V = kringles; P = protease domain; T = tail region. Reprinted with permission from [18].

Table 10.3 Lp(a) assays.	
Assay	**Upper limit of normal**
Quest	75 nmol/L
Lab Corp	30 mg/dL
VAP	10 mg/dL

associated with increased risk for MI and angina, with the greatest effect in individuals with high LDL-C [26]. In addition, the Women's Health Study found that high levels of Lp(a) (>90th percentile) were associated with increased cardiovascular risk especially in women with high LDL-C levels [27].

Lack of standardization of Lp(a) measurement has been a major barrier to both clinical research and defining the role of Lp(a) in clinical practice. Measurement of Lp(a) usually relies on immunological methods, and antibodies that react with the repeating kringle IV type 2 domain are sensitive to the apo(a) isoform size. Marcovina has developed an assay for Lp(a) using a monoclonal antibody to a unique epitope located in apo(a) kringle IV type 9 that does not repeat [28]. This assay was shown to reclassify 5–15% of individuals [29]. In the Physicians' Health Study, baseline Lp(a) assessed by this method was associated with the subsequent development of angina whereas Lp(a) assessed by a commercial assay was not associated with subsequent angina [30]. Because this method is not affected by apo(a) size, Lp(a) values are less likely to be over- or underestimated than with other immunological methods. The units and cut-points of three widely used assays for Lp(a) are shown in Table 10.3. Clinical situations in which measurement of Lp(a) level may be useful are listed in Table 10.4.

Statins do not reduce Lp(a) level. In patients with extremely elevated Lp(a) levels, LDL-C reduction with statin therapy may be less than expected ("statin resistant") because of the remaining high concentration of Lp(a) particles. Although some studies have shown apo(a) isoforms to be associated with cardiovascular

Table 10.4 Clinical situations in which Lp(a) testing may be useful.

- Intermediate-risk individuals for better risk stratification
- Familial history of cardiovascular disease
- Established coronary heart disease with a "normal" lipid profile
- Hypercholesterolemia refractory to therapy
- History of recurrent restenosis

disease independent of Lp(a) concentration [30,31], this association has not been consistently found in other studies [32,33]. Furthermore, measurement of apo(a) isoform size is not standardized.

Low-density lipoprotein particle size and number

LDL particles are heterogeneous in size and composition. Considerable in vitro evidence indicates that small dense LDL is more atherogenic than large buoyant LDL. Small dense LDL particles can enter the arterial wall more easily than large buoyant LDL [34]. Studies have shown that small dense LDL particles are more susceptible to oxidation, exhibit increased toxicity to vascular endothelial cells [35,36], have greater affinity for glycoproteins of the arterial wall, and bind more readily to scavenger receptors than to the classic LDL receptor [37,38]. The distribution of LDL subfractions is determined by both genetic and environmental factors [39,40]. However, the single most important determinant of the LDL particle size is the size of the pool of triglyceride-rich lipoproteins (ie, VLDL). Therefore, it is not surprising that small dense LDL concentration is highly correlated with triglyceride concentration and is increased in individuals with an atherogenic lipoprotein profile, e.g., patients with diabetes and patients with the metabolic syndrome [41]. Although LDL can be separated on the basis of size into as many as seven subclasses by electrophoresis [42], LDL is most commonly separated into two phenotypes. These phenotypes are commonly known as "pattern A" (characterized by a preponderance of large buoyant LDL particles) and "pattern B" (characterized by a preponderance of small dense LDL particles) [43].

Small dense LDL has been found to be associated with increased risk for vascular disease in cross-sectional studies [44–46] as well as prospective observational studies [47–49]. Furthermore, several clinical trials have shown that lipid-lowering therapy slowed the rate of progression of CHD, which was associated with a decrease in small dense LDL concentration [50–53]. However, in most of these studies, small dense LDL did not remain an independent risk predictor when adjusted for other cardiovascular risk factors such as triglyceride and total cholesterol/HDL-C ratio. The Québec Cardiovascular Study showed that the presence of small dense LDL did not substantially increase the risk of CHD in subjects that did not have an increased number of LDL particles [49]. However, in subjects who had an increased number of LDL particles as well as small dense LDL present (pattern B), the risk for CHD was increased 6-fold [13]. Furthermore, in contrast to LDL size, LDL particle number as measured by nuclear magnetic resonance (NMR) spectroscopy has more consistently been shown to be an independent predictor of CHD [54]. Taken together, these data indicate that it is the combination of increased numbers of LDL particles and the presence of small dense LDL that is highly atherogenic [55].

These findings have sparked debate regarding the importance of LDL particle size versus LDL particle number. Some investigators have argued that measurement of LDL particle size does not add independently (statistically) to the risk prediction of CHD when LDL particle number is assessed either by measuring apo B or by NMR spectroscopy [56]. However, a number of imaging studies [50,57] have demonstrated that the therapeutic modification of LDL size or the number of small dense LDL particles is associated with reduced progression of atherosclerosis. It is currently not known whether the increased cardiovascular risk associated with small dense LDL is a consequence of its increased atherogenicity or is instead caused by a broader underlying dyslipidemic pathophysiology. Although some have argued that changes in LDL particle size may be a target of therapy, additional research is necessary, as some therapies that increase LDL particle size (CETP inhibition, rosiglitazone) have not reduced CHD risk.

A number of laboratory techniques have been used to measure LDL particle size distribution in plasma, including gradient-gel electrophoresis, density-gradient ultracentrifugation, vertical automated profile (VAP) [58], and NMR spectroscopy. Each of these techniques has a number of limitations. Gradient-gel electrophoresis is a relatively complex technique that allows for LDL size measurements but cannot determine the number of LDL particles. NMR provides information on LDL particle size as well as concentration, and the technique is relatively fast compared with other methodologies. However, NMR requires expensive laboratory equipment as well as a high level of expertise in instrument operation and data analysis; therefore, analysis of LDL subclasses by NMR will most likely remain limited to specialized laboratories. In addition, there are large variations between measurements obtained by different methods [59], leading to reservations about the usefulness of LDL subclass analysis in clinical practice [60]. A novel precipitation method allows for measurement of small dense LDL particle concentration and can be adapted for most automated chemistry analyzers.

To date there are no standardized assays available for measurement of LDL particle size and concentration that are routinely available for use in clinical labs. The lack of standardization and reference values severely hampers the usefulness of these methodologies for general clinical practice. Based on the available data at the time of preparation of this chapter, assessment of LDL particle number appears to have greater promise, as this may potentially be useful in deciding when to treat and also may serve as a secondary goal in a manner similar to non–HDL-C and apo B levels. However, additional studies in outcomes trials would be necessary to determine whether LDL particle concentration adds significant incremental value beyond non–HDL-C and apo B for risk assessment in clinical practice.

High-density lipoprotein subclasses
In contrast to the atherogenic properties of LDL, HDL is considered cardioprotective, and low plasma HDL-C level is recognized as a risk factor for cardiovascular disease [2,61]. Cardioprotective functions of HDL include its involvement in the reverse cholesterol transport pathway, antioxidant effects, particularly in

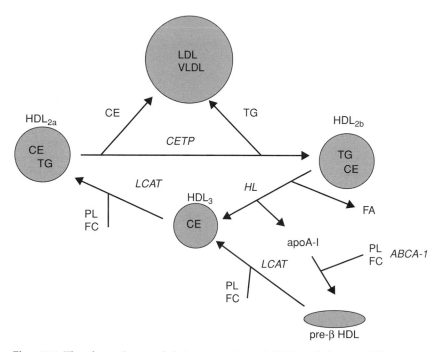

Fig. 10.3 The formation and interconversion of HDL subclasses. *Abbreviations:* ABCA1 = ATP-binding cassette transporter A1; CE = cholesteryl esters; CETP = cholesteryl ester transfer protein; FA = fatty acids; FC = free cholesterol; HL = hepatic lipase; LCAT = lecithin:cholesterol acyltransferase; PL = phospholipids; TG = triglycerides [62].

protecting LDL from oxidation, anti-inflammatory effects, and improvement of vascular endothelial cell functions. The Framingham Heart Study demonstrated that HDL-C is a stronger predictor of risk for CHD than LDL-C [61]. Furthermore, clinical trials of statin therapy have shown that low HDL-C levels remain highly predictive of cardiovascular events despite successful lowering of LDL-C levels [12].

HDL is a heterogeneous class of lipoprotein particles comprised of subspecies that differ in density, size, shape, composition, charge, and biological functions. The formation of different HDL subpopulations is a result of the metabolic remodeling of HDL particles through their interactions with lipases as well as cellular receptors and lipid transporters (Fig. 10.3). HDL was first isolated based on density using ultracentrifugation and later by gel electrophoresis, identifying three major HDL subclasses, referred to as pre-β HDL, HDL2, and HDL3. However, with the advent of high-resolution procedures, several additional HDL subpopulations have been identified, including pre-β1 HDL, pre-β2 HDL, pre-β3 HDL, HDL2a, HDL2b, HDL3a, HDL3b, and HDL3c [63]. Furthermore, HDL can be differentiated into two subclasses based on apolipoprotein composition: lipoprotein A-I (LpA-I), which contains apo A-I but not apo A-II, and LpA-I/A-II, which contains both apo A-I and apo A-II. However, it is important to point out that although distinct HDL subfractions can be isolated based on their physiochemical properties by the various methodologies, the individual HDL subfractions remain heterogeneous in nature due to the constant remodeling of HDL particles in the circulation, as well as the association of numerous proteins and nonprotein factors with different HDL subfractions. The distribution of HDL subfractions is gender dependent [64], and individuals with low HDL-C levels (<40 mg/dL) have selectively lower circulating levels of large HDL subfractions compared to individuals with HDL-C >40 mg/dL [65]. Furthermore, associations between apo A-I gene polymorphisms and the distribution of HDL subfractions have been reported [66]. Several clinical studies have found associations of HDL particle size with CHD risk [67,68]. A recent study reported that decreased levels of HDL2b and pre-β HDL correlated with increased carotid intima–media thickness in families with low HDL [69]. Generally, these studies have shown the large LpA-I subfraction to be more anti-atherogenic than the smaller LpA-I/A-II particles [70,71]. However, a recent report from combined analyses in the Framingham Offspring Study and Veterans Affairs HDL Intervention Trial (VA-HIT) showed that LpA-I and LpA-I/A-II were not associated with CHD prevalence or recurrence of cardiovascular events [72]. The apparent discrepancy between studies may be a result of differences in methodologies used to isolate HDL subfractions or may reflect the fact that individual HDL subfractions are heterogeneous and contain a variety of different HDL species. In an attempt to avoid these complications, several studies have investigated the use of molar ratios of apo A-I/apo A-II to estimate the relative proportion of α- and pre-β HDL particles as a risk factor for CHD [73,74]. The current lack of standardized methodologies and the inherent heterogeneous nature of distinct HDL subfractions hamper their efficacy in cardiovascular risk prediction.

Apo A-I

Because apo A-I is the major protein constituent of anti-atherogenic HDL particles, it is not surprising that plasma apo A-I levels are inversely correlated with risk for CHD. However, the relationship between apo A-I and HDL-C is not as straightforward as that of apo B and atherogenic lipoproteins, because unlike atherogenic lipoproteins, which each contain 1 apo B molecule per particle, the number of apo A-I molecules per HDL particle varies from 2 to 4. Therefore, the apo A-I concentration does not represent the HDL particle concentration. Although some studies have suggested that apo A-I concentration is a stronger predictor of cardiovascular events than HDL-C concentration [75], this has not been shown in several large epidemiological studies [14].

Plasma apo A-I levels can be measured in the nonfasting state by standardized commercial assays and reference intervals have been established. Furthermore, the apo B/apo A-I ratio has been shown to be a strong predictor of cardiovascular risk and benefit of therapy.

Lipoprotein-associated phospholipase A$_2$ (Lp-PLA$_2$)

Lp-PLA$_2$ is a biomarker that has received Food and Drug Administration (FDA) approval for use in conjunction with clinical evaluation for risk assessment in prediction of CHD and stroke. Lp-PLA$_2$ is an enzyme that is principally produced by macrophages but is also produced by monocytes, platelets, and mast cells and circulates bound to LDL (~80%) and HDL (~15–20%) [76,77].

The serine-dependent, calcium-independent Lp-PLA$_2$ is a member of the phospholipase A$_2$ family and is thought to play a role in atherosclerosis by potentiating the inflammatory cascade in the intima of the vessel wall. The oxidation of LDL renders its phospholipid susceptible to hydrolysis by Lp-PLA$_2$. The result of this hydrolysis is the production of lysophosphatidylcholine (LPC) and nonesterified fatty acid (NEFA), which have been described to have various proinflammatory activities including chemoattraction of monocytes [78], upregulation of adhesion molecules and CD40 ligand on endothelial cells, and smooth muscle cell migration [79,80] all important components in atherogenesis. Lp-PLA$_2$ activity has been found to be higher in small dense LDL [81]. Increased expression of Lp-PLA$_2$ has been described in the necrotic core and surrounding macrophages of ruptured atherosclerotic plaques and in plaques with a thin cap, suggesting a role in plaque instability [82]. Hence, there is strong pathological and biological evidence that links Lp-PLA$_2$ to atherosclerosis and its complications (Fig. 10.4) [77]. However, the role of Lp-PLA$_2$ in cardiovascular disease may be more complex. Lp-PLA$_2$ is also known as platelet-activating factor–acetylhydrolase (PAF-AH). PAF, a phospholipid, has been shown to lead to degranulation and aggregation of platelets [83], and by hydrolyzing PAF, Lp-PLA$_2$ may have a potential anti-atherogenic or antithrombotic role. Similarly, Lp-PLA$_2$ that is associated with HDL is thought to be anti-atherogenic as well [84], and has been reported to protect LDL against oxidation [77]. Although one may consider the possibility that the net effect of Lp-PLA$_2$ depends on the relative amounts that are bound to LDL and HDL, current data seem to support a more proatherogenic role for Lp-PLA$_2$.

Lp-PLA$_2$ in clinical studies

Lp-PLA$_2$ has been studied in various populations (Table 10.5) [85]. In a nested case–control analysis from the West of Scotland Coronary Prevention Study (WOSCOPS) [86], Lp-PLA$_2$ level in the highest quintile at baseline was associated with an approximately 2-fold higher risk for adverse coronary events even after adjusting for traditional risk factors and inflammatory biomarkers, including CRP, fibrinogen, and leukocyte count. In the Women's Health Study [87], although baseline Lp-PLA$_2$ was significantly higher in CHD cases than controls, the association was not significant after adjustment for other risk

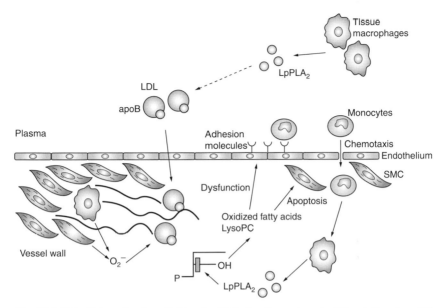

Fig. 10.4 Potential mechanisms linking Lp-PLA$_2$ to atherosclerosis. *Abbreviations:* LysoPC = lysophosphatidylcholine; O$_2^-$ = oxygen free radical; OH = hydroxy group; P = phosphate; SMC = smooth muscle cell. Reprinted with permission from [77].

factors. In a case-cohort study from ARIC that compared Lp-PLA$_2$ in 608 cases with incident CHD and 740 noncases, Lp-PLA$_2$ was significantly associated with incident CHD; individuals with Lp-PLA$_2$ in the highest tertile ($\geq$422 μg/L) had a hazard ratio (HR) of 1.78 (95% CI 1.33–2.38) compared with the lowest tertile (<310 μg/L) in a model adjusted for age, sex, and ethnicity, but the association did not remain significant after also adjusting for smoking status, systolic blood pressure, LDL-C, HDL-C, diabetes, and CRP [88]. However, in the subset of individuals with LDL-C <130 mg/dL (ie, among whom LDL-C–lowering may be optional depending on risk status), Lp-PLA$_2$ in the highest tertile was associated with a significantly higher HR compared with those in the lowest tertile (HR 2.08, 95% CI 1.20–3.62), even after full multivariable adjustment. Other studies have shown an association between Lp-PLA$_2$ and severity of CHD [89–91]. In addition, increased production of Lp-PLA$_2$ and LPC have been reported in the coronary circulation of patients with mild coronary atherosclerosis compared with controls, despite similar systemic levels of Lp-PLA$_2$, indicating local coronary production of Lp-PLA$_2$ and LPC in early coronary atherosclerosis [92].

The association between Lp-PLA$_2$ and stroke has also been examined in a number of studies. In the ARIC study, Lp-PLA$_2$ levels in the highest tertile were associated with an increased risk for incident ischemic stroke (HR 1.97, 95% CI 1.16–3.33) after adjusting for smoking status, LDL-C, HDL-C, systolic

Table 10.5 Studies evaluating the association between Lp-PLA$_2$ and CHD and stroke [85].

Population	Study	Design	Assay	Cases/noncases, n	Endpoint/Follow-up, y	Comparison of Lp-PLA$_2$	Adjusted HR
Primary prevention	WOSCOPS [86]	nested case–control	mass	580/1160	CHD death, MI, revascularization/5	per 1-SD increase	1.18 (1.05–1.33)
Primary prevention	WHS [87]	nested case–control	mass	123/123	CHD death, MI, stroke/3	highest vs lowest quartile	1.17 (0.45–3.05)
Primary prevention	ARIC [88]	case–cohort	mass	608/740	CHD death, MI, revascularization/6	highest vs lowest tertile	1.15 (0.81–1.63)
Primary prevention	ARIC [93]	case–cohort	mass	194/766	ischemic stroke/6	highest vs lowest tertile	1.93 (1.14–3.27)
Primary prevention	MONICA [89]	cohort	mass	97/837	CHD death, MI/14	per 1-SD increase	1.23 (1.02–1.47)
Primary prevention	Rotterdam [90]	case–cohort	activity	308/1822	CHD death, MI/7	highest vs lowest quartile	1.97 (1.28–3.02)
						per 1-SD increase	1.20 (1.04–1.39)
Primary prevention	Rotterdam [90]	case–cohort	activity	110/1822	ischemic stroke/6	highest vs lowest quartile	1.97 (1.03–3.79)
						per 1-SD increase	1.24 (1.02–1.52)
Acute coronary syndrome	PROVE IT [98]	clinical trial cohort with available samples	activity	3648 (baseline) 3265 (30-day)	death, MI, revascularization, stroke, unstable angina/2	highest vs lowest quintile	baseline: 1.08 (0.86–1.36); 30-day: 1.33 (1.01–1.74)
Secondary prevention	Koenig et al. [99]	patients with CAD	mass and activity	1051	cardiovascular events/4	highest vs lowest tertile	mass: 2.65 (1.47–4.76); activity: 2.40 (1.35–4.29)

blood pressure, diabetes, and CRP [93]. Individuals with both Lp-PLA$_2$ levels in the highest tertile and CRP >3 mg/L had the highest risk for stroke (HR 11.38, 95% CI 3.13–41.41; absolute 10-year risk 5.8%) compared with those with Lp-PLA$_2$ levels in the lowest tertile and CRP <1 mg/L (absolute 10-year risk 0.8%). Similarly in the Rotterdam study, Lp-PLA$_2$ activity was an independent predictor of ischemic stroke over a median follow-up period of 6.4 years [90].

As previously noted, the FDA has approved Lp-PLA$_2$ as a marker for prediction of CHD and ischemic stroke. For a marker to improve risk stratification and therefore be useful in routine screening in clinical practice, it must be additive to current risk prediction tools. The conventional way to evaluate predictive value is to look at 1) the ability of a marker to improve the area under a receiver operating characteristic curve (AUC) and 2) the ability of a marker to reclassify patients when added to traditional risk scores. Adding Lp-PLA$_2$ to standard risk factor models in the ARIC study significantly increased the AUC for prediction of CHD but by only 0.006 [94]. On the other hand the addition of CRP and Lp-PLA2 significantly improved the AUC for prediction of stroke in the ARIC study [95] with CRP increasing the AUC by 0.011 and Lp-PLA2 increasing it by 0.018 and the combination of CRP and Lp-PLA2 and its interaction term increasing the AUC by 0.039. Further, the addition of CRP, Lp-PLA$_2$, and the interaction between CRP and Lp-PLA$_2$ to the traditional risk factor model reclassified 4% of the low-risk category, 37% of the intermediate-risk category, and 34% of the high-risk category. However, while <1% shifted from the high-risk to the low-risk category, 26% of the moderate-risk category was reclassified as low risk and 11% as high risk. On the basis of these analyses, the authors concluded that routine measurement of Lp-PLA$_2$ was not warranted for CHD prediction while the measurement of Lp-PLA$_2$ and CRP may be useful in individuals in the intermediate-risk category for stroke prediction but not in those in the low- or high-risk categories.

Conclusion and recommendations

Currently, all adults should have a routine lipid panel measured as recommended by ATP III. Although LDL-C level remains the primary target of therapy, non–HDL-C level is a secondary target of therapy in patients with high triglycerides, as non–HDL-C level better captures the total "atherogenic" particles.

Apo B also measures total atherogenic lipoproteins and is a good predictor of CHD risk but only modestly improves risk assessment compared with the standard lipid profile; therefore, apo B should not be routinely measured for global risk assessment. Although measuring apo B may be useful as an alternative to calculating non–HDL-C for monitoring the efficacy of lipid-modifying therapy in patients with elevated triglycerides, the incremental benefit and cost-effectiveness have not been established. Apo B/apo A-I ratio may be useful as an alternative to total cholesterol/HDL-C ratio in assessing CHD risk.

LDL particle concentration, particularly in patients with elevated triglycerides, may help to identify patients at increased risk for CHD and may be useful in examining response to therapy. However, the incremental benefit of measuring particle concentration in addition to assessment of non–HDL-C or apo B level, both of which are well standardized, has not been shown. Therefore, measurement of particle concentration is not recommended for general practice.

Although LDL particle size has been associated with CHD risk, the data have not clearly indicated a benefit in risk prediction compared with traditional risk assessment and therefore routine assessment is not recommended. The usefulness of LDL particle size for monitoring response to lipid-modifying therapy has not been established. Although a number of methods are available for measuring LDL particle size, standardization is needed before this technology becomes useful in general clinical practice.

Lp(a) screening is not recommended for primary prevention or routine risk assessment, and assessment of apo(a) isoforms is not recommended for the general population. However, Lp(a) measurement may be useful in patients with a strong family history of premature cardiovascular disease to identify individuals with a genetic predisposition for cardiovascular disease. The usefulness of Lp(a) level as a target of therapy has not been established.

Lp-PLA$_2$ screening is not recommended for initial risk assessment. However, in patients at intermediate risk for whom the relative benefits and risks of preventive therapies such as statins or aspirin are uncertain, Lp-PLA$_2$ measurement may be used to inform clinical decisions about treatment. The suggested cutpoint for plasma or serum levels of Lp-PLA$_2$ that identify cardiovascular risk is ≥ 235 ng/mL (i.e., $\geq$ the 50th percentile) [96].

References

1 Ridker PM. Evaluating novel cardiovascular risk factors: can we better predict heart attacks? *Ann Intern Med* 1999; **130**: 933–937.
2 National Cholesterol Education Program. Third Report of the National Cholesterol Education Program (NCEP) Expert Panel on Detection, Evaluation, and Treatment of High Blood Cholesterol in Adults (Adult Treatment Panel III) final report. *Circulation* 2002; **106**: 3143–3421.
3 Arad Y, Goodman KJ, Roth M, Newstein D, Guerci AD. Coronary calcification, coronary disease risk factors, C-reactive protein, and atherosclerotic cardiovascular disease events: the St. Francis Heart Study. *J Am Coll Cardiol* 2005; **46**: 158–165.
4 Keevil JG, Cullen MW, Gangnon R, McBride PE, Stein JH. Implications of cardiac risk and low-density lipoprotein cholesterol distributions in the United States for the diagnosis and treatment of dyslipidemia: data from National Health and Nutrition Examination Survey 1999 to 2002. *Circulation* 2007; **115**: 1363–1370.
5 Greenland P, Smith SC, Jr., Grundy SM. Improving coronary heart disease risk assessment in asymptomatic people: role of traditional risk factors and noninvasive cardiovascular tests. *Circulation* 2001; **104**: 1863–1867.

6 Cui Y, Blumenthal RS, Flaws JA, Whiteman MK, Langenberg P, Bachorik PS, Bush TL. Non–high-density lipoprotein cholesterol level as a predictor of cardiovascular disease mortality. *Arch Intern Med* 2001; **161**: 1413–1419.

7 Ridker PM, Rifai N, Cook NR, Bradwin G, Buring JE. Non-HDL cholesterol, apolipoproteins A-I and B_{100}, standard lipid measures, lipid ratios, and CRP as risk factors for cardiovascular disease in women. *JAMA* 2005; **294**: 326–333.

8 Sniderman A, Vu H, Cianflone K. Effect of moderate hypertriglyceridemia on the relation of plasma total and LDL apo B levels. *Atherosclerosis* 1991; **89**(2–3): 109–116.

9 St-Pierre AC, Cantin B, Dagenais GR, Mauriege P, Bernard PM, Despres JP, Lamarche B. Low-density lipoprotein subfractions and the long-term risk of ischemic heart disease in men: 13-year follow-up data from the Quebec Cardiovascular Study. *Arterioscler Thromb Vasc Biol* 2005; **25**: 553–559.

10 Benn M, Nordestgaard BG, Jensen GB, Tybjaerg-Hansen A. Improving prediction of ischemic cardiovascular disease in the general population using apolipoprotein B: the Copenhagen City Heart Study. *Arterioscler Thromb Vasc Biol* 2007; **27**: 661–670.

11 Gotto AM Jr. Whitney E, Stein EA, Shapiro DR, Clearfield M, Weis S, Jou JY, Langendörfer A, Beere PA, Watson DJ, Downs JR, de Cani JS. Relation between baseline and on-treatment lipid parameters and first acute major coronary events in the Air Force/Texas Coronary Atherosclerosis Prevention Study (AFCAPS/TexCAPS). *Circulation* 2000; **101**: 477–484.

12 Simes RJ, Marschner IC, Hunt D, Colquhoun D, Sullivan D, Stewart RA, Hague W, Keech A, Thompson P, White H, Shaw J, Tonkin A. Relationship between lipid levels and clinical outcomes in the Long-term Intervention with Pravastatin in Ischemic Disease (LIPID) Trial: to what extent is the reduction in coronary events with pravastatin explained by on-study lipid levels? *Circulation* 2002; **105**: 1162–1169.

13 Lamarche B, Moorjani S, Lupien PJ, Cantin B, Bernard PM, Dagenais GR, Despres JP. Apolipoprotein A-I and B levels and the risk of ischemic heart disease during a five-year follow-up of men in the Quebec Cardiovascular Study. *Circulation* 1996; **94**: 273–278.

14 Sharrett AR, Ballantyne CM, Coady SA, Heiss G, Sorlie PD, Catellier D, Patsch W. Coronary heart disease prediction from lipoprotein cholesterol levels, triglycerides, lipoprotein(a), apolipoproteins A-I and B, and HDL density subfractions: the Atherosclerosis Risk in Communities (ARIC) Study. *Circulation* 2001; **104**: 1108–1113.

15 Ballantyne CM, Andrews TC, Hsia JA, Kramer JH, Shear C, for the ACCESS study group. Correlation of non–high-density lipoprotein cholesterol with apolipoprotein B: effect of 5 hydroxymethylglutaryl coenzyme A reductase inhibitors on non–high-density lipoprotein cholesterol levels. *Am J Cardiol* 2001; **88**: 265–269.

16 Grundy SM. Low-density lipoprotein, non-high-density lipoprotein, and apolipoprotein B as targets of lipid-lowering therapy. *Circulation* 2002; **106**: 2526–2529.

17 Koschinsky ML, Marcovina SM. Structure-function relationships in apolipoprotein(a): insights into lipoprotein(a) assembly and pathogenicity. *Curr Opin Lipidol* 2004; **15**: 167–174.

18 McLean JW, Tomlinson JE, Kuang WJ, Eaton DL, Chen EY, Fless GM, Scanu AM, Lawn RM. cDNA sequence of human apolipoprotein(a) is homologous to plasminogen. *Nature* 1987; **330**: 132–137.

19 Rath M, Niendorf A, Reblin T, Dietel M, Krebber HJ, Beisiegel U. Detection and quantification of lipoprotein(a) in the arterial wall of 107 coronary bypass patients. *Arteriosclerosis* 1989; **9**: 579–592.

20 Rader DJ, Cain W, Ikewaki K, Talley G, Zech LA, Usher D, Brewer HB, Jr. The inverse association of plasma lipoprotein(a) concentrations with apolipoprotein(a) isoform size is not due to differences in Lp(a) catabolism but to differences in production rate. *J Clin Invest* 1994; **93**: 2758–2763.

21 Boerwinkle E, Leffert CC, Lin J, Lackner C, Chiesa G, Hobbs H. Apolipoprotein(a) accounts for greater than 90% of the variation in plasma lipoprotein(a) concentrations. *J Clin Invest* 1992; **90**: 52–60.

22 Utermann G, Menzel HJ, Kraft HG, Duba HC, Kemmler HG, Seitz C. Lp(a) glycoprotein phenotypes: inheritance and relation to Lp(a)-lipoprotein concentrations in plasma. *J Clin Invest* 1987; **80**: 458–465.

23 Marcovina SM, Albers JJ, Wijsman E, Zhang Z, Chapman NH, Kennedy H. Differences in Lp[a] concentrations and apo[a] polymorphs between black and white Americans. *J Lipid Res* 1996; **37**: 2569–2585.

24 Danesh J, Collins R, Peto R. Lipoprotein(a) and coronary heart disease: meta-analysis of prospective studies. *Circulation* 2000; **102**: 1082–1085.

25 Ohira T, Schreiner PJ, Morrisett JD, Chambless LE, Rosamond WD, Folsom AR. Lipoprotein(a) and incident ischemic stroke: the Atherosclerosis Risk in Communities (ARIC) study. *Stroke* 2006; **37**: 1407–1412.

26 Luc G, Bard JM, Arveiler D, Ferrieres J, Evans A, Amouyel P, Fruchart JC, Ducimetiere P. Lipoprotein (a) as a predictor of coronary heart disease: the PRIME Study. *Atherosclerosis* 2002; **163**: 377–384.

27 Suk Danik J, Rifai N, Buring JE, Ridker PM. Lipoprotein(a), measured with an assay independent of apolipoprotein(a) isoform size, and risk of future cardiovascular events among initially healthy women. *JAMA* 2006; **296**: 1363–1370.

28 Marcovina SM, Albers JJ, Gabel B, Koschinsky ML, Gaur VP. Effect of the number of apolipoprotein(a) kringle 4 domains on immunochemical measurements of lipoprotein(a). *Clin Chem* 1995; **41**: 246–255.

29 Marcovina SM, Koschinsky ML, Albers JJ, Skarlatos S. Report of the National Heart, Lung, and Blood Institute Workshop on Lipoprotein(a) and Cardiovascular Disease: recent advances and future directions. *Clin Chem* 2003; **49**: 1785–1796.

30 Rifai N, Ma J, Sacks FM, Ridker PM, Hernandez WJ, Stampfer MJ, Marcovina SM. Apolipoprotein(a) size and lipoprotein(a) concentration and future risk of angina pectoris with evidence of severe coronary atherosclerosis in men: the Physicians' Health Study. *Clin Chem* 2004; **50**: 1364–1371.

31 Emanuele E, Peros E, Minoretti P, D'Angelo A, Montagna L, Falcone C, Geroldi D. Significance of apolipoprotein(a) phenotypes in acute coronary syndromes: relation with clinical presentation. *Clin Chim Acta* 2004; **350**: 159–165.

32 Paultre F, Pearson TA, Weil HF, Tuck CH, Myerson M, Rubin J, Francis CK, Marx HF, Philbin EF, Reed RG, Berglund L. High levels of Lp(a) with a small apo(a) isoform are associated with coronary artery disease in African American and white men. *Arterioscler Thromb Vasc Biol* 2000; **20**: 2619–2624.

33 Wild SH, Fortmann SP, Marcovina SM. A prospective case-control study of lipoprotein(a) levels and apo(a) size and risk of coronary heart disease in Stanford Five-City Project participants. *Arterioscler Thromb Vasc Biol* 1997; **17**: 239–245.

34 Nordestgaard BG, Zilversmit DB. Comparison of arterial intimal clearances of LDL from diabetic and nondiabetic cholesterol-fed rabbits: differences in intimal clearance explained by size differences. *Arteriosclerosis* 1989; **9**: 176–183.

35 Sattar N, Petrie JR, Jaap AJ. The atherogenic lipoprotein phenotype and vascular endothelial dysfunction. *Atherosclerosis* 1998; **138**: 229–235.

36 Dejager S, Bruckert E, Chapman MJ. Dense low density lipoprotein subspecies with diminished oxidative resistance predominate in combined hyperlipidemia. *J Lipid Res* 1993; **34**: 295–308.

37 Hurt-Camejo E, Camejo G, Rosengren B, Lopez F, Wiklund O, Bondjers G. Differential uptake of proteoglycan-selected subfractions of low density lipoprotein by human macrophages. *J Lipid Res* 1990; **31**: 1387–1398.

38 Anber V, Griffin BA, McConnell M, Packard CJ, Shepherd J. Influence of plasma lipid and LDL-subfraction profile on the interaction between low density lipoprotein with human arterial wall proteoglycans. *Atherosclerosis* 1996; **124**: 261–271.

39 Austin MA. Genetic and environmental influences on LDL subclass phenotypes. *Clin Genet* 1994; **46**: 64–70.

40 Austin MA, Talmud PJ, Farin FM, Nickerson DA, Edwards KL, Leonetti D, McNeely MJ, Viernes HM, Humphries SE, Fujimoto WY. Association of apolipoprotein A5 variants with LDL particle size and triglyceride in Japanese Americans. *Biochim Biophys Acta* 2004; **1688**: 1–9.

41 Gazi I, Tsimihodimos V, Filippatos T, Bairaktari E, Tselepis AD, Elisaf M. Concentration and relative distribution of low-density lipoprotein subfractions in patients with metabolic syndrome defined according to the National Cholesterol Education Program criteria. *Metabolism* 2006; **55**: 885–891.

42 Krauss RM, Burke DJ. Identification of multiple subclasses of plasma low density lipoproteins in normal humans. *J Lipid Res* 1982; **23**: 97–104.

43 Austin MA, Hokanson JE, Brunzell JD. Characterization of low-density lipoprotein subclasses: methodologic approaches and clinical relevance. *Curr Opin Lipidol* 1994; **5**: 395–403.

44 Austin MA, Breslow JL, Hennekens CH, Buring JE, Willett WC, Krauss RM. Low-density lipoprotein subclass patterns and risk of myocardial infarction. *JAMA* 1988; **260**: 1917–1921.

45 Campos H, Genest JJ Jr., Blijlevens E, McNamara JR, Jenner JL, Ordovas JM, Wilson PW, Schaefer EJ. Low density lipoprotein particle size and coronary artery disease. *Arterioscler Thromb* 1992; **12**: 187–195.

46 Coresh J, Kwiterovich PO Jr., Smith HH, Bachorik PS. Association of plasma triglyceride concentration and LDL particle diameter, density, and chemical composition with premature coronary artery disease in men and women. *J Lipid Res* 1993; **34**: 1687–1697.

47 Gardner CD, Fortmann SP, Krauss RM. Association of small low-density lipoprotein particles with the incidence of coronary artery disease in men and women. *JAMA* 1996; **276**: 875–881.

48 Stampfer MJ, Krauss RM, Ma J, Blanche PJ, Holl LG, Sacks FM, Hennekens CH. A prospective study of triglyceride level, low-density lipoprotein particle diameter, and risk of myocardial infarction. *JAMA* 1996; **276**: 882–888.

49 Lamarche B, Tchernof A, Moorjani S, Cantin B, Dagenais GR, Lupien PJ, Despres JP. Small, dense low-density lipoprotein particles as a predictor of the risk of ischemic

heart disease in men. Prospective results from the Quebec Cardiovascular Study. *Circulation* 1997; **95**: 69–75.

50 Watts GF, Mandalia S, Brunt JN, Slavin BM, Coltart DJ, Lewis B. Independent associations between plasma lipoprotein subfraction levels and the course of coronary artery disease in the St. Thomas' Atherosclerosis Regression Study (STARS). *Metabolism* 1993; **42**: 1461–1467.

51 Miller BD, Alderman EL, Haskell WL, Fair JM, Krauss RM. Predominance of dense low-density lipoprotein particles predicts angiographic benefit of therapy in the Stanford Coronary Risk Intervention Project. *Circulation* 1996; **94**: 2146–2153.

52 Mack WJ, Krauss RM, Hodis HN. Lipoprotein subclasses in the Monitored Atherosclerosis Regression Study (MARS): treatment effects and relation to coronary angiographic progression. *Arterioscler Thromb Vasc Biol* 1996; **16**: 697–704.

53 Williams PT, Superko HR, Haskell WL, Alderman EL, Blanche PJ, Holl LG, Krauss RM. Smallest LDL particles are most strongly related to coronary disease progression in men. *Arterioscler Thromb Vasc Biol* 2003; **23**: 314–321.

54 Cromwell WC, Otvos JD. Low-density lipoprotein particle number and risk for cardiovascular disease. *Curr Atheroscler Rep* 2004; **6**: 381–387.

55 Otvos JD, Jeyarajah EJ, Cromwell WC. Measurement issues related to lipoprotein heterogeneity. *Am J Cardiol* 2002; **90**: 22i–29i.

56 Sacks FM, Campos H. Clinical review 163: Cardiovascular endocrinology: low-density lipoprotein size and cardiovascular disease: a reappraisal. *J Clin Endocrinol Metab* 2003; **88**: 4525–4532.

57 Rosenson RS, Otvos JD, Freedman DS. Relations of lipoprotein subclass levels and low-density lipoprotein size to progression of coronary artery disease in the Pravastatin Limitation of Atherosclerosis in the Coronary Arteries (PLAC-I) trial. *Am J Cardiol* 2002; **90**: 89–94.

58 Kulkarni KR, Garber DW, Schmidt CF, Marcovina SM, Ho MH, Wilhite BJ, Beaudrie KR, Segrest JP. Analysis of cholesterol in all lipoprotein classes by single vertical ultra-centrifugation of fingerstick blood and controlled-dispersion flow analysis. *Clin Chem* 1992; **38**: 1898–1905.

59 Ensign W, Hill N, Heward CB. Disparate LDL phenotypic classification among 4 different methods assessing LDL particle characteristics. *Clin Chem* 2006; **52**: 1722–1727.

60 Stein EA. Are LDL subclass measurements clinically relevant? *Nat Clin Pract Endocrinol Metab* 2006; **2**: 120–121.

61 Gordon T, Castelli WP, Hjortland MC, Kannel WB, Dawber TR. High density lipoprotein as a protective factor against coronary heart disease: the Framingham Study. *Am J Med* 1977; **62**: 707–714.

62 Langlois MR, Blaton VH. Historical milestones in measurement of HDL-cholesterol: impact on clinical and laboratory practice. *Clin Chim Acta* 2006; **369**: 168–178.

63 Li Z, McNamara JR, Ordovas JM, Schaefer EJ. Analysis of high density lipoproteins by a modified gradient gel electrophoresis method. *J Lipid Res* 1994; **35**: 1698–1711.

64 Li Z, McNamara JR, Fruchart JC, Luc G, Bard JM, Ordovas JM, Wilson PW, Schaefer EJ. Effects of gender and menopausal status on plasma lipoprotein subspecies and particle sizes. *J Lipid Res* 1996; **37**: 1886–1896.

65 Montali A, Vega GL, Grundy SM. Concentrations of apolipoprotein A-I-containing particles in patients with hypoalphalipoproteinemia. *Arterioscler Thromb* 1994; **14**: 511–517.

66 Jia L, Bai H, Fu M, Xu Y, Yang Y, Long S. Relationship between plasma HDL subclasses distribution and apoA-I gene polymorphisms. *Clin Chim Acta* 2005; **360**: 37–45.

67 Cheung MC, Brown BG, Wolf AC, Albers JJ. Altered particle size distribution of apolipoprotein A-I-containing lipoproteins in subjects with coronary artery disease. *J Lipid Res* 1991; **32**: 383–394.

68 Asztalos BF, Collins D, Cupples LA, Demissie S, Horvath KV, Bloomfield HE, Robins SJ, Schaefer EJ. Value of high-density lipoprotein (HDL) subpopulations in predicting recurrent cardiovascular events in the Veterans Affairs HDL Intervention Trial. *Arterioscler Thromb Vasc Biol* 2005; **25**: 2185–2191.

69 Watanabe H, Soderlund S, Soro-Paavonen A, Hiukka A, Leinonen E, Alagona C, Salonen R, Tuomainen TP, Ehnholm C, Jauhiainen M, Taskinen MR. Decreased high-density lipoprotein (HDL) particle size, prebeta-, and large HDL subspecies concentration in Finnish low-HDL families: relationship with intima-media thickness. *Arterioscler Thromb Vasc Biol* 2006; **26**: 897–902.

70 Fruchart JC, Ailhaud G. Apolipoprotein A-containing lipoprotein particles: physiological role, quantification, and clinical significance. *Clin Chem* 1992; **38**: 793–797.

71 Asztalos BF, Roheim PS, Milani RL, Lefevre M, McNamara JR, Horvath KV, Schaefer EJ. Distribution of apoA-I-containing HDL subpopulations in patients with coronary heart disease. *Arterioscler Thromb Vasc Biol* 2000; **20**: 2670–2676.

72 Asztalos BF, Demissie S, Cupples LA, Collins D, Cox CE, Horvath KV, Bloomfield HE, Robins SJ, Schaefer EJ. LpA-I, LpA-I:A-II HDL and CHD-risk: The Framingham Offspring Study and the Veterans Affairs HDL Intervention Trial. *Atherosclerosis* 2006; **188**: 59–67.

73 Rosseneu M, De Backer G, Caster H, Hulstaert F, Bury J. Distribution and composition of HDL subclasses in students whose parents suffered prematurely from a myocardial infarction in comparison with controls. *Atherosclerosis* 1987; **63**: 231–234.

74 Asztalos BF, Batista M, Horvath KV, Cox CE, Dallal GE, Morse JS, Brown GB, Schaefer EJ. Change in α_1 HDL concentration predicts progression in coronary artery stenosis. *Arterioscler Thromb Vasc Biol* 2003; **23**: 847–852.

75 Walldius G, Jungner I, Holme I, Aastveit AH, Kolar W, Steiner E. High apolipoprotein B, low apolipoprotein A-I, and improvement in the prediction of fatal myocardial infarction (AMORIS study): a prospective study. *Lancet* 2001; **358**: 2026–2033.

76 Stafforini DM, McIntyre TM, Carter ME, Prescott SM. Human plasma platelet-activating factor acetylhydrolase. Association with lipoprotein particles and role in the degradation of platelet-activating factor. *J Biol Chem* 1987; **262**: 4215–4222.

77 Caslake MJ, Packard CJ. Lipoprotein-associated phospholipase A2 as a biomarker for coronary disease and stroke. *Nat Clin Pract Cardiovasc Med* 2005; **2**: 529–535.

78 Quinn MT, Parthasarathy S, Steinberg D. Lysophosphatidylcholine: a chemotactic factor for human monocytes and its potential role in atherogenesis. *Proc Natl Acad Sci USA* 1988; **85**: 2805–2809.

79 Zhu Y, Lin JH, Liao HL, Verna L, Stemerman MB. Activation of ICAM-1 promoter by lysophosphatidylcholine: possible involvement of protein tyrosine kinases. *Biochim Biophys Acta* 1997; **1345**: 93–98.

80 Macphee CH, Moores KE, Boyd HF, Dhanak D, Ife RJ, Leach CA, Leake DS, Milliner KJ, Patterson RA, Suckling KE, Tew DG, Hickey DM. Lipoprotein-associated phospholipase A$_2$, platelet-activating factor acetylhydrolase, generates two bioactive products during the oxidation of low-density lipoprotein: use of a novel inhibitor. *Biochem J* 1999; **338**: 479–487.

81 Karabina SA, Liapikos TA, Grekas G, Goudevenos J, Tselepis AD. Distribution of PAF-acetylhydrolase activity in human plasma low-density lipoprotein subfractions. *Biochim Biophys Acta* 1994; **1213**: 34–38.

82 Kolodgie FD, Burke AP, Skorija KS, Ladich E, Kutys R, Makuria AT, Virmani R. Lipoprotein-associated phospholipase A2 protein expression in the natural progression of human coronary atherosclerosis. *Arterioscler Thromb Vasc Biol* 2006; **26**: 2523–2529.

83 Lepran I, Lefer AM. Ischemia aggravating effects of platelet-activating factor in acute myocardial ischemia. *Basic Res Cardiol* 1985; **80**: 135–141.

84 Mackness MI, Durrington PN. HDL, its enzymes and its potential to influence lipid peroxidation. *Atherosclerosis* 1995; **115**: 243–253.

85 Nambi V, Ballantyne CM. Lipoprotein-associated phospholipase A$_2$: pathogenic mechanisms and clinical utility for predicting cardiovascular events. *Curr Atheroscler Rep* 2006; **8**: 374–381.

86 Packard CJ, O'Reilly DS, Caslake MJ, McMahon AD, Ford I, Cooney J, Macphee CH, Suckling KE, Krishna M, Wilkinson FE, Rumley A, Lowe GD, for the West of Scotland Coronary Prevention Study Group. Lipoprotein-associated phospholipase A2 as an independent predictor of coronary heart disease. *N Engl J Med* 2000; **343**: 1148–1155.

87 Blake GJ, Dada N, Fox JC, Manson JE, Ridker PM. A prospective evaluation of lipoprotein-associated phospholipase A$_2$ levels and the risk of future cardiovascular events in women. *J Am Coll Cardiol* 2001; **38**: 1302–1306.

88 Ballantyne CM, Hoogeveen RC, Bang H, Coresh J, Folsom AR, Heiss G, Sharrett AR. Lipoprotein-associated phospholipase A$_2$, high-sensitivity C-reactive protein, and risk for incident coronary heart disease in middle-aged men and women in the Atherosclerosis Risk in Communities (ARIC) Study. *Circulation* 2004; **109**: 837–842.

89 Koenig W, Khuseyinova N, Lowel H, Trischler G, Meisinger C. Lipoprotein-associated phospholipase A$_2$ adds to risk prediction of incident coronary events by C-reactive protein in apparently healthy middle-aged men from the general population: results from the 14-year follow-up of a large cohort from southern Germany. *Circulation* 2004; **110**: 1903–1908.

90 Oei HH, van der Meer IM, Hofman A, Koudstaal PJ, Stijnen T, Breteler MM, Witteman JC. Lipoprotein-associated phospholipase A2 activity is associated with risk of coronary heart disease and ischemic stroke: the Rotterdam Study. *Circulation* 2005; **111**: 570–575.

91 Brilakis ES, McConnell JP, Lennon RJ, Elesber AA, Meyer JG, Berger PB. Association of lipoprotein-associated phospholipase A2 levels with coronary artery disease risk factors, angiographic coronary artery disease, and major adverse events at follow-up. *Eur Heart J* 2005; **26**: 137–144.

92 Lavi S, McConnell JP, Rihal CS, Prasad A, Mathew V, Lerman LO, Lerman A. Local production of lipoprotein-associated phospholipase A2 and lysophosphatidylcholine in

the coronary circulation: association with early coronary atherosclerosis and endothelial dysfunction in humans. *Circulation* 2007; **115**: 2715–2721.

93 Ballantyne CM, Hoogeveen RC, Bang H, Coresh J, Folsom AR, Chambless LE, Myerson M, Wu KK, Sharrett AR, Boerwinkle E. Lipoprotein-associated phospholipase A$_2$, high-sensitivity C-reactive protein, and risk for incident ischemic stroke in middle-aged men and women in the Atherosclerosis Risk in Communities (ARIC) study. *Arch Intern Med* 2005; **165**: 2479–2484.

94 Folsom AR, Chambless LE, Ballantyne CM, Coresh J, Heiss G, Wu KK, Boerwinkle E, Mosley TH Jr., Sorlie P, Diao G, Sharrett AR. An assessment of incremental coronary risk prediction using C-reactive protein and other novel risk markers: the Atherosclerosis Risk in Communities Study. *Arch Intern Med* 2006; **166**: 1368–1373.

95 Nambi V. Inflammatory biomarkers LpPLA2 and CRP for prediction of first ischemic stroke. Paper presented at: Society for Vascular Medicine and Biology 18th Annual Scientific Sessions; June 7, 2007; Baltimore, Maryland.

96 Lanman RB, Wolfert RL, Fleming JK, Jaffe AS, Roberts WL, Warnick GR, McConnell JP. Lipoprotein-associated phospholipase A2: review and recommendation of a clinical cut point for adults. *Prev Cardiol* 2006; **9**: 138–143.

97 Grundy SM, Cleeman JI, Bairey Merz CN, Brewer HB, Jr., Clark LT, Hunninghake DB, Pasternak RC, Smith SC Jr., Stone NJ, for the Coordinating Committee of the National Cholesterol Education Program. Implications of recent clinical trials for the National Cholesterol Education Program Adult Treatment Panel III guidelines. *Circulation* 2004; **110**: 227–239.

98 O'Donoghue M, Morrow DA, Sabatine MS, Murphy SA, McCabe CH, Cannon CP, Braunwald E. Lipoprotein-associated phospholipase A$_2$ and its association with cardiovascular outcomes in patients with acute coronary syndromes in the PROVE IT-TIMI 22 (PRavastatin Or atorVastatin Evaluation and Infection Therapy-Thrombolysis In Myocardial Infarction) trial. *Circulation* 2006; **113**: 1745–1752.

99 Koenig W, Twardella D, Brenner H, Rothenbacher D. Lipoprotein-associated phospholipase A$_2$ predicts future cardiovascular events in patients with coronary heart disease independently of traditional risk factors, markers of inflammation, renal function, and hemodynamic stress. *Arterioscler Thromb Vasc Biol* 2006; **26**: 1586–1593.

PART IV

A Look to the Future

Chapter 11

Moving toward personalized medicine

David A. Morrow, Marc S. Sabatine, and James A. de Lemos

Introduction

Personalized medicine has been described as "the use of marker-assisted diagnosis and targeted therapy derived from an individual's [biochemical and] molecular profile" [1]. This promising paradigm has reached a contemporary formulation framed by substantial advances in the epidemiology and technology surrounding protein and molecular profiling (Fig. 11.1). However, the notion of using non-invasive testing to individualize therapy to maximize therapeutic benefit and minimize risk is fundamental to clinical medicine, as long-standing as microscopic examination of sputum in a patient with suspected pneumonia, and as pervasive as using testing of cholesterol to guide cardiovascular risk modification. Nevertheless, the goals of "personalized medicine" have expanded substantially from tailoring therapy around a single pathogen or cause, such as in pneumococcal pneumonia or pernicious anemia, to characterizing much more complex and heterogeneous disease states such as heart failure and acute coronary syndromes. This effort has its basis in the potential to apply newer genomic, proteomic, and imaging strategies to evaluate the individual patient. These same discovery efforts also offer the opportunity to identify new targets for which novel pharmacologic approaches may be developed. Consistent with the topic of this book, the discussion in this chapter will focus on protein biomarkers, as well as their possible integration with genomic and imaging techniques. The chapter will begin by drawing on the contemporary application of biomarkers in acute coronary syndromes (ACS) as an example to illustrate both early modest successes as well as failures of multiple biomarker profiling to realize the promise of personalized medicine in cardiovascular disease.

Biomarkers in Heart Disease, 1st edition. Edited by James A. de Lemos.
© 2008 American Heart Association, ISBN: 978-1-4051-7571-5

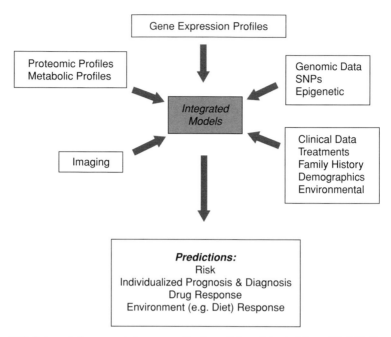

Fig. 11.1 Integrated approach to personalized medicine. Adapted from West M. *Genome Res* 2006; **16**: 559–566.

The remainder of the chapter will be devoted to future investigation, including criteria for assessment of novel biomarkers, newer strategies for biomarker discovery through proteomics and metabolomics, and integration with other clinical tools.

Multimarker strategies in ACS: A window to early experience with personalized medicine

The application of biomarkers for the evaluation of patients at risk for or presenting with atherothrombosis is one purpose for which there has been substantial evolution toward the paradigm of personalized medicine [2]. In particular, the use of biomarkers to comprehensively profile the individual patient presenting with suspected ACS has garnered intense investigational effort. As is true for most domains of personalized medicine, major advances in the understanding of the pathogenesis and consequences of acute coronary atherothrombosis have provided a stimulus for development of new biomarkers aimed at detecting underlying contributors to a complex syndrome. The emergence of numerous novel and pathobiologically diverse biomarkers has created the opportunity for an expanded role of multiple biomarkers in the diagnosis, classification of risk, and selection of treatment in ACS [2].

Mechanisms of Acute Coronary Ischemia

- Progressive mechanical obstruction
- Acute thrombosis on pre-existing plaque
- Dynamic obstruction (coronary spasm or vasoconstriction)
- Inflammation and/or infection
- Secondary unstable angina

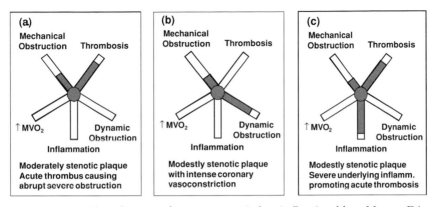

Fig. 11.2 Principal mechanisms of acute coronary ischemia. Reprinted from Morrow DA, Antman E (2005) The Pathobiology of Acute Coronary Syndromes: Mechanisms and Implications for Therapy. In: Becker RC, Harrington R, (eds), *The Practice of Clinical, Interventional, and Investigational Thrombocardiology*, Marcel Dekker, New York, with permission. MVO_2 = myocardial oxygen demand; inflamm. = inflammation

Characterizing pathogenesis and prognosis in ACS

ACS is a heterogeneous syndrome with multiple potential etiologies [3]. It follows that therapy is likely to be most effective when directed at the primary underlying contributors. Braunwald described five principal causes of ACS: 1) plaque rupture with acute thrombosis; 2) progressive mechanical obstruction; 3) inflammation; 4) secondary unstable angina; and 5) dynamic obstruction (coronary vasoconstriction) [4]. It is rare that any one of these processes exists in isolation, and inflammation appears to be a common thread in the majority patients with atherothrombosis. Thus, individual patients with ACS may vary substantially with respect to the predominance of contributions from each of these major mechanisms (Fig. 11.2) [4]. In addition, the risk of subsequent death and/or recurrent ischemic events also varies widely in this population, depending on the extent of irreversible myocyte injury, the hemodynamic sequelae of ischemia, and the severity and stability of atherosclerotic vascular disease. As such, patients presenting with ACS are excellent candidates for an individualized approach to care. To achieve this objective it is necessary to have both the means to discriminate the underlying pathobiology in the individual patient and the availability of appropriate therapeutic strategies.

Role of biomarkers

The emergence of novel biomarkers of inflammation, platelet activation, plaque vulnerability, and hemodynamic stress, along with more sensitive biomarkers of necrosis has fulfilled, in part, the need for tools to non-invasively profile the pathobiology, while at the same time refining the assessment of the patient's risk for recurrent cardiovascular events [2].

Cardiac-specific troponin has exemplified the potential for a protein biomarker to guide therapy. In addition to identifying patients at higher risk for recurrent ischemic events, an elevated concentration of cardiac troponin in the blood of patients with ACS is associated with the presence of intracoronary thrombus, distal embolization of platelet microaggregates, and impaired myocardial microvascular flow [5,6]. At the same time, potent anti-thrombotic agents and a strategy of early invasive management have been shown to provide particular benefit for patients with non-ST elevation ACS and elevated cardiac troponin (see chapter 2) [7,8]. As such, cardiac troponin has provided the prototype for use of biomarkers in personalizing therapy for patients with ACS. At the same time, the fact that cardiac troponin is also elevated in clinical settings outside of ACS in which very different therapy is warranted (see chapter 3) is a compelling caution against complete reliance on biomarker-guided therapy, and highlights the need to integrate other clinical data as well as clinical judgment.

As described in detail in other sections of this text, newer markers of inflammation, ischemia, thrombosis, and hemodynamic stress add to cardiac troponin for the evaluation of the patient with atherosclerosis, supporting the exploration of approaches that include a profile of multiple biomarkers. In particular, biomarkers of inflammation and hemodynamic stress have emerged as robust, independent predictors of outcome in patients with chronic and acute atherothrombosis (see chapter 4). Specifically, elevated levels of C-reactive protein (hs-CRP) are associated with poor short- and long-term prognosis in patients with ACS [9,10]. In addition, the concentrations of B-type natriuretic peptide (BNP) and the N-terminal fragment of pro-BNP (NT-proBNP) correlate with left ventricular dilatation, remodeling, and dysfunction, as well as the risk of congestive heart failure and death in patients presenting with ACS [11,12,13–17]. These observations set the stage for a combined assessment in multimarker strategies.

Enhanced risk stratification with simple multimarker approaches

Based upon their strong relationship with cardiovascular outcomes in patients with ACS and their diverse pathobiology, hs-CRP and BNP or NT-proBNP have been the first newer biomarkers to be formally evaluated along with cardiac troponin in a multimarker approach to the patient with suspected ACS. For example, our group evaluated a strategy that combined testing for hs-CRP and cardiac troponin T in patients with non-ST elevation ACS and found that the dual marker strategy provided more comprehensive risk assessment [9]. These

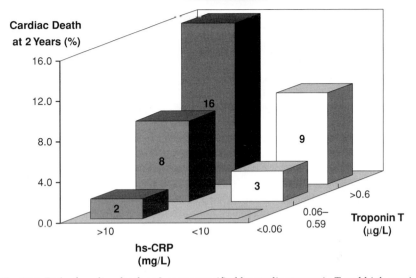

Fig. 11.3 Risk of cardiac death at 2 years stratified by cardiac troponin T and high sensitivity testing for C-reactive protein among patients with non-ST elevation ACS (N = 917) enrolled in the Fragmin during Instability in Coronary artery disease (FRISC) trial. Data from [10].

results were subsequently confirmed with respect to cardiac mortality through 2 years in 917 patients with non-ST elevation ACS, among whom CRP was associated with a higher 2-year risk of death regardless of troponin strata (Fig. 11.3) [10]. The assessment of dual marker strategies using a cardiac troponin and a natriuretic peptide has produced very similar results. BNP and NT-proBNP levels are elevated in 10–30% of patients with unstable angina (i.e., without myonecrosis) [13,16,18] and are associated with an increased risk of death and heart failure in this group (see chapter 4). When assessed in non-ST elevation ACS, BNP offers significant prognostic information independently of cTnI, identifying patients at significantly higher mortality risk among those with either negative (OR 6.9; 95% CI 1.9–25.8) or positive (OR 4.1; 95% CI 1.9–9.0) baseline troponin results. Thus, similar to that for hs-CRP, the combined use of BNP and cTnI improves risk assessment, enabling discrimination of patients with negative BNP or troponin who are at increased risk of death or myocardial infarction (MI).

   Building on this experience with dual-marker testing, our group evaluated a simple multimarker strategy combining BNP, CRP, cTnI, and assigning one point for each elevated marker. We found that use of 3 markers revealed a more than 10-fold gradient of mortality risk (1% to 18%) among patients with non-ST elevation ACS [19]. This strategy provided consistent risk prediction at both 30 days and 6 to 10 months, as well as across 2 independent data sets

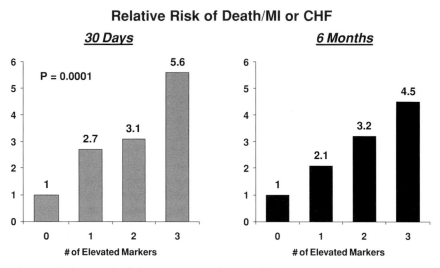

Fig. 11.4 Relative risk of the composite end-point of death, MI, or new CHF at 30 days and 6 months of follow-up in TACTICS-TIMI 18 stratified using the combination of cTnI, BNP, and hs-CRP. Data are from [19].

(Fig. 11.4). Although the risk relationships were not entirely homogeneous, a graded pattern of risk was present for the individual end-points of death, MI, and heart failure (Table 11.1). After adjustment for age, diabetes, ST deviation, history of heart failure, and prior MI, each multimarker category (1, 2, or 3 markers elevated) was independently associated with the risk of death, MI, or new heart failure at 6 months. These observations provided an important proof of concept for the value of a multimarker strategy for risk stratification using a practical approach that can be applied using widely available biomarkers [2].

Together with evidence demonstrating the complementary mechanistic information offered by a marker of hemodynamic stress, a marker of inflammation, and a marker of myocyte necrosis, this substantial evidence base has established the value of a multimarker profile for characterizing the clinical risk of the patients with ACS (Fig. 11.5). Moreover, it is likely that ongoing investigation with other novel biomarkers (chapter 5) or more sophisticated methods for integrating the information from multiple biomarkers may improve upon these preliminary simple strategies for risk assessment. Despite this encouraging evolution, the usefulness of such strategies for personalizing therapy, beyond the appropriate matching of aggressiveness to risk, is dependent on the ability of specific therapies to modify the risk associated with specific biomarker profiles. In addition, several important potential barriers to optimal clinical integration have also been revealed by this early development of multimarker strategies in ACS and warrant discussion.

Table 11.1 Relative risk of clinical events using a multimarker strategy.

End-points	# of Elevated Biomarkers (cTnI, BNP, hs-CRP)				
	0	1	2	3	p-value
30 Days					
MI	1.0	2.6	2.9	1.9	0.03
CHF	1.0	1.8	3.2	7.3	0.0046
D/MI	1.0	2.9	3.6	5.1	0.0001
6 Months					
MI	1.0	1.8	2.3	1.1	0.06
CHF	1.0	2.6	4.7	8.4	0.0001
D/MI	1.0	2.0	3.2	4.4	0.0001

MI = myocardial infarction; CHF = congestive heart failure; D/MI = composite of death or MI
Data are from [19].

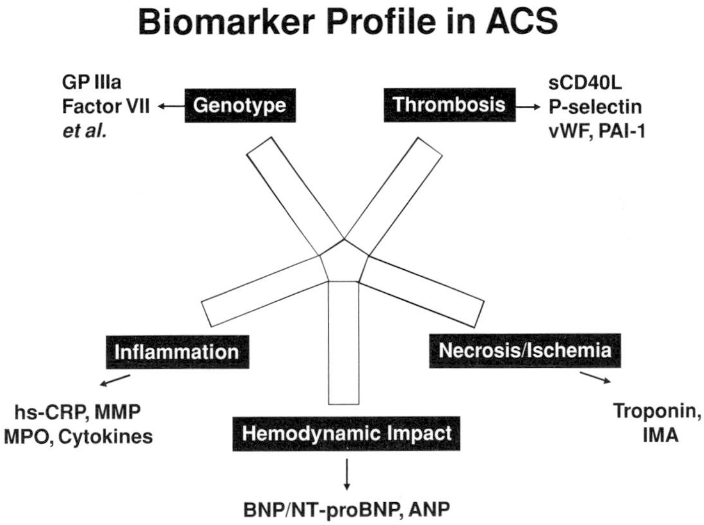

Biomarker Profile in ACS

Fig. 11.5 Conceptual application of a multimarker approach to characterization of the patient with acute coronary syndromes (ACS). ANP = atrial natriuretic peptide; BNP = B-type natriuretic peptide, GP = glycoprotein, hs-CRP = high sensitivity C-reactive protein, IMA = ischemia modified albumin, MMP = metalloproteinases, MPO = myeloperoxidase, PAI-1 = plasminogen activator inhibitor-1, sCD40L = soluble CD40 ligand, vWF = von Willebrand Factor. Adapted from [2].

Implications for therapy

Despite strong evidence for the prognostic value of the newer markers, such as BNP and CRP, their integration into clinical practice has not become widespread in ACS. The primary determinant of this pace of integration has been the absence of guidance regarding the appropriate therapeutic response. The established clinical value of cardiac troponin in targeting antithrombotic and invasive therapy to patients with ACS who have the most to gain and have the greatest probability of benefit has provided a clear example that biomarkers may be extremely useful to guide therapy (see chapter 2). However, to date there is not a consistent base of evidence to guide treatment in response to elevated levels of BNP, CRP, or other novel biomarkers of cardiovascular risk. In this regard, the promise of using expanded biomarker panels to personalize medical therapy is as yet unfulfilled and there is a need for additional investigation.

Owing to the overwhelming evidence that inflammation is a pervasive contributor to atherothrombosis, the effort to identify therapies directed at the inflammation underlying plaque instability has been particularly intense. Notably, examination of established treatments aimed at other contributors to atherothrombosis (e.g., aspirin, statins, fibric acid derivatives, angiotensin converting enzyme inhibitors, thiazolidinediones, and clopidogrel) has revealed anti-inflammatory actions [20]. In particular, the evidence for anti-inflammatory effects of statins is compelling, and supports intensive statin therapy as being particularly important for patients with evidence of inflammation [21]. However, it is not clear that patients with normal levels of inflammatory markers respond differentially to intensive statin therapy from those with elevated levels. Indeed, given the consistent safety and efficacy data supporting intensive LDL-lowering with statins following ACS, clear proof of an *absence of benefit* of intensive statin therapy among patients without inflammation may be needed before CRP can be used as a "gatekeeper" for the initiation or titration of statin therapy.

Similar research aimed at evaluating the potential of other newer biomarkers to direct therapy for patients at risk for or with established atherothrombosis is not as far advanced. It is notable that multiple randomized trials testing the use of natriuretic peptides to guide treatment of heart failure have been conducted with results that overall have provided support for the concept of using BNP/NT-proBNP to guide the pharmacotherapy of patients with heart failure. Studies in patients with acute or stable ischemic heart disease have been fewer and produced conflicting results (see chapter 4). Because blood concentrations of BNP and NT-proBNP are associated with left ventricular dysfunction and the extent of coronary artery disease, it is reasonable to hypothesize that early invasive evaluation and revascularization can reduce the risk linked to higher levels. Data from a nested substudy from one randomized trial support this hypothesis. However, findings from two other similar studies were neutral. Therefore, despite the strong relationship between BNP and NT-proBNP and outcome in

Table 11.2 Challenges in developing a multimarker strategy.

1. Requires adequate clinical and analytic validation of each individual biomarker, including determination of appropriate sample handling, analytic performance, biological variability, and clinical decision-limits

2. Relationship between the biomarker and the risk of specific clinical events may differ, i.e., not all biomarkers are associated with the same clinical events with equal strength

3. Dichotomization of biomarker results may be overly simple and even misleading with respect to the magnitude of risk

4. Complex modeling is likely to hinder clinical application; whereas, an overly simplified formulation may limit the validity and discriminatory capacity of the strategy

5. Evidence regarding the implications for therapy is critical to guiding clinical implementation

Reprinted from Morrow DA (2006) A Multimarker Approach to Risk Stratification in Acute Coronary Syndromes. In Morrow DA (ed), *Cardiovascular Biomarkers: Pathophysiology and Disease Management*. Humana Press, Totawa.

patients with ischemic heart disease, there is not yet conclusive data defining an appropriate therapeutic response to the finding. Data evaluating other newer and novel biomarkers of cardiovascular risk such as myeloperoxidase are even fewer.

Lessons learned: Facing the complexity of a multimarker strategy

As illustrated by the examples discussed in this chapter thus far, despite improvements in the ability to assess prognosis using multiple diverse biomarkers, there are a number of challenges that have yet to be navigated in developing multimarker strategies that are viable for clinical application to personalize care (Table 11.2). Two additional specific challenges are worthy of discussion.

Heterogeneity of risk relationships

Although composite clinical end-points are frequently used to provide statistical power in the evaluation of new biomarkers, the relationship between the biomarker and the risk of individual elements of that end-point are sometimes not homogenous. For example, troponin concentration has a near-linear relationship with the risk of death, but appears to have a non-monotonic relationship (inverted U-shape) with the risk of recurrent MI, such that those with the highest levels of troponin are at lower risk of recurrent MI [22]. Therefore, troponin shows a strong association with the risk of death and recurrent ischemic events that exhibits a threshold in the risk relationship at the lower

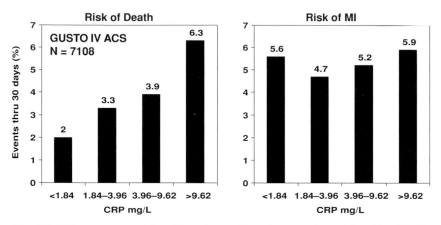

Fig. 11.6 Heterogeneous relationship between C-reactive protein and the risk of death compared with the risk of myocardial infarction in patients with acute coronary syndrome. Data from [24].

limit of detection [23]. As a second example, for BNP and CRP a relationship with the risk of recurrent ischemic events is less certain and the correlation with mortality is graded (with less of a clear-cut threshold than troponin) (see chapter 4) (Fig. 11.6) [16,17,24]. In light of this complexity, a multimarker strategy that is "positive" for one marker appears to have different clinical implications depending upon the marker that is elevated. For example, a patient with elevated levels of BNP and CRP is likely at significantly increased risk of death via mechanical failure but without a substantially increased risk of recurrent MI, whereas a patient with normal levels of CRP and BNP but a low-level troponin elevation is at relatively low risk for death but remains at high risk for recurrent ischemic events that may be mitigated by early invasive treatment. In addition to such differences in the relationship with alternative end-points, individual biomarkers may also exhibit a variety of patterns to the relationship (e.g., threshold, linear, or nonlinear). In the case of those with a linear relationship, application of a dichotomous cut-point does not appropriately capture the full prognostic potential for the biomarker. For example, given the step-wise relationship between increasing levels of the natriuretic peptides and death or heart failure, the clinician should be aware that absolute plasma concentration of the biomarker carries more information with respect to the magnitude of risk than a simple "positive" versus "negative" interpretation conveys (e.g., the 6-month mortality risk with BNP 80–100 pg/mL is 3.6% versus 10.9% for BNP 120–160 pg/mL).

Interpretation for therapeutic decision making
Although as yet untested, it may be possible to handle the complexity of varied risk relationships for individual biomarkers by weighting them differently for

specific end-points of interest and for different ranges of concentration. However, the advantages of such an approach are counterbalanced by the desire to maintain ease of application. In addition, strategies that use multiple biomarkers to arrive at a single composite risk estimate are not likely to be easily translated into appropriate clinical decisions. As highlighted in the two preceding sections, increased concentrations of different biomarkers carry different therapeutic implications. For example, only an elevated troponin has been shown to connote risk that is particularly responsive to more aggressive anti-thrombotic therapy, whereas elevated hs-CRP or BNP may someday warrant advancement of therapies promoting favorable cardiac remodeling. At least at this time, knowledge of individual biomarker results and familiarity with the base of evidence with respect to therapeutic interactions are necessary to integrate a multimarker strategy into clinical decision making.

Criteria for evaluating new biomarkers

In the face of the extremely rapid pace of biomarker discovery and testing, it has become increasingly important for researchers, manufacturers, regulators, and clinicians to critically appraise the value of new biomarkers as they emerge as candidates for further investigation and possible clinical application. The criteria for such evaluation follow from lessons learned along the path to clinical integration of currently available biomarkers, and include three basic questions for each candidate (Fig. 11.7) [25]: 1) Can the clinician measure it? 2) Does it add new information? and 3) Does it help the clinician better manage patients?

Can the clinician measure the biomarker?

To be clinically useful, analytical methods must be available that allow reliable measurement in the environment in which the biomarker is to be applied. Optimally, the methods should also provide prompt turnaround time and be available at reasonable cost. As such, each new biomarker and its assay(s) must undergo thorough evaluation of pre-analytical (conditions of measurement, sample handling, sample type, etc.), and analytical performance. Although these steps are preferably completed early in the development of a biomarker, they are often undertaken after initial epidemiologic studies bring attention to the new test. For example, although experimental and epidemiological data have established links between soluble CD40 ligand and atherothrombosis, further investigation has revealed important confounding influences of sample handling (timing of processing, temperature, and centrifugation steps) and sample type on its measured concentration [26].

Does the biomarker add new information?

Perhaps the most important criterion with respect to the assessing the clinical value of a candidate biomarker is the consistency and strength of the association

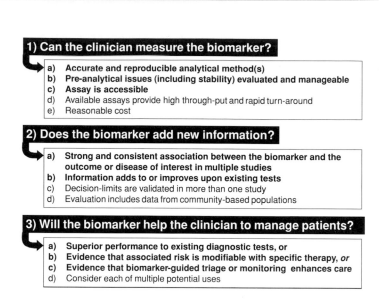

1) Can the clinician measure the biomarker?

a) **Accurate and reproducible analytical method(s)**
b) **Pre-analytical issues (including stability) evaluated and manageable**
c) **Assay is accessible**
d) Available assays provide high through-put and rapid turn-around
e) Reasonable cost

2) Does the biomarker add new information?

a) **Strong and consistent association between the biomarker and the outcome or disease of interest in multiple studies**
b) **Information adds to or improves upon existing tests**
c) Decision-limits are validated in more than one study
d) Evaluation includes data from community-based populations

3) Will the biomarker help the clinician to manage patients?

a) **Superior performance to existing diagnostic tests, or**
b) **Evidence that associated risk is modifiable with specific therapy, *or***
c) **Evidence that biomarker-guided triage or monitoring enhances care**
d) Consider each of multiple potential uses

Fig. 11.7 Criteria for assessment of novel cardiovascular biomarkers for clinical use. Statements in bold font are given the highest priority. Reprinted from [25] with permission.

with the outcome or disease of interest, and the extent to which the biomarker improves upon (either adding to or replacing) established tools. Because of obvious pressures on investigators and publishers considering reporting and publication of first-time observations, the first publication of data with a new marker is often dramatically "positive" and not necessarily representative of analyses that follow. For this reason, external validation is crucial in the development of any candidate biomarker. For prognostic application in patients with ACS, for example, we have previously recommended that this criterion include a consistent independent association with the risk of death, or death and nonfatal clinical events in multiple studies utilizing prospectively collected samples in patients with well-characterized clinical outcomes. Although validation in at least two adequately sized clinical studies may be regarded as a minimum requirement, most biomarkers recommended for routine clinical use by professional society guidelines draw on such evidence from 10 or more studies [27,28]. In addition, if specific decision-limits are recommended for a biomarker, these thresholds must be validated in multiple data sets.

There is no simple criterion for the magnitude of the risk relationship that will translate into clinical value. In addition, multiple metrics for the discriminatory and prognostic value of a marker are available and validated, with ongoing debate as to whether any single metric is optimal for assessing the incremental value of a new clinical risk indicator [29]. Such metrics include multivariable adjusted estimates of relative risk, the area under the receiver operating characteristics curve for a specific diagnosis or future clinical outcome, and reclassification analyses. Our experience is that each metric may reveal different advantages and disadvantages in the potential clinical application of a new marker. We and others have sometimes used a 2-fold higher adjusted relative risk as an initial litmus test in early decisions to pursue additional investigation of a prognostic biomarker. Nevertheless, many established risk indicators used in cardiovascular disease exhibit more modest association. As an example, tertiles of systolic blood pressure reveal only a 1.5-fold higher risk of a first coronary event with an area under the receiver operating characteristic curve of 0.64 [30]. Still, systolic blood pressure is appropriately deep-rooted in clinical guidelines and clinical practice because the associated risk is modifiable and useful to direct therapeutic interventions. In addition, there can be a particular need for new tools in subsets of patients for whom available methods have limitations [31].

As such, we propose that all of the available information, including preanalytical and analytical performance, unadjusted and adjusted relative risks, ROC analyses, reclassification, and performance in subgroups, should be used along with evidence regarding the possibility of modifying the risk associated with the biomarker to make an integrated assessment of the potential value of a biomarker. In addition, the settings in which the biomarker was studied and the outcomes analyzed must be considered in assessing the consistency of data and in formulating any recommendations for clinical use or regulatory approval. For example, the relationship between the inflammatory biomarker C-reactive protein (CRP) and outcome in patients with ACS is dependent on the timing of measurement and the end-point of interest. When measured early after presentation, CRP is associated with short- and long-term mortality risk but shows a more modest, if any, relationship with the risk of recurrent ischemic events [24]. However, when measured remotely after ACS, after the acute-phase response to the ACS has resolved, a relationship between CRP and recurrent myocardial infarction emerges [21]. Lastly, other physiologic characteristics that influence clearance or biologic variability of the marker should be determined. Such information is likely to be useful in anticipating potential limitation in specific groups of patients or the need for alternative cut-point values for those groups.

Will it help the clinician better manage patients?

Biomarkers have a variety of possible applications that may improve the clinical care of patients with cardiovascular disease [2]. As we have described previously [25], such uses include 1) early detection of otherwise subclinical disease; 2) diagnostic assessment of an acute or chronic clinical syndrome; 3) risk stratification of patients with a suspected or confirmed diagnosis; 4) selection of an appropriate therapeutic intervention; and 5) monitoring the response to therapy (Fig. 11.8). Each of these potential uses should be considered in assessing the possible value of a new biomarker.

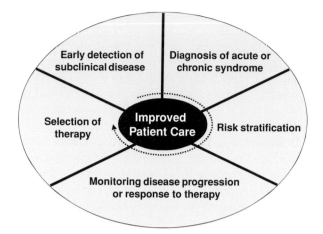

Fig. 11.8 Clinical applications of cardiovascular biomarkers. Reprinted from [25] with permission.

Those biomarkers that fill an unmet medical need are those that are most likely to be integrated into clinical care. In particular, those applications that directly enhance medical decision making have the most palpable value to the practitioner. As an example, because cardiac troponin is useful both for diagnosing myocardial infarction and for identifying patients who are most likely to benefit from specific therapies, such as administration of glycoprotein IIb/IIIa receptor inhibitors, more potent anti-thrombotic agents, and early invasive evaluation, this biomarker has become a cornerstone of evidence-based care for patients with suspected ACS [27,28]. At present, many newer markers, including some with regulatory approval for clinical use such as myeloperoxidase, have been shown to be independently associated with prognosis but have very little or no data regarding therapeutic considerations. The prognostic information gained from such biomarkers may still be used to guide triage, inform patients and their families, and to identify those patients at highest risk who have the most to gain in absolute terms from all effective interventions. Selective use of these biomarkers, such as BNP and hs-CRP, is reasonable in patients for whom a more complete assessment of the absolute risk is desired by the clinician [28]. However, recommendations for routine measurement in all patients with ACS are not likely to emerge unless data supporting the benefit of specific therapeutic interventions become available.

Pathobiologic considerations

A thorough understanding of the pathophysiology of a candidate novel marker is not essential to establishing its diagnostic or prognostic performance. However, this information may be very important in supporting the validity of epidemiologic observations, and directing investigation of possible diagnostic and therapeutic applications. It is also intuitive that biomarkers that reflect pathophysiologically distinct processes have the greatest promise to provide information that is incremental to other biomarkers or clinical tools [2]. We believe that insight into the biology of a candidate marker will help to ensure that all of its potential applications (and limitations) are fully considered.

Biomarker discovery: Proteomics and metabolomics

Most of the currently used cardiac biomarkers have developed out of studies either of known cardiac proteins (i.e., troponin and BNP) or from known systemic biomarkers of a relevant process (i.e., CRP as a reflection of inflammation). Although such an approach has been fruitful, recent advancements in protein display and identification technologies now permit one to characterize global alterations associated with disease conditions. First introduced in 1995, the term proteome refers to the entire group of *proteins* associated with a given *genome*.

In fact, proteomics is far more complex and ambitious than genomics. Whereas all cells of a given organism contain an equivalent genomic content, the proteome varies during development and differentiation and in response to external stimuli. Thus, one can speak not only of the general human proteome but also more specifically of the proteome of particular cells under specific physiologic or pathophysiologic conditions. Moreover, following transcription, a protein may undergo one or more posttranslational modifications, such as phosphorylation, glycosylation, acetylation, and sulfation.

Despite the complexity highlighted here, proteomics is uniquely positioned to offer insight into disease because proteins and their bio-enzymatic functions largely determine the phenotypic diversity that arises from a set of common genes and because the proteome is highly dynamic, in contrast to the stability of the genome. *This complexity is the basis of both its great informative potential and analytical challenge.*

Researchers have begun to apply protein profiling to cardiovascular disease, specifically investigating serum signatures of myocardial infarction. However, most of the protein peaks identified were abundant proteins whose differences may have been artifacts of sample handling, rather than being truly reflective of the pathobiology [32]. Many of the biologically interesting molecules relevant to cardiovascular disease are low abundance proteins. For example, troponin is found in the nanomolar (10^{-9}) range, insulin in the picomolar range (10^{-12}), and tumor necrosis factor (TNF)-α in the femtomolar (10^{-15}) range. In all, there are an estimated 10,000 unique proteins in the plasma, with concentrations spanning a 9-fold dynamic range. However, some hypothesize that the entire set of over 300,000 estimated human polypeptide species resulting from splice variants and posttranslational modifications is potentially represented in the plasma proteome.

Given the existing hurdles for proteomics, we have employed the far more tractable technologies of metabolomics (analogous to proteomics but examining metabolites rather than proteins) to patients undergoing exercise stress testing for suspected coronary artery disease. We found six metabolites that exhibited significant discordant regulation among those with versus without ischemia. Using a score reflecting the change for each of the six metabolites, we were able to differentiate ischemic cases from controls with a high degree of accuracy (P < 0.0001, cross-validated c-statistic = 0.83) [33].

Although many technological challenges still exist, we remain optimistic that proteomics and metabolomics have the potential to lead to the discovery of novel biomarkers. By focusing the experimental process, proteomics can target discovery of biomarkers to fill current unmet needs such as very early markers of injury, markers of myocardial ischemia in the absence of infarction, and so on. In addition, the biomarkers discovered using proteomics might provide insight into the cellular mechanisms of disease and uncover new proteins that might serve as targets for therapeutic intervention.

Research directions

In addition to the broad-based exploratory approaches of proteomic, metabolomic, and genomic strategies described in detail in the preceding section, hypothesis-based testing of specific candidate biomarkers is likely to play a central role in the discovery of new biomarkers. Continuing in the path of the past decade, advances in our understanding of the pathobiology of atherosclerosis, conduction disorders, and heart failure will inevitably direct us to participants in key pathophysiologic processes that when assayed may enable non-invasive detection of underlying disease. The integration of the cadre of biomarkers that will surface from these efforts with other clinical tools is likely to remain a major focus of research endeavors in the foreseeable future. The substrate for these efforts will include not only traditional clinical risk indicators and diagnostic data but also existing and new technologies for imaging the cardiovascular system.

Integration into clinical instruments

Simple clinical scoring systems and more computationally complicated prognostic instruments based upon clinical data routinely available have proven useful in guiding therapy. Incorporation of biomarkers into these instruments has precedent in tools for primary prevention, such as the use of cholesterol in the Framingham Risk Score, as well as for guiding secondary prevention, such as use of cardiac troponin in the TIMI Risk Score for Non–ST-Elevation ACS [34]. The inclusion of hs-CRP in the recently developed Reynolds Risk Score for evaluation of cardiovascular risk in apparently healthy women presages the expanding integration of other novel biomarkers into existing and new prognostic and diagnostic instruments [35]. Such efforts will require thoughtful assessment of the incremental value of adding newer biomarkers, particularly to less costly established tools, as well as external validation.

Integration with cardiovascular imaging

The interface between biomarkers and imaging technology has stimulated two initial directions for investigation and clinical application from which others are likely to develop. First, biomarkers and cardiovascular imaging may be combined as complementary tools in algorithms for diagnosis and risk assessment of cardiovascular disease [36]. For example, the use of natriuretic peptides as an initial screening tool to identify patients for whom non-invasive imaging for structural heart disease should be performed is under investigation. Second, biomarker discovery efforts have been linked to molecular imaging methods to target imaging to specific tissues and/or cell types [37]. This latter application of molecular imaging is a rapidly evolving discipline that includes the development of imaging agents and technologies to visualize specific molecular processes in vivo. Sharing a rationale similar to that for the development of multimarker strategies, molecular imaging aims to assess the biological properties of any given structural region of the cardiovascular anatomy; one example is the detection of atherosclerotic plaque vulnerable to rupture by imaging molecular attributes of inflammatory cells within the atheroma. The capacity to image specific biological aspects of atherosclerotic lesions could: 1) provide new diagnostic capabilities for detecting high-risk plaques before symptomatic; 2) guide the initiation and titration of therapy; and 3) also yield noninvasive surrogate end-points for clinical trials to assess the efficacy of novel therapeutics. As such, this application of technology has the possibility to meet the core goals of personalized medicine. The close ties of this field to biomarker discovery are readily illustrated by the most promising imaging targets (Table 11.3).

Clinical trials of biomarker-based strategies

Perhaps the most important direction for research in the coming years is the expansion of trials that will put the notion of biomarker-based personalized medicine to the test. There is a strong need to prospectively establish the value of biomarkers in targeting specific therapies through the design of randomized clinical trials. Such trials may take two basic forms.

First, randomized trials of specific therapeutic agents or strategies among candidates characterized by the biomarker of interest are requisite to establish evidence for use of biomarkers to identify candidates for therapy. In order to definitively establish that those with detectable elevation of the biomarker experience a greater therapeutic benefit than those with a negative result, patients with both positive and negative biomarker results must be enrolled. However, trials designed to test a hypothesis generated based upon previous evidence

Table 11.3 High priority imaging targets in atherosclerosis.

Biological Process	Class	Specific Molecular Targets
Macrophage activity	Surface receptors	SRA, CD36, dextran receptor (magnetic nanoparticles-MRI), others
	Metabolism	Hexokinase, GLUT-1 (FDG-PET)
	Proteases	MMP (1, 8, 9, 13), cathepsins-NIRF (B, S, K)
	Peroxidases	MPO
	Modified lipoproteins	OxLDL, others
Angiogenesis	Increased vascularity and leakage	Perfusion markers
	Endothelium	VCAM-1, $\alpha_v\beta_3$ (angiogenesis-MRI), E-selectin
Apoptosis	Cell membrane	Phosphatidylserine (Annexin A5–SPECT)
	Enzymes	Caspases, scramblases
Cell trafficking	Monocytes	
	Lymphocytes	
	Stem cells	

FDG = fluorodeoxyglucose; GLUT-1 = glucose transporter-1; MMP = matrix metalloproteinase; MPO = myeloperoxidase; MRI = magnetic resonance imaging; NIRF = near infrared fluorescence imaging; OxLDL = oxidized low-density lipoprotein; PET = positron emission tomography; SPECT = single-photon emission computed tomography; SRA = scavenger receptor A; VCAM = vascular cell adhesion molecule
From [37].

may also be informative in providing an evidence base for biomarker-guided therapy. For example, an ongoing clinical trial will test the efficacy of expanding the indication for early inhibition of the renin angiotensin aldosterone system to ACS patients without clinical heart failure or left ventricular dysfunction that have an elevated concentration of a natriuretic peptide.

Second, randomized trials of biomarker-based strategies for monitoring the success of therapy will be necessary to conclusively demonstrate the value of using biomarkers to guide the titration of therapy. Encouraging progress has been made in this regard with the implementation and completion of randomized trials testing natriuretic peptide-guided therapy versus standard of care for patients with chronic heart failure. Similar trials are needed in patients with atherosclerotic vascular disease.

Summary

Cardiac biomarkers provide a convenient and non-invasive means by which to more completely profile the patient with cardiovascular disease, gaining insight into the underlying causes and consequences that mediate the risk of future events and may be targets for therapeutic interventions. Steady progress in the discovery of new biomarkers and evolution toward more sophisticated clinical applications has offered promise to improve the care of patients through approaches tailored to the individual's risk and the underlying causes of disease. As yet, this promise is incompletely realized supporting the need for additional investigation. At the same time, the remarkable increase in the pace of emerging information demands even greater commitment to rigorous individual and comparative assessment.

References

1 Ginsburg GS, McCarthy JJ. Personalized medicine: revolutionizing drug discovery and patient care. *Trends Biotechnol* 2001; **19**: 491–496.

2 Morrow DA, Braunwald E. Future of biomarkers in acute coronary syndromes: moving toward a multimarker strategy. *Circulation* 2003; **108**: 250–252.

3 Braunwald E. Unstable angina. A classification. *Circulation* 1989; **80**: 410–414.

4 Braunwald E. Unstable angina: an etiologic approach to management. *Circulation* 1998; **98**: 2219–2222.

5 Morrow DA. Troponins in patients with acute coronary syndromes: biologic, diagnostic, and therapeutic implications. *Cardiovasc Toxicol* 2001; **1**: 105–110.

6 Wong GC, Morrow DA, Murphy S, Kraimer N, Pai R, James D et al. Elevations in troponin T and I are associated with abnormal tissue level perfusion: a TACTICS-TIMI 18 substudy. Treat Angina with Aggrastat and Determine Cost of Therapy with an Invasive or Conservative Strategy-Thrombolysis in Myocardial Infarction. *Circulation* 2002; **106**: 202–207.

7 Morrow DA, Antman EM, Tanasijevic M, Rifai N, de Lemos JA, McCabe CH et al. Cardiac troponin I for stratification of early outcomes and the efficacy of enoxaparin in unstable angina: a TIMI 11B substudy. *J Am Coll Cardiol* 2000; **36**: 1812–1817.

8 Hamm CW, Heeschen C, Goldmann B, Vahanian A, Adgey J, Miguel CM et al. Benefit of abciximab in patients with refractory unstable angina in relation to serum troponin T levels. c7E3 Fab Antiplatelet Therapy in Unstable Refractory Angina (CAPTURE) Study Investigators. *N Engl J Med* 1999; **340**: 1623–1629.

9 Morrow DA, Rifai N, Antman EM, Weiner DL, McCabe CH, Cannon CP et al. C-reactive protein is a potent predictor of mortality independently of and in combination with troponin T in acute coronary syndromes: a TIMI 11A substudy. Thrombolysis in Myocardial Infarction. *J Am Coll Cardiol* 1998; **31**: 1460–1465.

10 Lindahl B, Toss H, Siegbahn A, Venge P, Wallentin L. Markers of myocardial damage and inflammation in relation to long-term mortality in unstable coronary artery disease. FRISC Study Group. Fragmin during Instability in Coronary Artery Disease. *N Engl J Med* 2000; **343**: 1139–1147.

11 de Lemos JA, Morrow DA. Brain natriuretic peptide measurement in acute coronary syndromes: ready for clinical application? *Circulation* 2002; **106**: 2868–2870.

12 Richards AM, Nicholls MG, Yandle TG, Frampton C, Espiner EA, Turner JG et al. Plasma N-terminal pro-brain natriuretic peptide and adrenomedullin: new neurohormonal predictors of left ventricular function and prognosis after myocardial infarction. *Circulation* 1998; **97**: 1921–1929.

13 de Lemos JA, Morrow DA, Bentley JH, Omland T, Sabatine MS, McCabe CH et al. The prognostic value of B-type natriuretic peptide in patients with acute coronary syndromes. *N Engl J Med* 2001; **345**: 1014–1021.

14 Omland T, de Lemos JA, Morrow DA, Antman EM, Cannon CP, Hall C et al. Prognostic value of N-terminal pro-atrial and pro-brain natriuretic peptide in patients with acute coronary syndromes. *Am J Cardiol* 2002; **89**: 463–465.

15 Jernberg T, Stridsberg M, Venge P, Lindahl B. N-terminal pro brain natriuretic peptide on admission for early risk stratification of patients with chest pain and no ST-segment elevation. *J Am Coll Cardiol* 2002; **40**: 437–445.

16 Morrow DA, de Lemos JA, Sabatine MS, Murphy SA, Demopoulos L, DiBattiste P et al. Evaluation of B-type natriuretic peptide for risk assessment in unstable angina/non-ST elevation MI: BNP and prognosis in TACTICS-TIMI 18. *J Am Coll Cardiol* 2003; **41**: 1264–1272.

17 James SK, Wallentin L, Armstrong PW, Barnathan ES, Califf RM, Lindahl B et al. N-terminal pro brain natriuretic peptide and other risk markers for the separate prediction of mortality and subsequent myocardial infarction in patients with unstable coronary disease – a GUSTO IV substudy. *Circulation* 2003; **108**: 275–281.

18 Omland T, de Lemos JA, Morrow DA, Antman EM, Cannon CP, Hall C et al. Prognostic value of n-terminal pro-atrial and pro-brain natriuretic peptide in patients with acute coronary syndromes: a TIMI 11B substudy. *Am J Cardiol* 2002; **89**: 463–465.

19 Sabatine MS, Morrow DA, de Lemos JA, Gibson CM, Murphy SA, Rifai N et al. Multimarker approach to risk stratification in non-ST elevation acute coronary syndromes: simultaneous assessment of troponin I, C-reactive protein, and B-type natriuretic peptide. *Circulation* 2002; **105**: 1760–1763.

20 Libby P, Aikawa M. Stabilization of atherosclerotic plaques: new mechanisms andclinical targets. *Nat Med* 2002; **8**: 1257–1262.

21 Ridker PM, Cannon CP, Morrow D, Rifai N, Rose LM, McCabe CH et al. C-reactive protein levels and outcomes after statin therapy. *N Engl J Med* 2005; **352**: 20–28.

22 Lindahl B, Diderholm E, Lagerqvist B, Venge P, Wallentin L. Mechanisms behind the prognostic value of troponin T in unstable coronary artery disease: a FRISC II substudy. *J Am Coll Cardiol* 2001; **38**: 979–986.

23 Morrow DA, Cannon CP, Rifai N, Frey MJ, Vicari R, Lakkis N et al. Ability of minor elevations of troponin I and T to identify patients with unstable angina and non-ST elevation myocardial infarction who benefit from an early invasive strategy: Results from a prospective, randomized trial. *JAMA* 2001; **286**: 2405–2412.

24 James SK, Armstrong P, Barnathan E, Califf R, Lindahl B, Siegbahn A et al. Troponin and C-reactive protein have different relations to subsequent mortality and myocardial infarction after acute coronary syndrome: a GUSTO-IV substudy. *J Am Coll Cardiol* 2003; **41**: 916–924.

25 Morrow DA, de Lemos JA. Benchmarks for the assessment of novel cardiovascular biomarkers. *Circulation* 2007; **115**: 949–952.

26 Halldorsdottir AM, Stoker J, Porche-Sorbet R, Eby CS. Soluble CD40 ligand measurement inaccuracies attributable to specimen type, processing time, and ELISA method. *Clin Chem* 2005; **51**: 1054–1057.

27 The Joint European Society of Cardiology/American College of Cardiology Committee for the redefinition of myocardial infarction. Myocardial infarction redefined—a consensus document of The Joint European Society of Cardiology/American College of Cardiology Committee for the redefinition of myocardial infarction. *J Am Coll Cardiol* 2000; **36**: 959–969.

28 Morrow DA, Cannon CP, Jesse RL, Newby LK, Ravkilde J, Storrow AB et al. National Academy of Clinical Biochemistry Laboratory Medicine Practice Guidelines: Clinical Characteristics and Utilization of Biochemical Markers in Acute Coronary Syndromes. *Circulation* 2007; **115**: e356–e375.

29 Cook NR. Use and misuse of the receiver operating characteristic curve in risk prediction. *Circulation* 2007; **115**: 928–935.

30 Danesh J, Wheeler JG, Hirschfield GM, Eda S, Eiriksdottir G, Rumley A et al. C-reactive protein and other circulating markers of inflammation in the prediction of coronary heart disease. *N Engl J Med* 2004; **350**: 1387–1397.

31 Wiviott SD, Cannon CP, Morrow DA, Murphy SA, Gibson CM, McCabe CH et al. Differential expression of cardiac biomarkers by gender in patients with unstable angina/non–ST-elevation myocardial infarction: a TACTICS-TIMI 18 (Treat Angina with Aggrastat and determine Cost of Therapy with an Invasive or Conservative Strategy-Thrombolysis In Myocardial Infarction 18) substudy. *Circulation* 2004; **109**: 580–586.

32 Marshall J, Kupchak P, Zhu W, Yantha J, Vrees T, Furesz S et al. Processing of serum proteins underlies the mass spectral fingerprinting of myocardial infarction. *J Proteome Res* 2003; **2**: 361–372.

33 Sabatine MS, Liu E, Morrow DA, Heller E, McCarroll R, Wiegand R et al. Metabolomic identification of novel biomarkers of myocardial ischemia. *Circulation* 2005; **112**: 3868–3875.

34 Antman EM, Cohen M, Bernink PJ, McCabe CH, Horacek T, Papuchis G, et al. The TIMI risk score for unstable angina/non-ST elevation MI: A method for prognostication and therapeutic decision making. *JAMA* 2000; **284**: 835–842.

35 Ridker PM, Buring JE, Rifai N, Cook NR. Development and validation of improved algorithms for the assessment of global cardiovascular risk in women: the Reynolds Risk Score. *JAMA* 2007; **297**: 611–619.

36 Di Carli MF, Hachamovitch R. New technology for noninvasive evaluation of coronary artery disease. *Circulation* 2007; **115**: 1464–1480.

37 Jaffer FA, Libby P, Weissleder R. Molecular and cellular imaging of atherosclerosis: emerging applications. *J Am Coll Cardiol* 2006; **47**: 1328–1338.

Index

The AHA Clinical Series

SERIES EDITOR • ELLIOTT ANTMAN

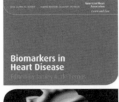

Biomarkers in Heart Disease
James A. de Lemos
9781405175715

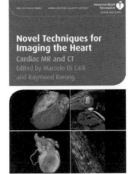

Novel Techniques for Imaging the Heart
Marcelo Di Carli & Raymond Kwong
9781405175333

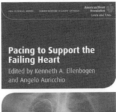

Pacing to Support the Failing Heart
Kenneth A. Ellenbogen
& Angelo Auricchio
9781405175340

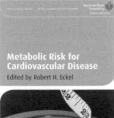

Metabolic Risk for Cardiovascular Disease
Robert H. Eckel
9781405181044

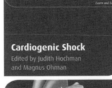

Cardiogenic Shock
Judith Hochman
& E. Magnus Ohman
9781405179263

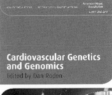

Cardiovascular Genetics and Genomics
Dan Roden
9781405175401

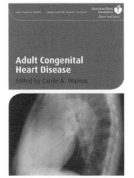

Adult Congenital Heart Disease
Carole A. Warnes
9781405178204

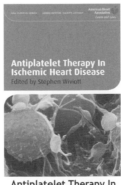

Antiplatelet Therapy In Ischemic Heart Disease
Stephen Wiviott
9781405176262

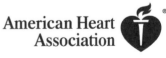